OXFORD MEDICAL PUBLICATIONS

Prevention of Cardiovascular Disease
An evidence-based approach

OXFORD GENERAL PRACTICE SERIES

Editorial Board

6. The consultation: an approach to learning and teaching
   David Pendleton, Theo Schofield, Peter Tate, and Peter Havelock
18. Health care for Asians
   Edited by Bryan R. McAvoy and Liam J. Donaldson
20. Geriatric problems in general practice (second edition)
   G. K. Wilcock, J. A. M. Gray, and J. M. Longmore
21. Efficient care in general practice
   G. N. Marsh
22. Hospital referrals
   Edited by Martin Roland and Angela Coulter
23. Prevention in general practice (second edition)
   Edited by Godfrey Fowler, Muir Gray, and Peter Anderson
25. Medical audit in primary health care
   Edited by Martin Lawrence and Theo Schofield
26. Gastrointestinal problems in general practice
   Edited by Roger Jones
27. Domiciliary palliative care
   Derek Doyle
28. Critical reading for primary care
   Edited by Roger Jones and Ann-Louise Kimonth
29. Research methods and audit in general practice
   David Armstrong and John Grace
30. Counselling in primary health care
   Edited by Jane Keithley and Geoffrey Marsh
31. Professional education for general practice
   Peter Havelock, John Hasler, Richard Flew, Donald McIntyre, Theo Schofield, and John Toby
32. Quality improvement by peer review
   Richard Grol and Martin Lawrence
33. Prevention of cardiovascular disease
   Edited by Martin Lawrence, Andrew Neil, David Mant, and Godfrey Fowler
34. Complementary medicine: an integrated approach
   George Lewith, Julian Kenyon, and Peter Lewis
35. A guide for new principals
   Mike Pringle, Jacky Hayden, and Andrew Procter
36. Paediatric problems in general practice (third edition)
   Michael Modell, Zulf Mughal, and Robert Boyd
37. Professional development in general practice
   Edited by David Pendleton and John Hasler
38. Teaching medicine in the community
   Edited by Carl Whitehouse, Martin Roland, and Peter Campion
39. Women's health (fourth edition)
   Edited by Ann McPherson and Deborah Waller
40. Infection
   Edited by Lesley Southgate, Cameron Lockie, Shelley Heard, and Martin Wood
41. Men's health
   Edited by Tom O'Dowd and David Jewell
42. Prescribing in primary care
   Edited by Richard Hobbs and Colin Bradley

Also avilable: Lawrence *et al.* Handbook of emergencies in general practice

Prevention of Cardiovascular Disease
An evidence-based approach

Oxford General Practice Series ● 33

Edited by

MARTIN LAWRENCE
ANDREW NEIL
DAVID MANT
and
GODFREY FOWLER

OXFORD NEW YORK TOKYO
OXFORD UNIVERSITY PRESS

Oxford University Press, Great Clarendon Street, Oxford OX2 6DP

Oxford New York

Athens Auckland Bangkok Bogota Bombay Buenos Aires
Calcutta Cape Town Dar es Salaam Delhi Florence Hong Kong
Istanbul Karachi Kuala Lumpur Madras Madrid Melbourne
Mexico City Nairobi Paris Singapore Taipei Tokyo Toronto Warsaw

and associated companies in
Berlin Ibadan

Oxford is a registered trade mark of Oxford University Press

Published in the United States by
Oxford University Press Inc., New York

First published 1996
Reprinted 1997, 1998

A catalogue record for this book is available from the British Library

Library of Congress Cataloging in Publication Data
Prevention of cardiovascular disease: An evidence-based approach / edited by
Martin Lawrence . . . [et al.].
(Oxford general practice series ; 33) (Oxford
medical publications)
Includes index.
1. Cardiovascular system—Diseases—prevention.   2. Primary care
(Medicine).   I. Lawrence, Martin.   II. Series.   III. Series: Oxford
medical publications.
[DNLM: 1. Cardiovascular Diseases—prevention & control.
2. Primary Health Care. W1 OX55 no.33 1996 / WG 120 P944 1996]
RC682.P72   1996   616.1'05—dc20   95–52217
ISBN 0 19 262397 4 (Pbk)

Printed in Great Britain by
Biddles Ltd,
Guildford and King's Lynn.

Foreword

Julian Tudor Hart

The definition of effective medical care is always difficult, and truths which appear self-evident to one generation are revalued by the next. By the middle 1970s, about half the variance in premature death from coronary heart disease was accounted for by known risk factors, mainly arterial pressure, blood cholesterol, and smoking. The next step was to try to control coronary disease by modifying these risk factors. Interventions on a population scale, such as the Finnish Karelia project, showed little change in outcome compared with control areas, perhaps because the control areas also changed. Interventions at a personal level, as in the OXCHECK study, have shown significant though marginal changes. It is hard to accept that assumptions about effective interventions must be modified.

The authors of this book, many of whom I have long known personally, are full of both enthusiasm and doubt. Enthusiasm is essential for success in all forms of significant innovation in primary care, and this book is all about innovation. They are also sceptics; they were before they began writing, and must be much more so now they have finished. No one could plough through all these references and sift all this contradictory and confusing evidence, and retain the credulity required to promote the uncritical health checks of the kind so popular in the 1980s. Instead they propose a new and rational programme.

It is beyond most of us to begin to cope with even a tenth of the existing literature on risk factors for premature vascular disease. Adding more facts to the same structure of ideas seems more likely to complicate than to simplify the present confusion. What is needed, and found here, is a new approach and a different sort of evidence.

This is essentially a resource book for practitioners who are ready to agree on explicit policies for clinical management, and need a reliable source book for relevant evidence and experience, from which to develop their own protocols. A framework for action is provided in the last chapter, with the recommendations based on the first sections of the book. Local circumstances, however, should lead to different priorities in different places. This book should help practitioners to think and act in new ways, applying continuing anticipatory care to their known populations. Any advances made are likely to be small, but that is the scale on which we work. We need not apologize but should at least ensure we do more good than harm.

It is a brave book, which deserves to succeed.

Preface

More than a third of men and women in the United Kingdom die from coronary heart disease or stroke. One in twelve men die from coronary heart disease before the age of 65. Yet this epidemic of premature death is reversible, indeed the death rate is already falling.

Medical research, especially in the past 10–15 years, has clarified the actions which are effective in reducing the risk of developing cardiovascular disease and the risk of death in patients with established disease. However, research is often difficult to interpret and sometimes conflicting. The issue facing general practitioners and primary health care teams is to decide how to respond to this research and to identify just what they should now be doing in practice, and why.

This book has been written to address this issue. Recommendations about what professionals in primary care should do to reduce cardiovascular disease are supported by full but concise evidence on which the recommendations are based. This evidence-based format is relatively unusual, but we believe it will become increasingly common.

The format accords with current views on the development of clinical guidelines—that they should be based so far as possible on evidence rather than consensus, wherever possible on randomized controlled trials and meta-analyses rather than observational studies, and that the evidence (or lack of it) for any recommendation should be open and available. It is important to remember that guidelines need to be adapted to local circumstances, and practical details need to be added, before they can be introduced as a practice policy or protocols.

HOW TO READ THIS BOOK

Recommendations for action are found in Part 3, especially Chapter 23, and primary care professionals may well prefer to read these first. The strength of the evidence for each statement is graded A, B, or C, and the reader can refer back to earlier chapters to find the basis for the recommendations made.

The first two parts provide the evidence: Part 1 focuses on clinical risk and its reduction, Part 2 on the effectiveness of implementation strategies. Each chapter is self-contained, and is designed to list and elucidate the main problems faced by primary care professionals. Taken together these chapters cover the key evidence concerning cardiovascular disease prevention, and should act as a reference source for practitioners and practices.

We trust that this book will be a useful guide for all those responsible for providing cardiovascular disease prevention in primary care, be they doctors, nurses or advisers. It also provides the evidence base needed by those entering this field of medical care, both medical students and vocational trainees.

Oxford   M.L.
February 1996   A.N.
                                                                                                                                    D.M.
                                                                                                                                    G.F.

Contents

Foreword   v

Preface   vii

List of Contributors   xiii

Part 1   Evidence for reducible risk   1

1   Smoking   3
      Godfrey Fowler

2   Hypertension   18
      Martin Lawrence and Kennedy Cruickshank

3   Lipids and lipoproteins   35
      Andrew Neil

4   Nutrition   54
      Margaret Thorogood

5   Exercise   67
      David Mant and Paul Little

6   Alcohol   81
      Peter Anderson

7   Personality and psychological environment   93
      John Muir

8   Diabetes   105
      Jim Mann

9   Social deprivation   120
      Angela Coulter and David Mant

10 Hormone replacement therapy   131
      Edel Daly and Martin Vessey

11 Haemostasis   143
      Chris Silagy

12   Antioxidants   154
Chris Silagy and David Mant

13   Prevention of stroke   162
Jonathan Mant

14   Secondary prevention of coronary heart disease   175
Tim Lancaster and Peter Sleight

15   Multiple risk   186
John Muir and David Mant

Part 2   Evidence for the effectiveness of implementation   201

16   Community-based interventions   203
Michael Rayner

17   Individual interventions and behaviour change   221
Theo Schofield

18   Taking the initiative: strategies and implications   231
Martyn Agass and David Mant

19   Issues in measurement   243

  19.1   Smoking   243
  Godfrey Fowler

  19.2   Blood pressure   249
  Martin Dawes

  19.3   Cholesterol   253
  Andrew Neil

  19.4   Diet   258
  Margaret Thorogood

  19.5   Fitness   266
  David Mant and Paul Little

  19.6   Alcohol   273
  Peter Anderson

  19.7   Diabetes   279
  Rury Holman

20　Screening policy　　　　　　　　　　　　　　　　283
　　　David Mant

Part 3　Implementation　　　　　　　　　　　　　　299

21　The population and individual strategies　　　　301
　　　Godfrey Fowler

22　Preparing the practice　　　　　　　　　　　　309
　　　Martin Lawrence

23　Principles of patient management　　　　　　　321
　　　Martin Lawrence, Andrew Neil, David Mant, and Godfrey Fowler

Index　　　　　　　　　　　　　　　　　　　　　331

Contributors

Martyn Agass. General Practitioner, Berinsfield Health Centre, Berinsfield, Oxfordshire, OX10 7NE.

Peter Anderson. World Health Organisation, WHO Regional Office for Europe, 8 Scherfigsvej, 2100 Copenhagen, Denmark.

Angela Coulter. Director, King's Fund Development Centre, 11–13 Cavendish Square, London W1M 0AN.

Kennedy Cruickshank. Senior Lecturer in Clinical Epidemiology and Honorary Consultant Physician, University of Manchester, Stopford Building, Oxford Road, Manchester, M13 9TP.

Edel Daly. Research Officer, University of Oxford, Department of Public Health and Primary Care, Gibson Building, Radcliffe Infirmary, Oxford, OX2 6HE.

Martin Dawes. General Practitioner, Hollow Way Surgery, Oxford, and Lecturer in General Practice, University of Oxford, Department of Public Health and Primary Care, Gibson Building, Radcliffe Infirmary, Oxford, OX2 6HE.

Godfrey Fowler. Clinical Reader in General Practice and Honorary Director of the ICRF General Practice Research Group, University of Oxford, Department of Public Health and Primary Care, Gibson Building, Radcliffe Infirmary, Oxford, OX2 6HE.

Rury Holman. Honorary Consultant Physician, Diabetes Research Laboratories, University of Oxford, Radcliffe Infirmary, Oxford OX2 6HE.

Tim Lancaster. General Practitioner, Jericho Health Centre, Oxford and Research Fellow, ICRF General Practice Research Group, University of Oxford, Department of Public Health and Primary Care, Gibson Building, Radcliffe Infirmary, Oxford, OX2 6HE.

Martin Lawrence. General Practitioner, West Street Surgery, Chipping Norton, Oxfordshire, and University Lecturer in General Practice, University of Oxford, Department of Public Health and Primary Care, Gibson Building, Radcliffe Infirmary, Oxford, OX2 6HE.

Paul Little. General Practitioner and Wellcome Training Fellow, University of Southampton, Department of Primary Medical Care, Aldermoor Health Centre, Southampton SO15 6ST.

Jim Mann. Professor of Human Nutrition, University of Otago, Department of Human Nutrition, PO Box 56, Dunedin, New Zealand.

David Mant. Professor of Primary Care Epidemiology, University of Southampton, Department of Primary Medical Care, Aldermoor Health Centre, Southampton, SO1 6ST.

Jonathan Mant. Clinical Lecturer and Honorary Senior Registrar in Public Health Medicine, University of Oxford, Department of Public Health and Primary Care, Gibson Building, Radcliffe Infirmary, Oxford, OX2 6HE.

John Muir. General Practitioner, The Surgery, Woburn, Bedfordshire, MK17 9PX and Senior Research Fellow, ICRF General Practice Research Group, University of Oxford, Department of Public Health and Primary Care, Gibson Building, Radcliffe Infirmary, Woodstock Road, Oxford, OX2 6HE.

Andrew Neil. University Lecturer in Clinical Epidemiology, University of Oxford, Department of Public Health and Primary Care, and Honorary Consultant Physician, Department of Diabetes, Endocrinology and Metabolism, Radcliffe Infirmary, Oxford, OX2 6HE.

Michael Rayner. Research Officer, University of Oxford, Department of Public Health and Primary Care, Gibson Building, Radcliffe Infirmary, Oxford OX2 6HE.

Theo Schofield. General Practitioner, The Medical Centre, Badger Crescent, Shipston-on-Stour, Warwickshire and Lecturer in General Practice, University of Oxford, Department of Public Health and Primary Care, Gibson Building, Radcliffe Infirmary, Oxford, OX2 6HE.

Chris Silagy. Professor of General Practice, Flinders University of South Australia, Department of General Practice, G.P.O. Box 2100, Adelaide, SA 5001, Australia.

Peter Sleight. Field Marshal Alexander Professor Emeritus of Cardiovascular Medicine, University of Oxford, John Radcliffe Hospital, Oxford OX3 9DU.

Margaret Thorogood. Senior Lecturer, Health Promotion Sciences Unit, London School of Hygiene and Tropical Medicine, Keppel Street, London WC1E 7HT.

Martin Vessey. Professor of Public Health, University of Oxford, Department of Public Health and Primary Care, Gibson Building, Radcliffe Infirmary, Oxford, OX2 6HE.

Part 1
Evidence for reducible risk

1 Smoking

Godfrey Fowler

INTRODUCTION

Tobacco smoking has been identified by the World Health Organisation as the most important preventable cause of disease and premature death.[1] Moreover, contrary to popular belief (which perceives lung cancer as the predominant smoking risk), much of this avoidable morbidity and mortality is cardiovascular.

The proportion of males in the population in Britain who smoke reached a peak at the end of the Second World War when about two thirds of men were smoking; by the 1970s, smoking had also peaked in women, when almost half were smoking. Since then, smoking has been declining in both sexes and in all age groups, but the decline has been less steep in women than in men[2] (Fig. 1.1). In 1992, 29 per cent of men and 28 per cent of women were current cigarette smokers.[2]

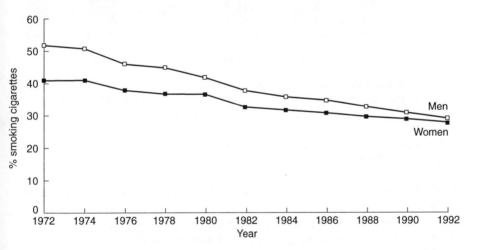

Fig. 1.1 Prevalence of cigarette smoking among adults, 1972–92, Great Britain. (Based on Office of population census and surveys, 1994 and previous editions; General household survey. London: HMSO, 1992.)

There have also been changes in the social class distribution of smoking. Until about 1960, smoking was more or less equally common in all social classes. Since then, smoking has declined fairly steeply in upper socio-economic groups, but less so in lower social classes (Fig. 1.2). In 1992, less than one in seven professional men and women were cigarette smokers, compared with about two-fifths of those in manual occupations.[2] Only about one in eight general practitioners currently smoke and fewer than half of these smoke cigarettes.[3]

Many children try smoking at an early age, boys usually earlier than girls. In 1992, nearly a third of those who had ever tried smoking had done so by the time they were 11 years old; the proportion of regular smokers (at least one cigarette a day) in the 11–15 year age group has not declined in recent years and in 1992 was 9 per cent in boys and 10 per cent in girls.[4]

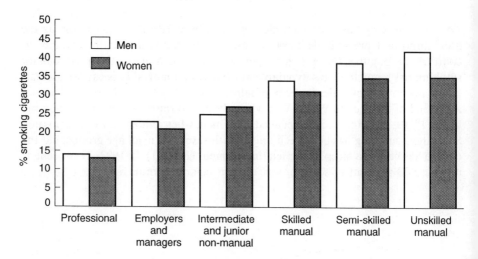

Fig. 1.2 Prevalence of cigarette smoking by sex and socio-economic group, 1992, Great Britain. (Based on Office of population census and surveys, 1994; General household survey. London: HMSO, 1992.)

In assessing the relationship of smoking to arterial disease, this chapter will address the following questions:

1. **What is the nature and strength of the evidence that cigarette smoking is a risk factor for arterial disease?**
2. **How important are cigar and pipe smoking as risk factors for arterial disease?**
3. **What are the mechanisms by which the risk is mediated?**
4. **What are the benefits from stopping smoking and how quickly are these achieved?**
5. **Is passive smoking important?**
6. **Is smoking cessation intervention effective and, if so, how should it be done and who should do it?**

WHAT IS THE NATURE AND STRENGTH OF THE EVIDENCE THAT SMOKING IS A RISK FACTOR FOR ARTERIAL DISEASE?

Although the relationship between smoking and lung cancer was established first,[5,6] cardiovascular disease, and especially coronary heart disease, is more important in terms of attributable deaths. This is because, although the relative risk of lung cancer death is much greater for smokers than non-smokers than is the relative risk of coronary heart disease death, coronary heart disease deaths are much more common than lung cancer deaths. It is estimated[7] that about a quarter of the 160 000 UK coronary heart disease deaths each year are attributable to smoking and that about half of the approximately 100 000 smoking-related deaths each year in Britain are from some form of arterial disease.

Coronary heart disease

Numerous cohort studies of smokers, non-smokers and ex-smokers have demonstrated the relationship between smoking and coronary heart disease. One of these is the *British Doctors Study*. This was established by Richard Doll and Bradford Hill in 1951 and the cohort is still being followed up. All 59 600 doctors on the British Medical Register were surveyed and over 40 000 responders provided a cohort which has been the source of much knowledge about smoke-related diseases. For coronary heart disease, the overall relative risk of death was shown to be about doubled, for both men and women, with a greater relative risk at a younger age and a dose response effect.[8,9] (Fig. 1.3).

As is discussed elsewhere in this book, the interaction between smoking and other risk factors is very important in relation to coronary heart disease. The relationship between smoking and coronary heart disease is much weaker in countries with a generally low incidence of coronary heart disease[10] and in individuals with relatively low levels of other coronary heart disease risk factors.[11] In women, studies with 'first generation pills' showed interaction between smoking and oral contraception, especially with increasing age,[12] but this may not be true with newer, 'low dose' oral contraceptives. Sudden cardiac death, especially in younger men, is strongly associated with smoking.[13]

Cerebrovascular disease (stroke)

The relationship between smoking and stroke has been less easily established than that of coronary heart disease. Many of the cohort studies have shown a small increase in the relative risk; for example the *British Doctors Study*[8] showed a risk ratio of 1.34. A recent meta-analysis of 32 studies[14] showed an overall relative risk of stroke associated with cigarette smoking of 1.5. There were considerable differences in relative risks amongst stroke subtypes; for cerebral infarction 1.9, for cerebral haemorrhage 0.7, and subarachnoid haemorrhage 2.9. An effect of age on overall relative risk was also noted; under 55 years 2.9, 55–74 years 1.8, and over 75 years 1.1. A dose–response relationship between the number of cigarettes smoked and relative risk was also found, and there was a smaller increased risk in women compared with men.

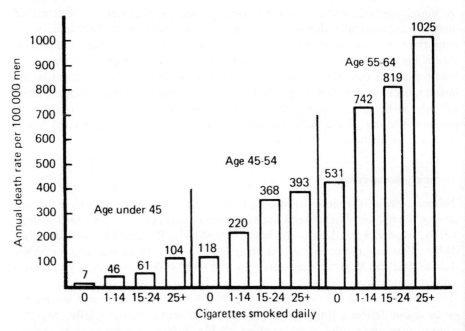

Fig. 1.3 British doctors study. Mortality from coronary heart disease in male non-smokers and current smokers by age and smoking category. With rising age the relative risk to smokers compared with non-smokers gets less although the number of deaths associated with smoking increases. (From Royal College of Physicians, Smoking or health, Pitman Medical, London, 1977.)

Other arterial disease

Aortic aneurysm is much more common in smokers than in non-smokers. In the *British Doctors Study*[8] the death rate from aortic aneurysm in smokers was more than six times that of non-smokers and ten times as high in those smoking more than 25 cigarettes a day.

Cigarette smoking is an important factor in the development of peripheral arterial disease[15] and very few patients with intermittent claudication are lifelong non-smokers. If patients with intermittent claudication continue to smoke, rest pain or gangrene, leading to amputation, are much more likely and symptoms are more likely to develop in previously asymptomatic limbs.[16] Occlusion of bypass grafts inserted for treatment of arterial disease is more common in continuing smokers.[17]

HOW IMPORTANT ARE CIGAR AND PIPE SMOKING AS A RISK FACTOR FOR ARTERIAL DISEASE?

The classical epidemiological studies[18,8] showed that, although pipe and cigar smoking generally confer an increased risk of cardiovascular disease, the attributable risk is substantially less than that for cigarette smoking.[19]

In these studies, pipe and cigar smokers were defined as those who had never smoked cigarettes; they were 'primary' cigar and pipe smokers who tend not to inhale. Now, most pipe and cigar smokers are ex-regular cigarette smokers who have switched but transferred their inhaling habit. Such 'secondary' cigar and pipe smokers are unlikely to reduce their excess cardiovascular risk substantially by this change.[20]

WHAT ARE THE MECHANISMS BY WHICH THIS RISK IS MEDIATED?

In spite of the mass of epidemiological evidence relating smoking to vascular disease, the mechanisms through which tobacco smoke produces its effects are largely unknown, in part because tobacco smoke is a mixture of several thousand components. But there is evidence that smoking contributes to both the atherosclerotic[21] and thrombotic processes (through effects on platelet survival,[22] platelet aggregation[23], and increased fibrinogen levels[24]). There is also an increased incidence of cardiac arrythmias in response to catecholamines.[25] Post mortem studies consistently show more extensive and severe atherosclerosis in smokers than in non-smokers,[26] and smoking appears to contribute to the generation of atherosclerotic plaques.

Experimental work on atheromatous lesions induced in cholesterol-fed rabbits exposed to tobacco smoke suggested that carboxyhaemoglobin was the harmful link;[27] but the relevance of such studies to man is questionable. Nicotine may also play a role in the pathogenesis of cardiovascular disease. It causes release of catecholamines from the adrenal gland[28] and this, in turn, influences cardiac output and risk of cardiac arrhythmias. The adverse effect of carbon monoxide on the oxygen carrying capacity of the blood[29] could mean that the combined actions of nicotine and carbon monoxide may be to increase myocardial oxygen demand and to limit supply, precipitating ischaemia. Recent evidence from animal experiments indicate that cigarette smoke causes arterial endothelial damage with oedema and bleb-like microvilli, and consequent platelet adhesion.[26] The presence of free radicals in cigarette smoke has been known for a long time[30] and there is an association between lipid peroxidation and endothelial damage, but differential levels of blood antioxidants between smokers and non-smokers may reflect diet rather than smoking and it remains debatable whether this is an important mechanism by which smoking causes arterial disease.

The epidemiological evidence shows a lack of correlation between type of cigarette and cardiovascular risk.[31,32] Although the introduction of filter/low tar/ low nicotine cigarettes and progressive reductions in the yield of tar and nicotine over the last 30 years have (along with decline in smoking prevalence) contributed to a fall in the death rate of smokers,[33] there is little evidence that these changes have reduced the coronary heart disease death rate in smokers. Data from the *Framingham Study* indicate that smokers of filter cigarettes suffer as many heart attacks as smokers of non-filter cigarettes.[34] Furthermore, nicotine levels are highest in pipe smokers—the smoking group with the lowest cardiovascular risk.[35]

WHAT ARE THE BENEFITS FROM STOPPING SMOKING HOW QUICKLY ARE THESE ACHIEVED?

Numerous epidemiological studies[36,8] have looked at the effect on cardiovascular risk of stopping smoking. These generally show a rapid reduction in risk, especially in younger men. In the *British Doctors Study*, excess risk was halved within the first two or three years following cessation, and by 10 years the risk level had returned to that of a non-smoker (Fig. 1.4). But in the *British Regional Heart Study*,[37] which has followed up since 1980 a cohort of 7735 men aged 40–59 years, disappearance of this excess risk was slower and even men who had given up smoking for more than 20 years still had an increased risk (Fig. 1.5).

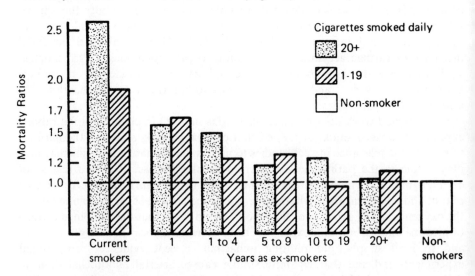

Fig. 1.4 Diminished risk of death from coronary heart disease in former light and heavy smokers. Both light and heavy smokers show a steady decline in risk after stopping until, after 10 to 20 years, it is little different from the risk of non-smokers. (From Royal College of Physicians, Smoking or health, Pitman Medical, London, 1977.)

Stopping smoking after myocardial infarction is associated with reduced risk of death. In one observational study[38] stopping smoking more than halved the number of deaths over a 13 year follow-up (Fig. 1.6). Also the one UK trial of smoking cessation advice that ascertained the incidence of ischaemic heart disease, in 1445 smokers, showed a (non-significant) 13 per cent difference in cumulative coronary heart disease deaths after 20 years follow-up in the intervention group, compared with the control group.[39] Smoking cessation is particularly important in secondary prevention of arterial disease and patients with established, manifest disease should be specifically targetted for help.

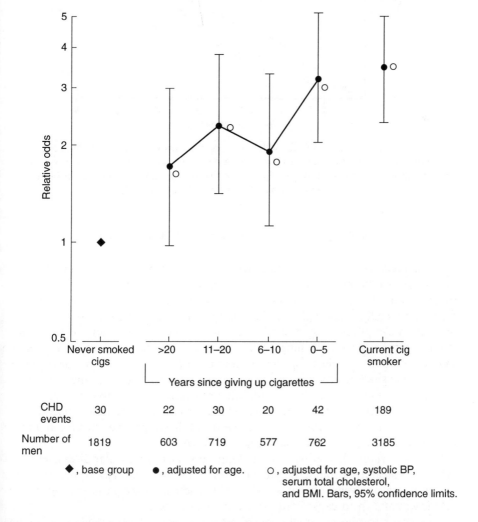

Fig. 1.5 Relative odds of a major coronary heart disease event in relation to years since stopping smoking cigarettes. (From Cook DG, Pocock SJ, Shaper AG, Kussick SJ. Giving up smoking and the risk of heart attacks. Lancet 1986; **2**: 1376-80.)

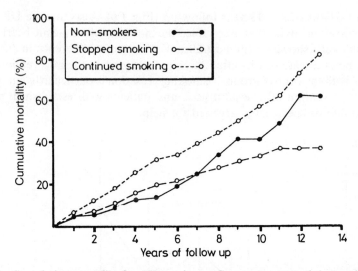

Fig. 1.6 Cumulative mortality for 498 survivors of a coronary attack by smoking habit. Life table curves start two years after attack. Average annual mortality was 6.5 per cent in non-smokers, 3.7 per cent in those who stopped smoking, and 10.2 per cent in those who continued smoking. (From Daly LE et al.[38])

IS PASSIVE SMOKING IMPORTANT?

There is much current concern and debate about the possible harmful effects of passive or involuntary smoking. In a study in middle aged men and women[40] lung function was shown to be impaired in non-smokers working in smoky environments and children brought up in smoky homes were shown to have more respiratory symptoms than others.[41] But it was a study from Japan,[42] demonstrating the increased risk of lung cancer amongst non-smoking wives of heavy smokers, which stimulated alarm. A number of case-control and prospective studies have since clearly demonstrated an increased risk of lung cancer of about 30 per cent in non-smokers living with smokers compared with non-smokers living with non-smokers.[43] It has been estimated that several hundred lung cancer deaths in non-smokers, annually in the UK, are attributable to passive smoking and that the number may be as many as 3000 in the USA.

It is less certain whether passive smoking caused cardiovascular disease but the evidence is steadily accumulating that it does.[44] It should, perhaps, be remembered that it was several years after it was shown that active smoking causes lung cancer that it was shown to cause cardiovascular disease also.

There have now been a number of cohort studies which have linked smoke in the home with heart disease in non-smoking spouses. But there are problems of possible misclassification of non-smokers and smokers in these studies and also of possible confounding by factors such as dietary differences of the non-smoking spouses of smokers and non-smokers. Moreover, measures of passive smoking are generally indirect, usually based on questionnaires. Nevertheless, collectively these cohort studies show substantial consistency and suggest a positive association between passive smoking and death from heart disease with relative risks ranging from 1.2 to 2.7; pooling 44 of all studies yields a relative risk of 1.3. There is also some evidence of a dose–response effect. In a case-control study of Chinese women,[45] the relative risk of non-fatal mycardial infarction from passive smoking at work was found to be greater (1.8) then from exposure to their husbands smoke at home (1.2).

Extrapolating the putative risks of passive smoking to attributable coronary heart disease deaths is very imprecise but one estimate attributes 62 000 ischaemic heart disease deaths a year in the USA to passive smoking.[46] From a public health view, a relationship between passive smoking and coronary heart disease is a serious and common disease—much commoner than lung cancer or respiratory disease.

IS SMOKING CESSATION INTERVENTION EFFECTIVE AND, IF SO, HOW SHOULD IT BE DONE AND WHO SHOULD DO IT?

Doctors who are themselves non-smokers are more likely than doctors who smoke to advise and help their patients to stop[47] and, fortunately, the great majority of UK general practitioners (almost 90 per cent) are now non-smokers.[3] Many smokers say they would stop smoking if advised to do so by their doctors,[48] and the role of the general practitioner as an exemplar should not be underestimated.[49]

The effectiveness of smoking cessation interventions, especially in primary care, has been extensively investigated through randomized controlled trials. The landmark study was done by Russell and colleagues in the 1970s in general practices in South London.[50] In this trial, 2138 cigarette smokers who were consulting their general practitioners about illness were recruited to a study of the effect of brief anti-smoking advice. They were allocated to one of four groups: a non-intervention control group with whom smoking was not discussed, a group simply given a questionnaire about smoking, a group who were also given brief advice to stop smoking, and a fourth group who in addition to this advice were given a self-help leaflet, and were warned they would be followed up. All participants were invited to provide follow-up information at one month and one year with 88 per cent (1884) and 73 per cent (1567) respectively doing so. The proportions who reported they had stopped smoking at one month and were still not smoking at one year were 0.3 per cent in the control group and 1.6 per cent, 3.3 per cent and 5.1 per cent respectively in the three intervention groups (p < 0.001). Although self-reported cessation was biochemically validated in a small proportion only, there was no evidence of major deception or differences between the groups. The results of the study are illustrated in Fig. 1.7.

This study has been replicated many times with similar results[51] and in one similar study, demonstration to the smoker of the level of carbon monoxide in expired breath was shown to enhance the effect of advice.[52] In specialist settings, such as smoking cessation clinics, higher success rates have been achieved. This may be because such programmes selectively recruit smokers who are highly motivated to stop but also because interventions are more intensive.[53] However, the general applicability of such programmes, compared to minimal interventions with those who have not specifically sought smoking cessation advice is questionable.

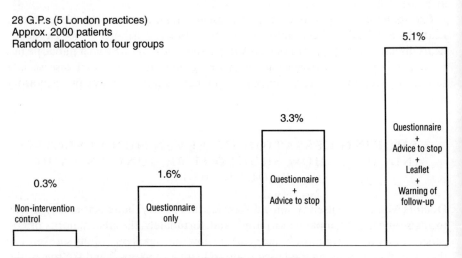

28 G.P.s (5 London practices)
Approx. 2000 patients
Random allocation to four groups

%= proportion who stopped smoking during the first month and were still not
smoking one year later (p<0.001)
equivalent to 25 long term successes per G.P.each year

Fig. 1.7   Effects of GP's advice against smoking. (From Russell MAH, Wilson C, Taylor C, Baker CD. Effects of general practitioners' advice against smoking. BMJ; **2**: 231–5.)

In reviewing 39 controlled trials of smoking cessation interventions, Kottke[51] demonstrated that determinants of success were: type of intervention (face-to-face advice better than others), type of intervenor (advice from both physician and non-physician counsellor better than advice from either alone), the number and duration of re-inforcing sessions, and the numbers of modalities used. Evidence of the efficacy of advice from nurses alone is limited[54] but the combination of brief advice from a physician supplemented by nurse support and advice appears much better.[55]

Nicotine replacement therapy (NRT)

In recent years there has been increasing recognition of the importance of nicotine in maintaining the smoking habit and in impeding smoking cessation.[56] The 1988 US Surgeon General's report concluded that 'the pharmacological and behavioural processes that determine tobacco dependence are similar to those that determine addiction to other drugs such as heroin and cocaine'.

The principle underlying nicotine replacement therapy as an aid to stopping smoking is the temporary provision of nicotine from a source other than tobacco, while the smoking habit, as behaviour, is being broken. Once the behavioural component has been dealt with, then the pharmacological addiction is 'treated' by the gradual withdrawal of the substitute source of nicotine. Stopping smoking may therefore be achieved through a two-stage process: first by tackling the physical, psychological, and social habit, and second by weaning off nicotine.

Nicotine chewing gum has been available as nicotine replacement therapy since about 1980. Placebo-controlled trials demonstrated its efficacy in specialist smoking cessation clinics but similar trials in primary care gave equivocal results. This was probably because of difficulties in using the gum, poor explanation provided by doctors, and poor compliance with its use.[57] Nicotine skin patches have become available more recently and randomized controlled trials of their use in primary care have demonstrated their efficacy.[58–61]

Two large meta-analyses[62,63] of nicotine replacement therapies in smoking cessation, together with a review,[64] have now demonstrated conclusively that these products can play a valuable part in helping motivated smokers to stop smoking. Use of either nicotine gum or nicotine patches approximately doubles cessation rates when compared with control interventions and the benefit is greater in those with high levels of nicotine dependence. On the other hand, intensity of additional support provided does not appear to influence substantially the relative effectiveness though it does influence the absolute probability of abstinence, which is much greater with the use of high intensity programmes. For this reason—and also because they tend to recruit smokers who are more motivated to stop—specialist smoking cessation clinics offer higher cessation rates than those achieved in primary care settings. Comparison of patches with gum in the overviews suggests that both absolute and relative abstinence rates are somewhat higher with patches, though for highly nicotine dependent smokers, 4 mg gum may be the most effective form of nicotine replacement therapy. Overall, compliance with patch use seems better than with gum and the likelihood of long-term dependency is less.

A simple smoking cessation protocol is illustrated in Fig. 1.8.

SUMMARY

- The relationship between smoking and cardiovascular disease is well established, especially for cigarette smoking.
- CHD, stroke, major arterial disease and peripheral arterial disease are all smoking-related diseases in the causation of which smoking interacts with other risk factors.
- Primary pipe and cigar smoking is less harmful than cigarette smoking but changing from cigarettes to pipes and cigars is not associated with substantial risk reduction.
- The mechanisms of these cardiovascular effects are probably both atherosclerotic and thrombotic.

PROTOCOL FOR DOCTOR/NURSE INTERVENTION

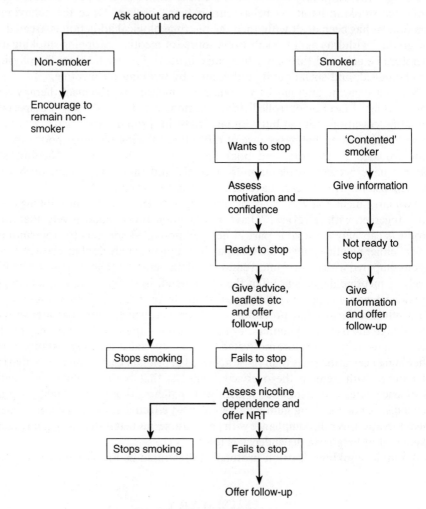

Fig. 1.8   Smoking cessation.

- Passive smoking may contribute to arterial disease but evidence so far is inconclusive.
- Stopping smoking confers benefits within 2–3 years.
- Smoking cessation is particularly important as part of a strategy for secondary prevention of cardiovascular disease.
- Simple advice (plus a patient leaflet) in general practice has been shown to increase sustained smoking cessation to about 5 per cent at one year.
- Nicotine replacement therapy (gum or skin patches) roughly doubles smoking cessation rates, compared with placebo, with one-year sustained abstinence rates of at least 10 per cent being achievable in primary care.

REFERENCES

1. World Health Organisation. Controlling the smoking epidemic. Technical Report Series 636, Geneva: WHO, 1979.
2. Thomas M, Goddard E, Hickman M, Hunter P. for OPCS. General Household Survey 1992. London: HMSO, 1993.
3. Fowler G, Mant D, Fuller A, Jones L. The 'Help your Patient Stop' initiative. Lancet 1989; **1**: 1253–5.
4. Thomas M, Holroyd S, Goddard E. for OPCS. Smoking amongst secondary school children in England in 1992. London: HMSO, 1994.
5. Doll R, Hill AB. Smoking and carcinoma of the lung. BMJ 1950; **2**: 739–48.
6. Wynder EL, Graham EA. Tobacco smoking as a possible etiological factor in bronchogenic carcinoma. J American Med Soc 1950; **143**: 329.
7. Royal College of Physicians. Health or Smoking? London: Pitman, 1983.
8. Doll R, Peto R. Mortality in relation to smoking: 20 years' observation of British male doctors. BMJ 1976; **4**: 1525–36.
9. Doll R, Gray R, Haffner B, Peto R. Mortality in relation to smoking: 22 years observations on female British doctors. BMJ 1980; **1**: 967–71.
10. Keys A. Coronary heart disease in seven countries. Circulation 1970; **41**: Supplement 1.
11. Reid DD, Hamilton PJS, McCartney P, *et al.* Smoking and other risk factors for coronary heart disease in British Civil Servants. Lancet 1976; **2**: 979–84.
12. Royal College of General Practitioners. Further analyses of mortality in oral contraceptive users. Lancet 1981; **1**: 541–6.
13. Kannel W, Doyle J, McNamara P, *et al.* Precursors of sudden coronary death. Circulation 1975; **51**: 606–13.
14. Shinton R, Beevers G. Meta-analysis of relation between cigarette smoking and stroke. BMJ 1989; **298**: 789–94.
15. Eastcott HH. Rarity of lower-limb ischaemia in non-smokers. Lancet 1962; **2**: 1117 (letter).
16. Hughson WG, Mann JI, Tibbs DJ, *et al.* Intermittent claudication: factors determining outcome. BMJ 1978; **1**: 1377–9.
17. Wray R, de Palma R, Hubar CH. Late occlusion of aorto-phemeral bypass grafts: influence of cigarette smoking. Surgery 1971; **70**: 969–73.
18. Hammond EC. Smoking in relation to the death rates of 1 million men and women. National Cancer Institute Monographs 1966, No. **19**: 127–204.
19. Levy LS and Martin PA. In: Nicotine Smoking and The Low Tar Programme. Wald N and Froggatt P (ed.) Oxford: Oxford University Press, 1989.
20. Higginbottom T, Shipley MS, Rose G. Cigarettes, lung cancer, and coronary heart disease: the effects of inhalation and tar yield. J Epidemiology and Community Health 1982; **36**: 113–17.
21. Auerbach O, Carter HW, Garfinkel L, Hammond EC. Cigarette smoking and coronary heart disease: a macroscopic and microscopic study. Chest 1976; **70**: 697–705.
22. Mustard JF, Murphy EA. Effect of smoking on blood coagulation and platelet survival in man. BMJ 1963; **i**: 846–9.
23. Hawkins RI. Smoking, platelets and thrombosis. Nature 1972; **263**: 450–2.
24. Meade TW, Imeson J, Sterling Y. Effects of changes in smoking and other characteristics on clotting factors and risk of ischaemic heart disease. Lancet 1987; **ii**: 986–8.
25. Lewis RP, Bondonlas H. Catecholamines, cigarette smoking, arrhythmias and acute myocardial infarction. Am Heart J 1974; **88**: 526–8.

26. Pittilo RM, Woolf N. Cigarette smoking, endothelial cell injury and atherosclerosis. J Smoking Related Disorders 1993; **4**: 17–25.
27. Astrup P. Some physiological and pathological effects of moderate carbon monoxide exposure. BMJ 1972; **4**: 447–52.
28. Armitage A. Effects of nicotine and tobacco smoke on blood pressure and release of catecholamines from the adrenal glands. British J Pharmacology 1965; **25**: 515–26.
29. Wright GR, Shepherd RGA. Physiological effect of carbon monoxide. International Review of Physiology 1979, **20**: 311–15.
30. Lyons MJ, Gibson JK, Ingram DJE. Free radicals produced in cigarette smoke. Nature 1958; **181**: 1003–4.
31. Lee PN, Garfinkel L. Mortality and type of cigarette smoked. J. Epidemiol Community Health 1981; **35**: 16–22.
32. Kaufman DW, Holmrich SP, Rosenberg L, *et al.* Nicotine and carbon monoxide content of cigarette smoke an risk of myocardial infarction in young men. N Engl J Med 1983; **308**: 409–13.
33. Hammond EC, Garfinkel H, Seidman M, *et al.* Tar and nicotine content of cigarette smoke in relation to death rates. Environmental Research 1976; **12**: 263–74.
34. Castelli WP, Garrison RJ, Dawber TR, *et al.* The filter cigarette and coronary heart disease. Lancet 1981; **2**: 109–13.
35. Wald NJ, Idle M, Boreham J. Serum cotinine levels in pipe smokers: evidence against nicotine as a cause of coronary heart disease. Lancet 1981; **1**: 775–7.
36. Hammond EC, Garfinkel L. Coronary heart disease, stroke and aortic aneurysm: factors in etiology. Archives of Environmental Health 1969; **19**: 167–71.
37. Cook DG, Pocock SJ, Shaper AG, Kussick SJ. Giving up smoking and the risk of heart attacks. Lancet 1986; **2**: 1376–80.
38. Daly LE, Mulcahy R, Graham IM, Hickey N. Long term effect on mortality of stopping smoking after unstable angina and myocardial infarction. BMJ 1983; **287**: 324–326.
39. Rose G, Colwell L. Randomised controlled trial of anti-smoking advice: final (20 year) results. J Epidemiol Community Health 1992; **46**: 75–7.
40. White JR, Froeb H. Small airways dysfunction in non-smokers chronically exposed to tobacco smoke. N Engl J Med 1980; **302**: 720–3.
41. Colley JRT. Respiratory symptoms in children and parental smoking. BMJ 1974; **2**: 201–4.
42. Hirayama T. Non-smoking wives of heavy smokers have a higher risk of lung cancer. BMJ 1981; **1**: 183–5.
43. Wald N, Nanchatal K, Thompson SG, Cuckle H. Does breathing other peoples' tobacco smoke cause lung cancer? BMJ 1986; **293**: 1217–22.
44. Beaglehole R. Does passive smoking cause heart disease? BMJ 1990; **301**: 1343–4.
45. He Y, Lam T, Li L, Du R, Jia J, Huang J, Zheng J. Passive smoking at work as a risk factor for coronary heart disease in Chinese women who have never smoked. BMJ 1994; **308**: 380–4.
46. Judson Wells A. Passive smoking as a cause of heart disease. J Am Coll Cardio 1994; **24**: 545–54.
47. Hallet R. Intervention against smoking and its relationship to general practitioners smoking habits. JRCGP 1983; **33**: 565–7.
48. Marsh A, Matheson J. Smoking attitudes and behaviour, London: HMSO, 1983.
49. Adriaanse H, van Reek J. Physicians' smoking and its exemplary effect. Scand J Primary Health Care 1989; **7**: 193–6.
50. Russell MAH, Wilson C, Taylor C, Baker CD. Effects of general practitioners' advice against smoking. BMJ 1979; **2**: 231–5.
51. Kottke T, Battisha R, DeFriese G, Brekke M. Attributes of successful smoking

cessation interventions in medical practice: a meta-analysis of 39 controlled trials. JAMA 1988; **259**: 2883–9.

52. Jamrozik K, Vessey M, Fowler G, *et al.* Controlled trial of three different anti-smoking interventions in general practice. BMJ 1984; **288**: 1499–1502.

53. Richmond RL, Austin A, Webster I. Three year evaluation of a programme by general practitioners to help patients stop smoking. BMJ 1986; **292**: 803–6.

54. Sanders D, Fowler G, Mant D, *et al.* Randomised controlled trial of anti-smoking advice by nurses in general practice. JRCGP 1989; **39**: 273–6.

55. Hollis J, Lichtenstein E, Vogt T, Stevens V, Biglan A. Nurse-assisted counselling for smokers in primary care. Ann Int Med 1993; **118**: 521–5.

56. US Department of Health and Human Sciences. The Health Consequences of Smoking: Nicotine Addiction. Report of Surgeon General 1988. Washington DC, 1989.

57. Lam W, Sachs H, Szep, Chalmers TC. Meta-analysis of randomised controlled trials of nicotine chewing gum. Lancet 1987; **2**: 27–9.

58. ICRF General Practice Research Group. Effectiveness of a nicotine patch in helping people stop smoking: results of a randomised trial in general practice. BMJ 1993; **306**: 1304–8.

59. Russell MAH, Stapleton JA, Feyeraband C, *et al.* Targetting heavy smokers in general practice: randomised controlled trial of transdermal nicotine patches. BMJ 1993; **306**: 1308–12.

60. Campbell IA (Editorial). Nicotine patches in general practice. BMJ 1993; **306**: 1284–5.

61. ICRF General Practice Research Group. Randomised trial of nicotine patches in general practice: results at one year. BMJ 1994; **308**: 1476–7.

62. Tang TL, Law M, Wald N. How effective is nicotine replacement therapy in helping people to stop smoking? BMJ 1994; **308**: 21–6.

63. Silagy C, Mant D, Fowler G, Lodge M. Meta-analysis on efficacy of nicotine replacement therapies in smoking cessation. Lancet 1994; **343**: 139–42.

64. Anon. Nicotine patches. Drug Ther Bull 1993; **31**: 95–6.

2 Hypertension

Martin Lawrence and Kennedy Cruickshank

INTRODUCTION

Severe hypertension as a risk factor for cardiovascular disease

It has long been recognized that high blood pressure is a major risk factor for overall mortality and for death from cardiovascular disease in particular. Untreated malignant hypertension has a mortality of over 80 per cent within a year from detection[1] and in 1959 treatment was first shown to reduce this at least six-fold.[2]

By 1967, in the first formal controlled trial by the *Veterans Administration team*, the control group of 70 untreated patients with diastolic blood pressure from 115–129 mm Hg ('severe' but not necessarily malignant hypertension), followed for an average of 18 months, showed major vascular events or death in 21 (30 per cent) compared with one stroke and no deaths in the actively treated group.[3] Following this unequivocal evidence of treatment effectiveness, subjects with diastolic blood pressure 90–114 mm Hg were randomized to active treatment or placebo for up to five years.[4] Among the 210 patients with diastolic blood pressure 105–114 mm Hg there was a 75 per cent reduction in major events in the treatment group (eight events versus 35). Further such placebo controlled trials in the range of diastolic blood pressure 105–129mm Hg would now be unethical.

Post-mortem studies in the 1960s demonstrated why severe hypertension is associated with such high morbidity and mortality. Apart from the findings of fibrinoid necrosis in blood vessels whose walls had been directly damaged by the pressure, a long-term observational study of mental hospital in-patients showed that atheroma, particularly of the proximal cerebral arteries, was closely associated with long-term raised blood pressure.[5] In a further post mortem study small aneurysms, originally described by Charcot and Bouchard as associated with cerebral haemorrhage, were shown to be common only in patients with diastolic pressures of greater than 110 mm Hg.[6]

Moderate hypertension as a risk factor for cardiovascular disease.

Actuarial data provide much of the evidence regarding the effect of blood pressure, because there is long term followup. These data show a steady increase in mortality with rising blood pressure. Men in the western world with blood pressures of 140/90 mm Hg have a mortality 50 per cent above average, at 145/95 mm Hg mortality is double, and at 160/100 mm Hg some three times higher than average.[7] Prospective observational studies, perhaps the most famous being the *Framingham Study*,[8] support these findings with a two to three fold difference in coronary disease between normotensives and hypertensives aged 45–64, and an eight-fold difference for stroke.

Observational studies suffer from the defect that the blood pressure may have been read only once at the start of observation. There is considerable evidence that initial readings tend to be high. In the MRC trial of mild hypertension, patients were admitted to the study only after readings of blood pressure on three separate occasions, twice by a nurse and once by a doctor, and if the mean of the diastolic blood pressure was in the required range 90–109 mm Hg. Despite, this the mean blood pressures of patients in the placebo group had fallen by the time of the first annual re-examination (Fig. 2.1), and indeed over 40 per cent of patients on placebo had diastolic blood pressure below 90 mm Hg at each of the five annual reviews.[9]

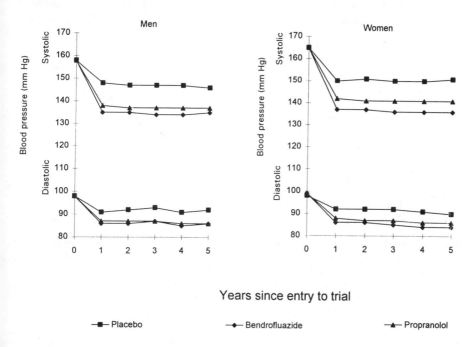

Fig. 2.1 Means levels of blood pressure in the Medical Research Council trial of mild hypertension. (Derived from MRC Working Party[9])

The result of this overestimation of the true blood pressure of subjects entering trials is to dilute the apparent effect of treatment. Despite this, it is remarkable how good and important a predictor of outcome such blood pressure readings can be. Nevertheless, trials in which blood pressure has been measured in this way substantially underestimate the real association of the 'true' blood pressure and outcome. This has been termed 'regression dilution bias'.

MacMahon and colleagues reviewed nine studies involving 418 000 subjects and corrected for this bias on the basis of remeasurements undertaken in the

Framingham study.[10] This analysis showed that the relative risk of both stroke and coronary heart disease (CHD) bear a log–linear relationship to blood pressure at all levels of blood pressure. The relative risk between the highest (mean usual diastolic blood pressure 105 mm Hg) and lowest (mean usual diastolic blood pressure 75 mm Hg) categories was 10–12 for stroke and 5–6 for CHD (Fig. 2.2). This means that there would be a 46 per cent reduction in stroke and a 29 per cent reduction in CHD if the usual diastolic blood pressure were 7.5 mm Hg lower (Fig. 2.3 (a) and (b)). These data from observational studies give a numerical estimate of the maximum benefit that could be expected from treatment (the 'attributable' benefit). Whether this benefit can be achieved by treatment is discussed below.

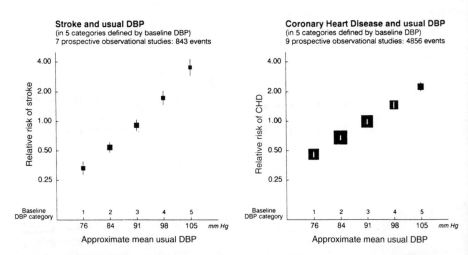

Fig. 2.2   Relative risks of stroke and of coronary heart disease, estimated from combined results. Estimates of the usual diastolic blood pressure (DBP) in each baseline DBP category are taken from mean DBP values four years post-baseline in the Framingham study. Solid squares represent disease risk in each category relative to risk in the whole study population; sizes of squares are proportional to the number of events in each DBP category; and 95 per cent confidence limits for estimates of relative risk are denoted by vertical lines.

The continuum of risk

Work in the early 1950s by Miall in community studies in south Wales and by Pickering and colleagues in hospital outpatients established that 'hypertension' is not a disease.[11] Blood pressures in the population form a continuum, and hypertension is defined as any pressure above some arbitrary point on that distribution. The risk of a stroke or myocardial infarction rises progressively with both systolic or diastolic blood pressure and not just from some arbitrary value used to define hypertension (Fig 2.4).[12] For these reasons, the best definition of hypertension is that of Rose:[13]

'the level of blood pressure above which treatment does more good than harm'.

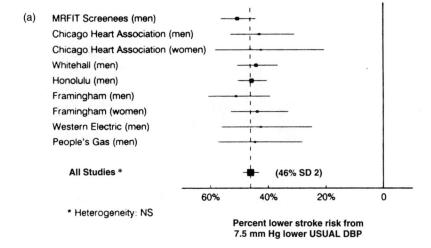

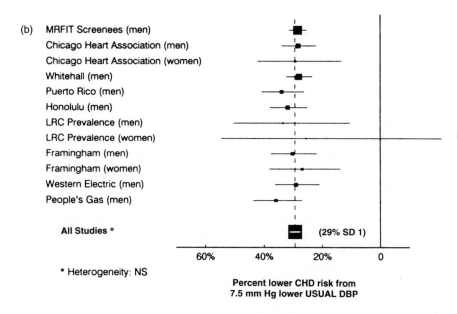

Fig. 2.3 (a) Estimates from seven studies of eventual difference in stroke risk associated with about a 7.5 mm Hg lower usual diastolic blood pressure. (b) Estimates from nine studies of eventual difference in coronary heart disease risk associated with about a 7.5 mm Hg lower usual diastolic blood pressure. Sizes of squares are proportional to the number of events in each study and 95 per cent confidence intervals for estimated differences in risk are denoted by horizontal lines.

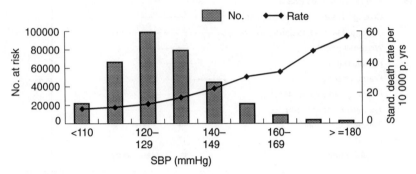

Fig. 2.4   MRFIT CHD death rate and number at risk by systolic blood pressure, 12 year follow-up.

In his final years' work Pickering focused on the key epidemiological point that most cases of disease relating to a risk factor arise in people at low but marginally increased risk, while those at high risk account for few of the total cases that occur. If ways could be found to reduce the blood pressure of the whole population by a little, many more events would be prevented than by just treating the high risk patients.

The effect of treating just the high risk patients is further reduced by the Rule of Halves. The rule states that, of those in a community with hypertension justifying treatment, only half are known, of that half only half are being treated, and of those treated only half are adequately controlled—that is 12.5 per cent of the potential total. Although this phenomenon was first recognised in the 1960s, the rule still applied in Scotland in the mid 1980s, almost exactly for men and only slightly better for women.[14]

There is also a concern that a common sequel to mild hypertension is slowly progressive cardiac failure. This is an end point beyond the duration of most trials of hypotensive therapy—but has clearly been shown in trials in the elderly—and it will command more attention as the early consequences of hypertension, myocardial infarction, and stroke, diminish.

MAJOR AREAS OF CONCERN IN THE MANAGEMENT OF HYPERTENSION

1. **Is it possible to achieve reduction of coronary heart disease and stroke by treatment of high blood pressure?**
2. **Do different groups, such as the elderly, women, different ethnic groups, or people with diabetes, need particular treatment policies?**
3. **What is the relative importance of systolic and diastolic blood pressure?**

4. **How frequently should we measure blood pressure, and what level of blood pressure should we aim for when introducing treatment?**
5. **How extensive are the side effects of treatment, and are there benefits in non-pharmacologic treatments?**

IS IT POSSIBLE TO ACHIEVE REDUCTION OF CORONARY HEART DISEASE AND STROKE BY TREATMENT OF HIGH BLOOD PRESSURE?

A source of confusion for many doctors and nurses interpreting research results has been the distinction between *observational* and *intervention* studies. The former provide evidence of risk; but association does not prove cause nor does it prove that reducing raised blood pressure would reduce risk. Randomized controlled trials are required to demonstrate the benefit of treatment.

There have been many trials of the management of moderate hypertension which provide evidence for the benefit of treatment in reducing stroke and CHD (Table 2.1).

Table 2.1   Trials of the management of moderate hypertension

DBP range	Trial	Date published	No in trial	Reference
90–104	HDFP	1979	7825	15
95–110	Australia	1980	3427	16
DBP <110 and SBP 140 – 180	Oslo	1980	785	17
90–115	MRFIT	1982	12866	18
90–109	MRC	1985	17354	9
SBP >160 and DBP <90	SHEP*	1991	4736	19, 20
SBP 180–230 or DBP 105–120	STOP*	1991	1627	21
SBP >160 and DBP<115	MRC*	1992	4396	22

* Trials in older adults

In the *Hypertension Detection And Follow Up Project* (HDFP)[15] there was a reduction in major events of 20 per cent in patients with a diastolic blood pressure of 90–104 mm Hg allocated to special treatment, and of 29 per cent in that subgroup without pre-existing CHD. The study has been criticized because it was really a trial of a health service rather than just blood pressure treatment since the randomization was either to special clinic care or to the patient's usual doctor. Since 29 per cent of the population was black, many of whom had no access to routine care, allocation to the intervention group may have conferred benefits in addition to the adequate treatment of blood pressure.

The *Australian Trial* [16] and the *Medical Research Council Trial of Mild Hypertension* (MRC)[9] included subjects of both sexes considered free of CHD at the outset. The Australian study showed a significant reduction in mortality with treatment, mainly due to a two thirds reduction in cardiovascular disease; the reduction in stroke was significant, but the confidence interval for reduction in CHD overlapped zero. In the first MRC trial there was no significant reduction in overall nor CHD mortality with treatment, but strokes were significantly reduced.[9]

Much has been made of the treatment years needed to save one stroke: 850 in the MRC trial, 490 in the Australian trial. However, as mentioned above, in the MRC trial 40 per cent of the subjects on placebo had diastolic blood pressure less than 90 mm Hg at each of the annual reviews. This implies that if corrected for bias due to regression to the mean, the results would be much more impressive than they appear.

The *Multiple Risk Factor Intervention Trial* (MRFIT)[18] involved intervention on several risk factors for cardiovascular disease, including blood pressure, smoking, and diet. After six years there was no significant difference in CHD or total deaths between intervention and control groups. However, the control group had also made major changes in risk factors (47 per cent were on hypotensive therapy) and the number of deaths was less than half that expected (219 vs 442).

These randomized trials were included in a meta-analysis by Collins, *et al*[23] (excluding the recent *Systolic Hypertension in Elderly Persons* (SHEP) and *MRC* elderly trials that were published later). In this overview the reduction in stroke was 42 per cent and in CHD 14 per cent (Fig. 2.5). This clinically important reduction in CHD was too small to be detected with statisical significance in the individual trials because they were too small and the follow-up period was often short. The relatively modest benefit for CHD also reflects the adverse metabolic (lipid and glucose) effects of the drugs, particularly at the doses then used.

Comparing the trials with the observational data it appears that almost all the expected benefit from treatment in respect of stroke takes place rapidly, but only about half that expected for CHD takes place within the first five years.

DO DIFFERENT GROUPS, SUCH AS THE ELDERLY, WOMEN, DIFFERENT ETHNIC GROUPS, OR PEOPLE WITH DIABETES, NEED PARTICULAR TREATMENT POLICIES?

The elderly

The case for vigorous screening and treatment for people over 65 with hypertension has now been clearly made. The 'elderly' trials provide the best evidence that treating hypertension, particularly with a low dose diuretic, reduces coronary mortality and morbidity. Until 1985, blood pressure treatment trials usually excluded patients over the age of 65. Then two trials, the *European Working Party on Hypertension in the Elderly* (EWPHE)[24] and the *Hypertension in the Elderly Project* (HEP),[25] produced impressively consistent reports of benefit.

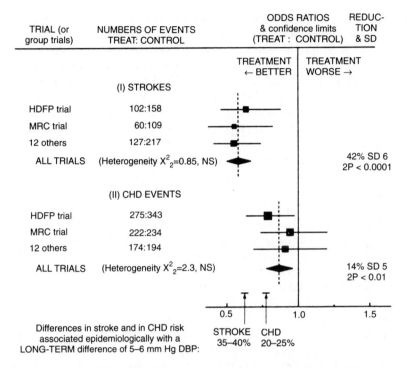

TRIAL (or group trials)	NUMBERS OF EVENTS TREAT: CONTROL	ODDS RATIOS & confidence limits (TREAT : CONTROL)	REDUC-TION & SD

TREATMENT ← BETTER | TREATMENT WORSE →

(I) STROKES

HDFP trial	102:158		
MRC trial	60:109		
12 others	127:217		
ALL TRIALS	(Heterogeneity X^2_2=0.85, NS)		42% SD 6 2P < 0.0001

(II) CHD EVENTS

HDFP trial	275:343		
MRC trial	222:234		
12 others	174:194		
ALL TRIALS	(Heterogeneity X^2_2=2.3, NS)		14% SD 5 2P < 0.01

0.5   1.0   1.5

Differences in stroke and in CHD risk associated epidemiologically with a LONG-TERM difference of 5–6 mm Hg DBP:

STROKE 35–40%   CHD 20–25%

Fig. 2.5 Reduction in the odds of stroke and of CHD in the HDFP trial, the MRC trial, and in all 12 other unconfounded randomized trials of anti-hypertensive therapy (mean diastolic blood pressure differences 5–6 mm Hg for five years). Sizes of squares are proportional to the number of events in each study and 95 per cent confidence intervals for estimated differences in risk are denoted by horizontal lines.

EWPHE was a multi-centre project in which 840 subjects of average age 72 were enrolled in 20 centres.[24] There was no exclusion of subjects with pre-existing cardiovascular disease and recruitment appears to have been unsystematic. Treatment was by diuretic versus placebo and results showed a 26 per cent drop in mortality with a 47 per cent fall in cardiac deaths, and a 43 per cent fall in stroke.

The *HEP Trial*[25] took place in 13 British general practices. Subjects were over 60 years with either diastolic blood pressure > 105 mm Hg or systolic blood pressure > 170 mm Hg on three successive readings and those with pre-existing cardio-vascular disease were excluded. Treatment was by atenolol with bendrofluazide added if necessary. The incidence of stroke fell by 40 per cent but overall mortality and myocardial infarction was unchanged. The incidence of congestive heart failure fell by 50 per cent, but this did not reach statistical significance owing to the small size of the study.

These two small trials suggested that the treatment of raised blood pressure in the elderly is highly effective, with one stroke or cardiovascular death prevented for every 50–100 treatment years. The results have since been confirmed by three larger studies.

The *American SHEP Trial* was aimed only at isolated systolic hypertension, specifically excluding those with diastolic blood pressure > 90 mm Hg; 4736 subjects over 60 years old were enrolled.[19] Treatment was with the long acting diuretic chlorthalidone,[20] initially at very low dose (12.5–25mg/day), adding atenolol if necessary to keep the systolic blood pressure < 160 mm Hg. The results were impressive and directly related to the degree of blood pressure reduction achieved. Stroke was reduced by 36 per cent (95 per cent confidence interval (CI), 18–50 per cent), coronary events by 25 per cent (6–40 per cent), and heart failure by 54 per cent (35–67 per cent).

The *Swedish Trial of Old Patients with Hypertension* (STOP)[21] also produced impressive results. Patients were aged 70 to 84 years. Treated patients were randomized to a beta blocker (atenolol, pindolol or metoprolol) or a hydrochlorthiazide 25mg plus amiloride 2.5mg combination diuretic. If blood pressure remained above 160/95 the alternative treatment was added, and 66 per cent of patients required a combination during the trial. Each agent was equally effective in treating diastolic blood pressure, but the diuretic was better for reducing systolic blood pressure. All cardiovascular disease endpoints fell from 94 in the placebo group to 58 in the treated group, a drop in relative risk of 40 per cent (95 per cent CI,15–57 per cent), strokes from 53 to 29, a drop of 47 per cent (14–67 per cent), and total mortality from 63 to 36, a drop of 43 per cent (13–63 per cent).

The *MRC's Older Adults Trial* results were equally impressive.[22] 226 general practices participated, screening 20 389 people aged 65–74 years of whom 4396 were randomized. The drugs used were again low dose diuretics (25mgs hydrochlorthiazide plus 2.5mgs amiloride) compared with 50mgs atenolol or placebo. Blood pressures were lowered effectively, although again systolic blood pressure slightly more so by the diuretic. The results were highly significant but only for diuretic therapy. Cardiovascular events were reduced by 44 per cent (95 per cent CI, 21–60 per cent), stroke 31 per cent (3–51 per cent) and all cardiovascular events 35 per cent (17–49 per cent). The beta-blocker had no significant effect on these endpoints. Total deaths were lowered in the diuretic group but were increased in the beta blocker group (but neither effect reached statisical significance).

Thus, there can be little doubt that a low dose diuretic should be the recommended first line therapy for all older patients with hypertension, aiming to reduce blood pressure to below 160/90 mm Hg if possible.

Women and blood pressure treatment

Men have higher risk than women of death and morbidity from cardiovascular disease—but does that mean that a less interventionist approach is needed in managing blood pressure in women?

The risk of stroke is similar in both sexes for a given blood pressure[8] but men have 2.5 times the incidence of myocardial infarction at all levels of blood pressure.[26] In subgroup analysis of treatment trials, the *HDFP Trial* reported significant benefit from treatment of black but not white women:[13] the Australian trial noted a reduction in trial end points for women who were treated (24 versus 36), which did not reach significance.[16] However, in the trials of elderly subjects and meta-analyses, results were equally positive for women and men.

There is evidence that women have more 'white coat' hypertension than men,[27] so special care should be taken to check women's blood pressure frequently before beginning treatment.Once treatment is started it should be conducted on the same basis in women as in men.

Ethnic groups at particular risk

People of west African descent, including Afro-Caribbeans and black Americans, appear to have higher levels of blood pressure at a given age and hence a higher prevalence of hypertension than other ethnic groups. However, many indigenous rural west Africans continue to have low levels of blood pressure, which tend to rise sharply in towns.

Despite this, the evidence that risk of a cardiovascular event is higher for a given level of blood pressure is poor.[28] Indeed, black subjects have shown particularly good responses to therapy in all the relevant treatment trials,[3,4,13,18,19] but appropriate therapy is essential. Mainly because plasma renin activity is lower in black than in white populations, treatment responses differ. Salt restriction and potassium supplementation, as simple fruit (juice) and lightly cooked vegetables, both lower blood pressure effectively.[29,30] Beta blockers and ACE inhibitors prescribed without diuretics are generally ineffective.[28,31]

There is no evidence that other ethnic groups—people of Indian, Chinese or other origin—have special needs in respect of hypertension, except for diligent treatment in Indians where risk of CHD and diabetes is high.

Diabetes

In view of the excellent long-term results from and minimal metabolic side-effects of low dose diuretics in the age groups affected by type II (non-insulin dependent) diabetes, these drugs should also be first choice for such patients, using the lowest dose possible. This may seem controversial advice but, without the results of planned trials for diabetic patients, no firm evidence is available. ACE inhibitors are promoted hard for patients with diabetes but, except for type I patients with early renal impairment, the evidence to date does not support their use for first line treatment. (Further discussion of CHD risk and diabetes will be found in Chapter 8).

WHAT IS THE RELATIVE IMPORTANCE OF SYSTOLIC AND DIASTOLIC BLOOD PRESSURE?

The earliest trials of treating raised blood pressure[3,4,13,18] used diastolic blood pressure as the main criterion. Since then studies have consistently shown that systolic blood pressure is slightly better than diastolic blood pressure as a predictor of the effect of blood pressure on CHD and stroke. The largest study to review this was the *Whitehall Study*[32] of 18 000 British Civil Servants which found that systolic blood pressure was a more powerful independent risk factor than diastolic blood pressure (systolic blood pressure corrected for diastolic blood pressure, relative risk (RR) 1.29; diastolic blood pressure corrected for systolic blood pressure, RR 1.09). Similarly, 15 per cent more of the men who died of CHD were in the upper quintile for systolic blood pressure than for diastolic blood pressure. There are difficulties, however, in following protocols using systolic blood pressure since it rises with age more steeply than diastolic blood pressure, and hence is more variable.

Observational studies have consistently shown that isolated systolic hypertension is associated with increased mortality. A study of 3901 Dutch Civil Servants and their spouses aged 40–65 started in the early 1950s showed that isolated systolic hypertension (systolic blood pressure > 160 mm Hg, diastolic blood pressure < 90 mm Hg) was present in three per cent of men and six per cent of women.[33] After 25 years of follow-up the all cause mortality for men was significantly higher (odds ratio 3.2; 95 per cent CI, 1.3–8.0) but only slightly raised for women (odds ratio 1.7; 95 per cent CI, 0.96–3.0). The value of treating isolated systolic hypertension has now been firmly established by the SHEP results and subgroup analysis of the MRC trial.

HOW FREQUENTLY SHOULD WE MEASURE BLOOD PRESSURE, AND WHAT LEVEL OF BLOOD PRESSURE SHOULD WE AIM FOR WHEN INTRODUCING TREATMENT?

Blood presure rises steadily with age, and the need to remeasure it depends on the rate of rise. The clearest data was reported by Miall and Chinn following a survey in Wales over a 17 year period.[34] They found that, of subjects with diastolic blood pressure < 90 mm Hg, less than four per cent had diastolic blood pressure > 100 mm Hg within 8–10 years. For those with initial diastolic blood pressure 90–99 mm Hg, 20 per cent had diastolic blood pressure > 100 within four years. These data support current practice by which routine measurement is not recommended more frequently than five yearly, but in patients with blood pressure that is borderline for treatment then remeasurement at between one and three yearly intervals is indicated. These data are supported by findings in the *Australian Therapeutic Trial of Mild Hypertension*, in which 198/1706 patients on placebo at entry had exceeded the entry band (95–109 mm Hg) within four years.[16]

In Miall's data 486 out of 499 deaths were in subjects over 35 years, and CHD deaths in subjects below 35 were 'too few to analyse'. Although blood pressure in youth is a predictor of blood pressure in older age, the likelihood of benefit from treatment suggests that regular screening only needs to begin by age 35.

Once treatment is started the full attributable risk of CHD may not be reversed, which is not surprising for a condition that develops over a lifetime. Results from the Australian study, confirmed by all the recent trial results, provide evidence that the risk of events during treatment corresponds more closely to the level of diastolic blood pressure achieved on treatment than to the entry diastolic blood pressure (Table 2.2).[16]

Table 2.2 Cardiovascular end points per 1000 patient years

diastolic blood pressure on treatment (mm Hg)	diastolic blood pressure at entry (mm Hg)		
	95–99	100–104	105–109
<90	12.1	17.6	12.2
90–94	24.8	14.4	19.9
95–99	69.8	38.4	58.4

Since the observed level of morbidity falls at all levels of blood pressure, it can reasonably be asked whether there is a point beyond which blood pressure reduction is no longer beneficial and may be deleterious. In an analysis of 13 separate trials Farnett *et al* have shown that there is a consistent trend by which CHD events and mortality rise, but stroke does not, if diastolic blood pressure is treated to below 85 mm Hg (Fig. 2.6).[35] However this J-shaped curve for achieved diastolic blood pressure may be due to patients' blood pressure falling as they become less well. It remains controversial and is the focus of a formal trial.

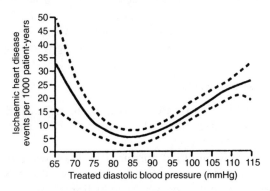

Fig. 2.6 Summary curve model derived by Farnett *et al* from analysis of 13 separate trials, 95 per cent confidence intervals are shown by the dashed curves.

HOW EXTENSIVE ARE THE SIDE-EFFECTS OF TREATMENT, AND ARE THERE BENEFITS IN NON-PHARMACOLOGICAL TREATMENTS?

Side effects

The incidence of side-effects from treatment is important, because if morbidity is directly related to the level of blood pressure then the threshold for treatment will be heavily dependent on side-effects. Side-effects fall into two categories: adverse effects on the physical health of the patient, and the psychological effect of being labelled as a patient.

All the early major trials were conducted using medication which is now regarded as out of date—mainly methyldopa, unselective beta blockers or diuretics in high doses. In the MRC trial of mild hypertension the rate of side-effects, in men on bendrofluazide 10mg daily, was 7.7, 12.4 and 12.6 per thousand patient years for diabetes, gout and impotence; and on propanolol was 3.4, 6.3 and 5.1 for diabetes, impotence and Raynaud's phenomenon.[9] If the rate of strokes avoided is 1.2 per thousand patient years for people under 65 years (above this age the benefits are much greater as described above), then the balance between benefits and disadvantages has to be carefully struck. More modern treatments with low dose diuretics, calcium channel antagonists, selective beta blockers and ACE inhibitors will alter this pattern.[36]

Being labelled as hypertensive may also cause disability. Haynes showed increased absenteeism from work after a diagnosis of hypertension had been made even when the subjects were not being treated,[37] and Jachuk noted that relatives report more psychiatric impairment in patients (decline in energy, irritability etc.) than the patients themselves.[38] On the other hand, Mann investigated change in the psychological state of participants in the first MRC trial and found significant falls in psychiatric morbidity which he attributed to the therapeutic supportive contact from interviews during follow-up.[39]

Non pharmacological treatments

If the decision to treat is determined by a balance between cardiovascular disease risk reduction and side-effects then non-pharmacological methods of treatment must be important as the first line.

The influence of *weight* on blood pressure is well known, although clouded by the false elevation of blood pressure readings due to a small cuff being used on a fat arm. Pooled data from studies of weight reduction show a decrease in systolic blood pressure of 21 mm Hg and of diastolic blood pressure of 13 mm Hg for a weight reduction of 12 kg.[40]

Salt intake appears to be influential on blood pressure on a population basis, and, in particular, low pressure communities have low salt intakes. There does however appear to be little evidence of an association between an individual intake and blood pressure within a community.[41] In terms of treatment, Morgan *et al* showed that a 'no added salt' regime (< 100 mmol/day) reduced diastolic blood pressure by 7 mm Hg[42]—more stringent salt restriction is more effective but usually intolerable to patients. An overview of intervention studies of reduction in salt intake showed a reduction of 5–7 mm Hg in systolic blood pressure and about half as much in diastolic blood pressure.[43] Salt restriction may well be beneficial, particularly because any adverse effects are minimal.[29]

Advising *increased potassium* intake from fresh fruit juice and lightly cooked vegetables also seems appropriate, again confirmed as effective in reducing blood pressure in an overview of trials.[30]

The Kaiser Permanente study showed no association between *alcohol* and blood pressure for an intake of less than two units per day, but a rise of 10 mm systolic blood pressure and 5 mm diastolic blood pressure as intake rose to 6 units per day.[44]

Patel has achieved substantial falls of blood pressure in a study of relaxation involving six weeks training and biofeedback.[45] Mean systolic blood pressure fell from 165 to 146 and diastolic blood pressure from 101 to 90 mm Hg, with no change in controls. Unfortunately this was not maintained over a year's follow-up.

SUMMARY

- There is clear evidence that high blood pressure is an independent risk factor for vascular disease, especially stroke, cardiac failure, and myocardial infarction.
- Treatment of patients with diastolic blood pressure > 110 mm Hg has been shown to decrease mortality tenfold in short (< 5 year) trials.
- There is clear evidence of the benefit of treatment in subjects with diastolic blood pressure 90–110 and systolic blood pressure > 160 mm Hg. Stroke is reduced by 42 per cent and coronary heart disease by 14 per cent for a 5–6 mm Hg drop in diastolic blood pressure.
- Because of the continuous relationship between blood pressure and cardiovascular disease, the threshold for treatment is limited by the adverse effects of treatment, and by the blood pressure level at which absolute risk is low. Once treatment is begun, systolic blood pressure should be reduced to 160 mm Hg if possible and diastolic blood pressure to 85–90 mm Hg.
- Life-style change which lowers blood pressure will be beneficial at all levels of blood pressure, and is generally free of side-effects.
- Systolic blood pressure is as good a measure of risk as diastolic, if not better. There is now evidence that treating isolated high systolic blood pressure, common in older people, is beneficial.
- Women benefit equally to men from the treatment of high blood pressure to avoid stroke. Their benefit from treatment with regard to CHD is less because of their lower incidence.
- People of Afro-Caribbean origin have a high prevalence of hypertension. Treatment with low dose diuretics is effective, but with beta blockers or ACE inhibitors alone is ineffective.

- The elderly benefit more than the young because they have a much higher absolute risk. Treatment should be gentle in view of the greater liability of the elderly to experience side effects.

REFERENCES

1. Leishman A W D. Hypertension—treated and untreated: a study of 400 cases. BMJ 1959; (i): 1361–8.
2. Harington M, Kincaid Smith P, McMichael J. Results of treatment of malignant hypertension: a 7-year experience in 94 cases. BMJ 1959; (ii): 969–72.
3. Veterans Administration Co-operative Study Group. Effects of treatment on morbidity in hypertension: Results on patients with diastolic blood pressure averaging 115 through 129mm Hg. JAMA 1967; 202: 116–22.
4. Veterans Administration Co-operative Study Group. Effects of treatment on morbidity in hypertension: Results in patients with diastolic blood pressure averaging 90 through 114 mm Hg. JAMA 1970; 213: 1143–52.
5. Evans P H. Relation of long standing blood pressure levels to atherosclerosis. Lancet 1965; (i): 516–19.
6. Cole F M, Yates P O. The occurrence and significance of intracerebral micro aneurysms. J Path Bacteriology 1967; 93: 393–411.
7. Lew E A. Blood pressure and mortality—life insurance experience. In Stamler J, Stamler R, Pullman T N.(ed.) The epidemiology of hypertension. New York: Grune & Stratton, 1967.
8. Kannel W B. Assessment of hypertension as a predictor of cardiovascular disease: the Framingham Study. In Burley D M, et al (ed.) Hypertension, its nature and treatment. Horsham, England: CIBA, 1975.
9. Medical Research Council Working Party. MRC trial of mild hypertension: principal results. BMJ 1985; 291: 97–104.
10. MacMahon S, Peto R, Cutler J, Collins R, Sorlie P, Neaton J, et al. Blood pressure, stroke, and coronary heart disease. Part I, prolonged differences in blood pressure: prospective observational studies corrected for the regression dilution bias. Lancet 1990; 335: 765–74.
11. Pickering G. High Blood Pressure, (2nd Edn). Churchill, London, 1968.
12. Stamler J, Stamler R, Newton J D. Blood pressure, systolic and diastolic, and cardiovascular risk. Arch Intern Med 1991; 153: 598–615.
13. Rose G A. Hypertension in the community, Ch.1, p1–14, Handbook of Hypertension, Vol. 6: Epidemiology of Hypertension. C J Bulpitt (ed.) Elsevier, 1985.
14. Smith W C S, Lee A J, Crombie I K, Tunstall-Pedoe H. Control of blood pressure in Scotland: the rule of halves. BMJ 1990; 300: 981–3.
15. Hypertension, Detection and Follow-up Programme (HDFP) Co-operative Group. The effect of treatment on mortality in 'mild' hypertension: Results of Hypertension, Detection and Follow-up Programme. N Engl J Med, 1982; 307: 976–80.
16. Management Committee. The Australian Therapeutic Trial in Mild Hypertension. Lancet 1980; (i): 1261–7
17. Helgeland A. Treatment of Mild Hypertension: A five year controlled drug trial (The Oslo Study). Am J Med 1980; 69: 725–32.
18. Multiple Risk Factor Intervention Trial Research Group. Risk factor changes and mortality results. JAMA 1982; 248: 1465–78.

19. SHEP Co-operative Research Group. Prevention of stroke by antihypertensive drug treatment in older persons with isolated systolic hypertension. JAMA 1991; **265**: 3255–64.
20. Hulley S B, Furberg CD, Gurland B, McDonald R, Perry HM, Schnape HW, *et al.* Systolic hypertension in the elderly programme (SHEP): anti-hypertensive efficacy of chlorthalidone. Am. J. Cardiol 1985; **56**: 913–20.
21. Dahlof B, Lindholm L, Hansson L, Schersten B, Ekbom T, Wester P-O. Morbidity and mortality in the Swedish Trial in Old Patients with Hypertension (STOP-Hypertension) Lancet 1991; **338**: 1281–5.
22. MRC Working Party. MRC trial of treatment of hypertension in older adults: principal results. BMJ 1992; **304**: 405–12.
23. Collins R, Peto R, MacMahon S, Hebert P, Fiebach NH, Ebertein KA, *et al.* Blood pressure, stroke and coronary heart disease. Part 2, short-term reductions in blood pressure: overview of randomized drug trials in their epidemiological context. Lancet 1990; **335**: 827–38.
24. European Working Party on High Blood Pressure in the Elderly. Mortality and morbidity results. Lancet 1985: 1349–54.
25. Coope J, Warrender C T. Randomised trial of treatment of hypertension in elderly patients in primary care. BMJ 1986; **293**: 1145–51.
26. Miall W E, Chinn S. Screening for hypertension: some epidemiological observations. BMJ 1973; **(iii)**: 595–600.
27. Pickering T G, James G D, Boddie C. 'How common is white coat hypertension?' JAMA 1988; **259**: 225–7.
28. Cruickshank JK. Natural history of blood pressure in black populations. Ch.31, p268–79. In Ethnic factors in health and disease (Ed. Cruickshank JK, Beevers DG.) London, Wright/Butterworths: 1989.
29. US HBPEP. Working group report on primary prevention of hypertension (Chair Whelton P K). NIH (number 93–2669): Washington, May 1993.
30. Cappuccio F, McGregor G. Meta-analysis of trials of K + supplementation and blood pressure reduction. J Hypert 1991; **9**: 465–74.
31. Cruickshank J K, Anderson N, Wadsworth J, Young SM, Hepson E, *et al.* Treating hypertension in black compared with white non-insulin dependent diabetics: a double-blind trial of verapamil and metoprolol. BMJ 1988; **297**: 1155–9.
32. Lichtenstein M J, Shipley M J, Rose G. Systolic and diastolic blood pressures as predictors of coronary heart disease mortality in the Whitehall study. BMJ 1985; **291**: 243–5.
33. Van den Ban G C, Campman E, Schouten E G, Kok F G, Van der Heide R M, Van der Heide Wessel C. Isolated systolic hypertension in Dutch middle aged and all cause mortality: a 25 year prospective study. Int. J. Epidemiol 1989; **18**: 95–9.
34. Miall W E, Chinn S. Screening for hypertension: some epidemiological observations. BMJ 1974; **3**: 595–600.
35. Farnett L, Mulrow CD, Linn WD, Lucey CR, Tuley MR. The J-curve phenomenon and treatment for hypertension. Is there a point beyond which pressure reduction is dangerous? JAMA 1991; **265**: 489–95.
36. Croog S, Levine S, Testa MA, Brown B, Bulpitt CJ, Jenkins CD, *et al.* The effects of anti hypertensive therapy on the quality of life. N Engl J Med 1986; **314**: 1657–64.
37. Haynes R B, Sackett D L, Taylor D W, Gibson E S, Johnson A L. Increased absenteeism from work after detection and labelling of hypertensive patients. N Engl J Med 1978; **299**: 741–4.
38. Jachuck S J, Brierley H, Jachuck S, Willcox P M. The effect of hypotensive drugs on the quality of life. J R Coll Gen Pract 1982; **32**: 103–5.

39. Mann A H. The psychological effects of a screening programme and clinical trial for hypertension upon the participants. Psychol Med 1977; **7**: 431–8.
40. Hovell M F. Experimental evidence for weight loss treatment for essential hypertension. Am J Public Health 1982; **72**: 359–86.
41. Law M R, Frost C D, Wald N J. By how much does dietary salt reduction reduce lower blood pressure? I & II-Analysis of observational data among and within populations. BMJ 1991; **302**: 811–5 and 815–8.
42. Morgan T, Adam W, Gillies A, Wilson M, Morgan G, Carney S. Hypertension treated by salt restriction. Lancet 1978; (i): 227–30.
43. Law M R, Frost C D, Wald N J. By how much does dietary salt reduction reduce lower blood pressure? III-Analysis of data from trials of salt reduction. BMJ 1991; **302**: 819–24.
44. Klatsky A L, Friedman G D, Siegelaub A B. Gerard M J. Alcohol consumption and blood pressure. N Engl J Med 1977; **296**: 1194–200
45. Patel C, Carruthers M, Coronary risk factor reduction through biofeedback aided relaxation and meditation. J R Coll Gen Pract 1977; **27**: 401–5.

3 Lipids and lipoproteins

Andrew Neil

INTRODUCTION

Cholesterol is a sterol which is essential for the synthesis of cell membranes and various hormones. It is transported in the plasma in macromolecular solubilizing complexes termed lipoproteins. The cholesterol concentration is an aggregate measure of the total amount of cholesterol carried in the various lipoproteins. About two-thirds of cholesterol in plasma is transported as low density lipoprotein (LDL) cholesterol. In excess it is potentially atherogenic which explains the relationship between elevated total cholesterol concentrations and coronary heart disease (CHD). High density lipoprotein (HDL) cholesterol accounts for 15–25 per cent of the total plasma cholesterol. It plays a major role in the mobilization and removal of tissue cholesterol and its concentration has been shown to be inversely related to the incidence of CHD. Very low density lipoprotein (VLDL) accounts for only about 10 per cent of total cholesterol but for over half of triglyceride concentration in the normal subject with the remaining triglycerides transported by other lipoproteins.

Strong evidence exists for a causal relationship between elevated blood cholesterol concentrations and CHD. Epidemiological, genetic, and experimental studies are consistent in showing this association. Using both pharmacological and non-pharmacological interventions, clinical trials have demonstrated that lowering total and LDL cholesterol concentrations results in a reduction in CHD and regression of angiographically visualized atherosclerotic plaques. It is perhaps, therefore, surprising that the identification and clinical management of hypercholesterolaemia remain such contentious issues. Much of this debate is due to a failure to appreciate the strengths and limitations of the evidence for cholesterol as a risk factor for CHD.

The aim of this chapter is to review this evidence, and to address the most important areas of uncertainty which are:

1. **The strength of the evidence for lipids and lipoproteins as risk factors for CHD**
2. **The evidence that lowering cholesterol reduces CHD incidence**
3. **The benefits and risks of lowering cholesterol**
4. **The appropriateness of lowering cholesterol in children, women, and the elderly**
5. **The level of cholesterol that warrants treatment.**

THE STRENGTH OF THE EVIDENCE FOR LIPIDS AND LIPOPROTEINS AS RISK FACTORS FOR CHD

Epidemiological evidence

Total cholesterol and CHD

There are marked geographic differences in the incidence of CHD both within and between countries. The United Kingdom, for example, has one of the highest CHD mortality rates in the world; by contrast, Japan has one of the lowest rates among industrialized countries despite its high prevalence of hypertension and cigarette smoking. In third world countries CHD is virtually unknown except where westernized diets and life-style have been adopted.

An early study of these interpopulation differences—*The Seven Countries Study*[1]—compared CHD mortality among 16 cohorts of 12 763 men aged 40–59 in seven different countries. It found a strong positive correlation on univariate analysis between CHD mortality and the percentage of calories consumed as fat, and a positive correlation between CHD rates and mean cholesterol concentrations (r = 0.80). From these and other data it is clear that high rates of CHD do not occur among populations with low mean cholesterol concentrations, and that low rates of CHD do not occur among populations with high mean cholesterol concentrations.

Migrant studies allow the influence of environmental and behavioural variables to be distinguished from genetic variability. The *NI–HON–SAN Study*[2] examined whether differences in CHD risk factors could explain the higher rates of CHD among Japanese men living in Honolulu and San Francisco than those living in Hiroshima and Nagasaki. The mean cholesterol concentrations of the cohorts living in Japan were approximately 1 mmol/l lower than Japanese men living in either Honolulu or San Francisco. This suggests that behavioural factors are at least as important as genetic in determining interpopulation differences in cholesterol concentrations.

Numerous prospective population studies have consistently shown that a high total cholesterol concentration can identify individuals within populations at an increased relative risk of CHD. Some observational studies provide information about the significance of elevated cholesterol concentrations that have persisted over a number of decades. *The Framingham Study*[3] provided some of the earliest evidence of this association by following-up some 5000 men and women aged between 30 and 59 years, who were recruited from a town of about 28 000 inhabitants, from 1948 onwards. However, the most powerful statistical data have accrued from the *Multiple Risk Factor Intervention Trial (MRFIT)*[4] which has followed for 12 years 361 667 men aged 35–57 years.

MRFIT demonstrated that there was a continuous, curvilinear, dose-related relationship between total cholesterol concentration and CHD incidence over the whole cholesterol distribution, and that an increased risk of CHD was not confined to cholesterol concentrations above a particular threshold level (Fig. 3.1). For 90 per cent of the men studied total cholesterol concentrations were in the range 4.1–7.3 mmol/l and among men in the top five per cent of the cholesterol measurements the mortality from CHD was more than five times higher than those in the lowest five per cent. Most CHD deaths, however, occur in individuals with only moderately increased cholesterol concentrations associated with a two- to three-fold increased relative risk, and in these individuals cholesterol is a poor predictor of individual risk, although it is a powerful determinant of differences in rates of CHD between populations. Nevertheless, it can be inferred from these data that lowering cholesterol levels might be expected to reduce CHD mortality regardless of the initial cholesterol concentration but, since the relationship is curvilinear, the largest reduction in the absolute risk of CHD for individuals might be expected to result from lowering the highest cholesterol concentrations.

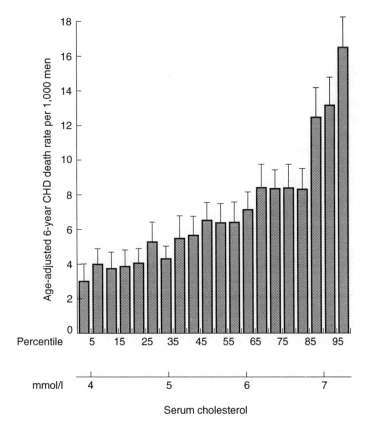

Fig. 3.1 Age-adjusted six year CHD death rate per 1000 men screened for MRFIT according to serum cholesterol percentile. (From Martin MJ *et al.* Lancet 1986: **ii**; 933-6.)

HDL cholesterol and CHD

Several prospective studies have found an inverse relationship between HDL cholesterol concentrations and CHD incidence which is independent of total or

LDL cholesterol concentrations. Unlike LDL cholesterol, the strength of this relationship does not appear to decline with age. It does, however, vary between studies and it is not clear whether a high level of HDL *per se* is protective, whether a low level is harmful or whether the concentration of HDL is a marker for some other risk factor. In *The British Regional Heart Study* [5], 7735 men aged 40–59 selected at random from the age–sex registers of general practices in England, Wales, and Scotland were examined and followed-up. After seven and a half years, it was found that men in the lowest fifth of the HDL cholesterol concentration (less than 0.93 mmol/l) had twice the risk of CHD compared with men in the highest fifth (greater than or equal to 1.33 mmol/l), after adjustment for total cholesterol concentration and other risk factors. A similar or more marked protective effect of high concentrations of HDL cholesterol has been reported in other studies[6]. However, the benefits of raising a low HDL cholesterol level (unlike lowering a high LDL cholesterol) have not been confirmed by randomized trials, and clinical intervention is generally not appropriate unless the total and LDL cholesterol concentrations are also raised.

Mean HDL cholesterol concentrations are usually about 0.25–0.40 mmol/l higher in women than men[7], which may partly explain the marked sex difference in the incidence of CHD in middle age. Only three of the prospective studies that have assessed the relationship between lipids and CHD in women also measured HDL cholesterol. In *The Framingham Study* [8] there was an inverse relationship between HDL cholesterol and CHD incidence in women aged 49–82 years which was similar to that reported for men.[5] In *The Follow-up Study of The Lipid Research Clinic Prevalence Study* [7] 3416 women aged at least 30 years were among the 8825 subjects followed up for a mean duration of 8.4 years. HDL cholesterol in these women was more closely related to cardiovascular disease than was LDL cholesterol. Interestingly, the *Donolo–Tel Aviv Study* [9] differed from these other two studies in finding that the total cholesterol concentration was not associated with the risk of CHD after adjustment for the HDL concentration.

On the basis of these studies, it appears that HDL cholesterol is an important determinant of the lipoprotein-mediated risk of CHD and, particularly in women, the risk of CHD may be overestimated when the total cholesterol concentration is elevated unless the HDL cholesterol concentration is known. A study of more than 4000 men and women aged 25–59 years screened in general practice[10] has shown that about 25 per cent of women and 8 per cent of men with raised total cholesterol concentrations of 6.5–7.8 mmol/l, and triglycerides of less than 2.3 mmol/l, have HDL cholesterol concentrations of more than 2.0 mmol/l which are associated with little or no excess risk of CHD.

Apolipoproteins, lipoprotein (a), and CHD

Apolipoproteins are genetically determined components of lipoproteins that influence the conformation, receptor binding, and metabolism of the lipoproteins. Interest has focused on whether they may better predict the risk of CHD since measurent of apolipoproteins, unlike lipoprotein concentrations, quantifies the number of particles. In a number of cross-sectional clinical studies, CHD has been shown to be positively associated with the concentration of apo B, the principal protein component of LDL, and inversely correlated with apo A-1, the principal protein of HDL. However, one of the few prospective studies that has measured apolipoproteins concentrations—*The Physicians' Health Study*[11]—found that they had little predictive value after taking account of conventional risk factors and the ratio of total to HDL cholesterol. The authors concluded that routine measurement of apolipoproteins as an indicator of risk could not yet be recommended.

Lipoprotein(a), usually termed Lp(a), comprises a molecule of LDL linked covalently to apolipoprotein(a) which is a protein homologous to plasminogen. Although the evidence from prospective studies is conflicting, it appears to be an independent risk factor for CHD[12], and raised levels are a common familial abnormality in patients with premature CHD and their children.[13] Most lipid-lowering drugs, however, do not reduce Lp(a) concentrations, and its measurement in routine clinical practice is not appropriate at present.

Triglycerides and CHD

The evidence for triglycerides as a risk factor for CHD is less convincing than for cholesterol. Case-control studies[14] have shown, on univariate analysis, that triglyceride concentrations are significantly higher in myocardial infarction survivors than in healthy control subjects. Triglycerides, however, are positively correlated with cholesterol, obesity, glucose intolerance, and hyperuricaemia, and are inversely correlated with HDL cholesterol levels. After adjustment for these risk factors using multivariate analysis, the association of triglycerides with CHD usually no longer remains statistically significant. However, the large variability in triglyceride measurement will result in underestimation of any statistical association with CHD. The process of adjustment using multivariate analysis has also been criticized because of the way in which it handles variables that are highly intercorrelated, and because of uncertainty as to which of these highly correlated factors is related to CHD independently of the other.

It is important to appreciate that there are few prospective data to suggest that triglycerides are independent risk factors for CHD. Considerable attention has focused on *The Stockholm Prospective Study* [15] of over 3000 men and 3000 women which is one of the few studies to show such a relationship. Some caution is needed in interpreting these data because HDL cholesterol was not measured, nor was it measured in the *Gothenburg Study*[16] which found that, in women, triglyceride concentration and abdominal adiposity were independent risk factors for total and CHD mortality. Plasma triglyceride concentrations were found to predict coronary events in The *Cerphilly and Speedwell Prospective Studies* [17] of nearly 5000 middle aged men after adjusting for HDL cholesterol, although by contrast *The Framingham Study*[8] found that triglycerides were a significant independent risk factor only in women aged over 50 years. It is possible that the lipid risk profile may be different in men and women, and there may be different risks associated with different triglyceride containing lipoproteins. At present, the role of triglycerides as a risk factor for CHD remains poorly defined, although markedly elevated triglyceride levels exceeding at least 10 mmol/l are well recognized to be associated with a risk of pancreatitis. Measurement of triglycerides is needed to classify lipoprotein abnormalities and to determine the most appropriate treatment.

Genetic evidence

Polygenic hypercholesterolaemia

It has been estimated that about 60 per cent of the variability in total cholesterol between individuals is attributable to genetic variation, which is thought to be largely polygenic, and that the remaining variability is due to environmental influences, which are mainly dietary, but recent evidence suggests that intrauterine nutrition may also be relevant.[18] The interaction between multiple genetic and environmental factors, such as diets high in saturated fat, is thought to be responsible for the mild to moderate hypercholesterolaemia (about 5.5–8 mmol/l) which is often termed 'common' or 'polygenic' hypercholesterolaemia. It is, however, a relatively poor predictor of individual risk of CHD in the absence of either pre-existing CHD or other cardiovascular risk factors.

Monogenic disorders

Monogenic disorders exert a major effect on serum cholesterol and may be present in up to 1 per cent of the population.[19] Familial hypercholesterolaemia is the most important example of such a disorder. It is an autosomal dominant condition characterized by mutations of the specific cell surface receptor which combines and internalises LDL cholesterol. This results in accumulation of LDL and total cholesterol with levels commonly of around 9 mmol/l or more in the untreated heterozygote and from 15–30 mmol/l in the homozygote. Homozygous familial hypercholesterolaemia is an extremely rare disorder occurring in about one in a million of the United Kingdom population while heterozygous familial hypercholesterolaemia occurs in about one in five hundred of the population (about the same prevalence as insulin-dependent diabetes).

Familial hypercholesterolaemia provides a model of the role of LDL cholesterol in CHD. In the heterozygous form the risk of myocardial infarction and sudden cardiac death is substantially increased, with one study of heterozygous patients finding that 51 per cent of men and 12 per cent of women had experienced a fatal or non-fatal myocardial infarction by the age of 50 years.[20] In young patients—aged 20–39 years—the excess risk of CHD may be increased nearly 100 times although this risk appears to decrease with age.[21] The response to diet is almost invariably inadequate and lipid-lowering drug therapy is then required. About three per cent of survivors of a myocardial infarction will have familial hypercholesterolaemia.[22] To exclude an inherited disorder of lipoprotein metabolism, cholesterol should be measured in patients with a personal or a strong family history of premature CHD. If the diagnosis is confirmed, screening of family members is required to identify secondary cases. In familial hypercholesterolaemia the age of onset of CHD is strongly correlated within families, but the prognosis differs widely between families possibly reflecting differences in LDL receptor activity associated with different mutations. Consequently, screening first-degree-relatives of index-cases with markedly premature CHD is likely to identify secondary cases at most risk of CHD.

Experimental evidence

The evidence from clinical trials is described below but animal experimental and physiological studies will not be reviewed in detail. It should, however, be stressed that the results are consistent with epidemiological, genetic, and clinical trial evidence in man. Atheroma has been produced experimentally in a number of animal species by diet-induced hypercholesterolaemia, and on withdrawal of the dietary stimulus there is gradual regression of the atheromatous lesions. In genetically hyperlipidaemic rabbits, arterial disease has been almost entirely prevented by administration of a cholesterol-lowering drug early in life.

THE EVIDENCE THAT LOWERING CHOLESTEROL REDUCES CHD INCIDENCE

Clinical trials

Clinical trials of cholesterol lowering using pharmacological and non-pharmacological interventions have shown that a reduction in total and LDL cholesterol can reduce the morbidity and mortality from CHD, and result in regression of atherosclerosis. More than 30 such trials have been conducted: most were trials of secondary prevention (aimed at reducing CHD events in subjects with clinically established disease), and a smaller number were trials of primary prevention (aimed at preventing the development of CHD). The most reliable estimates of the effect of cholesterol lowering are provided by meta-analyses (overviews) which combine the results of related trials and enable the size of the effect to be estimated with increased confidence.

Primary prevention trials

Primary prevention trials have demonstrated that lowering cholesterol by diet or drugs can significantly reduce the incidence of total CHD (fatal and non-fatal myocardial infarction). However, it is important to be aware of the limitations of these trials. They have mostly been restricted to middle-aged men with cholesterol concentrations in the upper part of the frequency distribution. This ensures an adequate number of clinical end-points (fatal and non-fatal myocardial infarctions) to provide the statistical power needed to detect differences in the incidence of myocardial infarction between active treatment and placebo groups. The results cannot be generalized with absolute certainty to older men or to women, and the trials were not large enough to demonstrate a significant decrease in total mortality because a reduction in the number of coronary deaths would be expected to produce a smaller percentage reduction in total mortality than coronary mortality.

Most trials lasted no more than five years and so may under-estimate the potential effect of a prolonged reduction in cholesterol concentration. In addition, they may under-estimate the reduction in the incidence of CHD associated with cholesterol lowering since the decrease in cholesterol achieved was generally about 10 per cent whereas the expected reduction would be nearer 25 per cent with the newer HMG CoA reductase inhibitor group of drugs (statins). Indeed, the recently published *West of Scotland Coronary Prevention Study*[23] randomly assigned 6595 men aged 45 to 64 years with a mean plasma cholesterol of 7.0 mmol/l to receive pravastatin or placebo and, over a mean follow-up period of 4.9 years, there was a 20 per cent reduction in plasma cholesterol in the statin treated group and a 22 per cent reduction in total mortality which was just short off statistical significance (95 per cent confidence intervals 0–40, p = 0.051). The absolute risk of mortality was low, about 0.8 per cent annually, and the indication for intervention remains doubtful.

Secondary prevention and angiographic trials

There have been far more secondary than primary prevention trials, but most secondary prevention trials had small numbers. Overall, the data demonstrate that cholesterol lowering results in a significant reduction in CHD mortality, and there is now conclusive evidence from the *Scandanavian Simvastatin Survival Study* [24] that treatment reduces total mortality as well as reducing cardiovascular end-points and cardiovascular mortality. This trial randomized 4444 patients with a total cholesterol concentration of 5.5–8.0 mmol/l and angina pectoris or a previous myocardial to simvastatin or placebo. Over a mean follow-up period of 5.4 years there was a mean reduction in total cholesterol of 25 per cent, and the relative risks of death from all causes and CHD were highly significantly reduced by 30 per cent and 42 per cent respectively.

Serial angiography has been used in a number of trials to demonstrate that regression of coronary atherosclerosis occurs with cholesterol lowering. The more recent trials have used computerized quantitative angiography to avoid the imprecision of visual assessment used in earlier studies. Because of differences in study design and outcome assessment, no quantitative meta-analysis of luminal changes has been performed but the results of the principal studies[25–27] are consistent in showing that within two years intensive lipid lowering therapy significantly reduces the frequency of progression of coronary lesions and in-creases the frequency of regression. The extent of regression of atherosclerosis, however, is small, and the decrease in coronary events observed may be explained by the restoration in atherosclerotic arteries of endothelial-dependent vasodilata-tion with treatment of hypercholesterolaemia, and the prevention of development of unstable plaques. A particularly important feature of these trials was that the benefit of treatment was evident across the whole range of cholesterol values found at entry and even among patients without clearly elevated total cholesterol concentrations.

THE BENEFITS AND RISKS OF LOWERING CHOLESTEROL

The benefits of lowering cholesterol

The best estimate of the reduction in CHD incidence resulting from lowering cholesterol is provided by a meta-analysis of 10 prospective (cohort) observational studies, three international studies in different communities, and 28 unconfounded randomized clinical trials.[28] The overview of observational cohort studies was based on half a million men and 18 000 ischaemic heart disease events. It showed that a reduction in serum cholesterol concentration of 0.6 mmol/l (about 10 per cent) was associated with a decrease in incidence of ischaemic heart disease of 54 per cent at age 40 years, 39 per cent at age 50, 27 per cent at 60, 20 per cent at 70, and 19 per cent at 80. The overview of randomized trials was based on 45 000 men and 4000 ischaemic heart disease events and demonstrated a reduction in incidence of ischaemic heart disease in men (for ages 55–64 years) of seven per cent in the first two years, 22 per cent from two to five years, and 25 per cent after five years, the last estimate being close to the estimate of 27 per cent for the long-term reduction from the observational cohort studies. The data for women were more limited but indicated a similar effect.

The estimate of a 20–25 per cent reduction in CHD incidence associated with a 10 per cent reduction in cholesterol may underestimate the potential benefit of lowering cholesterol. It does not allow for the 'regression dilution bias' which is due to the random fluctuations in cholesterol measurement over time. Repeated measurement of cholesterol results in observations at the top and bottom of the distribution moving towards the average value. The effect of this bias is to systematically underestimate the strength of the real association between plasma cholesterol and CHD. After allowing for this effect, it is likely that a 10 per cent reduction in total cholesterol would result in about a 30 per cent reduction in the incidence of CHD.[29]

The results of community programmes to control cardiovascular disease show that when mean plasma cholesterol levels of populations fall, there is a resultant reduction in CHD mortality rates. For example, in North Karelia, Finland, a comprehensive community programme to control cardiovascular disease was conducted from 1972 onwards. Although the programme did not achieve the expected difference between intervention and control populations, between 1972 and 1992 there was a 13 per cent reduction in the mean total cholesterol concentration from 6.78 to 5.90 mmol/l in men, and a larger reduction of 17 per cent in women, which was associated with a decline in CHD mortality of 55 per cent in men and 68 per cent in women.[30] Most of the decline in mortality could be explained by changes in the three main coronary risk factors, and the results are consistent with the three per cent mortality decline for a one per cent reduction in cholesterol predicted above.

The risks of lowering cholesterol

A number of observational cohort studies have shown a J-shaped relationship between serum cholesterol concentration and total mortality. For example, data from the 12 year *MRFIT Follow up Study* [31] of over a third of a million men screened aged 35–57 years demonstrated that a total cholesterol concentration of less than 4.14 mmol/l was associated with a significantly increased risk of death from haemorrhagic stroke; cancer of the liver and pancreas; digestive diseases, particularly hepatic cirrhosis; suicide; and alcohol dependence. However, the meta-analysis described above[28,32] which analysed data from 10 cohort studies found pronounced differences in the risk of non-circulatory causes of death between cohort studies of employed men who were likely to be healthy at recruitment, and studies of subjects in community settings that necessarily included some men with existing disease. The employed cohorts showed no excess mortality but there was an inverse association between low cholesterol concentrations and non-cardiovascular causes of death in the community cohorts. This can be explained by both low cholesterol concentrations and non-cardiovascular diseases being a consequence of other factors, or, in some instances, by low serum cholesterol concentrations being a metabolic consequence of various disease processes.

The most likely explanation of the apparent relationship between a low serum cholesterol concentration and cancer is that the nutritional and metabolic effects of occult cancer include lowering cholesterol, the so-called 'pre-clinical cancer' effect. This is consistent with the observation in prospective studies[31] that the relationship usually either diminishes or disappears with time. A small but important clinical study[33] of lipoprotein metabolism in prostatic cancer supports this explanation by demonstrating a significantly higher fractional catabolic rate for LDL cholesterol in patients with metastases than in either patients without metastases, or in a control group. Epidemiological evidence is consistent with this explanation and demonstrates that populations such as the Chinese and Japanese, with mean total cholesterol concentrations below 4.4 mmol/l,[34] have no higher overall cancer rates than Europeans. In summary, there is little evidence that naturally low cholesterol concentrations are harmful.

The effect of cholesterol-lowering drug treatment appears, in some clinical trials, to be associated with an increase in non-cardiovascular mortality. Attention first focused on this issue in 1978 with the publication of the results of *The WHO Cooperative Trial on Primary Prevention of Ischaemic Heart Disease* [35] which observed a 25 per cent excess of deaths from non-cardiovascular disease in the clofibrate-treated group. This excess was only partly explained by the mortality associated with a twofold increase in gall-bladder disease due to the lithogenic effect of clofibrate. Attention should not, however, be focused on a single trial since quantitative overviews provide a more reliable estimate of the effect of cholesterol lowering. In the meta-analysis (described above[28,32]), for the eight primary prevention trials which included men without ischaemic heart disease at entry there was a small excess of deaths due to causes other than ischaemic heart disease

(Table 3.1) although this was not large enough to be statistically significant (p = 0.07). There was no excess mortality in the dietary trials, but in the 18 drug trials there was a significant excess mortality (odds ratio 1.20, 95 per cent confidence intervals 1.02–1.40, p = 0.02) which the authors attributed to the inclusion of the apparently anomalous findings from four trials. Overall, for the 28 trials included in the meta-analysis there was no excess all cause or non-cardiovascular mortality.

Table 3.1 Combined results from randomised trials of reduction of serum cholesterol concentration; relative odds of death in treated/control groups per 0.6 mmol/l (10%) reduction in cholesterol according to type of trial.

Cause of death	No of trials	No of deaths	Odds of death in treated/control groups (95% confidence interval	P value
Ischaemic heart disease	28	2618	0.90 (0.84 to 0.97)	0.004
All other causes other than ischaemic heart disease*:				
All trials	28	1330	1.07 (0.97 to 1.18)	0.16
Drug trials	18	636	1.20 (1.02 to 1.40)	0.02
Dietary trials	9	660	1.01 (0.88 to 1.15)	>0.2
Surgery trial	1	34	0.99 (0.50 to 1.97)	>0.2
Subjects without ischaemic heart disease	8	990	1.11 (0.99 to 1.24)	0.07
Subjects with known ischaemic heart disease	21	339	0.99 (0.83 to 1.18)	>0.2
All cause mortality‡:				
All trials	28	4042	0.96 (0.90 to 1.02)	>0.2
Drug trials	18	2537	0.97 (0.89 to 1.05)	>0.2
Dietary trials	9	1394	0.97 (0.88 to 1.07)	>0.2
Surgery trial	1	111	0.75 (0.50 to 1.13)	>0.2
Subjects without ischaemic heart disease†	8	1555	1.06 (0.97 to 1.17)	>0.2
Subjects with ischaemic heart disease	21	2482	0.90 (0.84 to 0.07)	0.008

* Five trials recorded no deaths other than from ischaemic heart disease.
† One trial, with one death from cause other than ischaemic heart disease and four deaths from ischaemic heart disease could not be classified.
‡ Includes 94 deaths of unknown cause.

Although the overall evidence from these 28 clinical trials suggests that lipid lowering treatment is not harmful, an alternative interpretation of these results is that the subset analyses described above are valid and that the outcome depends on whether cholesterol is lowered by diet or drugs and the initial level of risk. In other words, lowering serum cholesterol with drugs produces greater benefit for men at high initial risk of ischaemic heart disease than for those at low initial risk for whom the potential adverse effects of lipid-lowering drug treatment may outweigh the benefits. It is not clear whether this might be a class effect of particular drugs, but it has been argued that lipid-lowering drug therapy should be restricted to patients with an initial annual CHD mortality risk exceeding three per cent in whom treatment was shown in a further meta-analysis[36] to result in a significant reduction in total mortality.

Use of a three per cent annual CHD mortality risk as the criterion for drug treatment is not, however, consistent with the results of recently published trials[23,24] which suggest that patients at lower absolute risk of CHD would benefit from treatment with statins. In The *Scandinavian Simvastatin Survival Study*[24] – a secondary prevention trial – there was a 30 per cent reduction in total mortality in the group treated with simvastatin. The annual CHD mortality in the placebo group was only 1.5 per cent, and the numbers-needed-to-treat (NNT) for five years to prevent one death were about 30 patients. In *The West of Scotland Coronary Prevention Study*[23] – a primary prevention trial – there was a 22 per cent reduction in total mortality in the group treated with pravastatin. In this study the annual CHD mortality in the placebo group was only about 0.4 per cent, and the NNT for five years to prevent one death were much higher at about 110 patients. Since the risk of fatal myocardial infarction is, of course, highest in men with existing CHD[37], priority should be given to lowering cholesterol after myocardial infarction[24], coronary artery by-pass grafting, or angioplasty, particularly in younger patients.

THE APPROPRIATENESS OF LOWERING CHOLESTEROL IN CHILDREN, WOMEN, AND THE ELDERLY

Lowering cholesterol in children

The indications for lowering cholesterol in children are less clearly defined than in adults, and there is often uncertainty about 'normal' lipid levels in childhood. Age and sex-specific frequency distributions in children are available from *The Lipid Clinics Prevalence Study*[38] which was conducted in North America between 1972 and 1976, and included 12 403 white males and females aged less than 20. Mean cord blood total cholesterol levels are 1.7–2.0 mmol/l and no interpopulation differences are apparent. Cholesterol levels rise in the first year of life to a mean of 4.1 mmol/l (95th percentile 5.2 mmol/l) which persists until the mid-teens. Levels are similar in boys and girls until adolescence when they both fall slightly. Thereafter they are higher in boys but increase in both sexes by about 0.5 mmol/l by the mid-twenties. Cholesterol levels in early childhood are only moderately predictive of early adult levels but by age 9–11 years they are good predictors (tracking coefficient, 0.7).[39] The long-term outcome for individuals with polygenic hypercholesterolaemia identified in childhood is uncertain. Treatment consists of giving dietary advice which follows recommendations accepted for the general population.[40]

Familial hypercholesterolaemia is the most important genetically determined abnormality of lipoprotein metabolism to be expressed in childhood. Other conditions, such as familial combined hyperlipidaemia, usually do not show full penetrance until late adolescence or early adulthood, and hypertriglycerideamia is rare. Familial hypercholesterolaemia cannot be confidently diagnosed until after the first year of life because earlier than this there are relatively low levels of LDL cholesterol, and variations in HDL cholesterol have more impact on total cholesterol concentrations. Where one parent is heterozygous for the condition the diagnosis should be made in childhood as soon as treatment is practical. Identification of the LDL receptor gene mutation is impractical except for research studies, and the recommended diagnostic criteria for use in children, aged less than 16 with an affected first degree relative, are a total cholesterol concentration of more than 6.7 mmol/l and an LDL cholesterol concentration of more than 4.0 mmol/l[41]. These criteria may misdiagnose about five per cent of children and serial measurements may be needed, particularly in those with borderline levels.

There are no data to show how the prognosis of familial hypercholesterolaemia is modified by treatment in childhood. However, atherosclerotic lesions occur in childhood and patients with this condition may experience coronary events in their early twenties. Identification of familial hypercholesterolaemia by selective screening of children with a positive family history of hypercholesterolaemia or premature CHD, and treatment to lower cholesterol levels, is therefore likely to be worthwhile. Drug treatment in childhood is very rarely indicated.

Lowering cholesterol in women

The evidence for treating high blood cholesterol levels in women is less impressive than for men. Few prospective studies have included women and most have studied only small populations. Evidence from clinical trials is almost entirely absent, and recommendations for treatment depend mainly on extrapolating from trials performed in middle-aged men.

Overall mortality rates from CHD are three to four times higher for men than women, but the sex difference declines with age. The extremely low incidence of myocardial infarction in pre-menopausal women is evident from a Swedish study which estimated it as only 14 per 100 000 per annum at age 38 years, increasing to 39 per 100 000 at age 50 years, and 63 per 100 000 at age 54 years.[42] Treatment of raised cholesterol levels in women must take account of the lower absolute risk of CHD in pre-menopausal women, and lipid-lowering drug therapy should be restricted to patients with major genetically determined abnormalities of lipoprotein metabolism, such as familial hypercholesterolaemia, or with either marked multiple CHD risk factors, or established CHD. It is important to remember that mean HDL cholesterol levels are higher in women than men, and that measurement of total cholesterol alone may overestimate CHD risk. Drug treatment can seldom be justified in pre-menopausal women unless they have familial hypercholesterolaemia and should be discontinued at least a month prior to conception, and during pregnancy. The long term significance of polygenic hypercholesterolaemia in pre-menopausal women is uncertain and it is not clear how closely pre-menopausal and post-menopausal cholesterol levels track in individuals.

The incidence of CHD increases dramatically after the menopause and mean cholesterol levels also increase. In *The Lipid Research Clinics Follow-up Study* [7] the mean cholesterol increased from 5.0 mmol/l at the age 40–45 years to 6.0 mmol/l at the age 55–59 years. Drug therapy is therefore somewhat easier to justify in post-menopausal women but evidence for a benefit of treatment depends on extrapolating from trials performed in middle-aged men. However, the logistic implications of treating hypercholesterolaemia in post-menopausal women are considerable. About 70 per cent of women aged 55–64 years have cholesterol levels exceeding 6.5 mmol/l and 30 per cent have levels exceeding 7.8 mmol/l.[43] In post-menopausal women, hormone replacement therapy (HRT) may become an established adjunct to other treatment of hypercholesterolaemia. A recent meta-analysis[44] (see Chapter 10) identified at least 32 observational studies that have evaluated the relationship between HRT use and CHD, and the pooled estimate of the relative risk of CHD for women who have ever used oestrogen compared with those who have never used oestrogen was 0.65 (95 per cent confidence intervals 0.59–0.71). Unfortunately, observational studies may be misleadingly positive since women who take HRT may be healthier than the average. A further difficulty is that there are few data on the effect of combined oestrogen and progestogen therapy on CHD risk.

Lowering cholesterol in the elderly

Much less is known about the appropriateness of lowering cholesterol in the elderly than in the middle aged population. The absolute risk of CHD increases with age, and people aged more than 65 years account for about two-thirds of the 140 000 annual deaths from CHD in the UK. However, although the absolute risk of CHD increases substantially with age, the relative risk due to cholesterol is attenuated by age. For example, in *The MRFIT Study* [45] the relative risk of fatal CHD was increased about eight times in men aged 35–39 years in the top 20 per cent of the cholesterol distribution, but by the age 55–57 years had fallen to about 2.5 times, and in the *Framingham Study* [46] the relative risk of fatal CHD in men and women with a high total cholesterol had fallen below 1.0 before the age of 80 years. Indeed, in elderly women mortality rates appear in some studies to be lower in those with high total cholesterol concentrations than in those with moderate levels.[47]

Because no sizeable trials have been performed in patients aged more than 65 years, it is necessary to extrapolate from trials of cholesterol lowering in middle-aged men to assess the possible benefits of treatment. If the treatment of elevated cholesterol levels is as effective in reducing the risk of CHD in elderly men as it is in middle-aged men, a greater reduction in mortality would be expected in the elderly because of their high CHD mortality rates.[48] Given the limitations of the available data, offering dietary advice to elderly patients may be reasonable but there is inadequate evidence to justify the use of lipid-lowering drug therapy, except possibly in patients with known CHD. It is, however, important to remember that clinical trials show that it is necessary to lower cholesterol for at least two years before any significant reduction in CHD incidence can be demonstrated.

THE LEVEL OF CHOLESTEROL THAT WARRANTS TREATMENT

Use of a particular cholesterol concentration as a clinical decision point for initiating lipid-lowering therapy is, necessarily, to some extent arbitrary because there is a continuous, curvilinear and dose-dependent relationship between cholesterol concentrations and the incidence of CHD over the whole cholesterol distribution, without evidence of a threshold effect. The most important consideration is to take account of clinical trial evidence in determining whether treatment is likely to be of net benefit.

Published guidelines

The recommendations for the management of hyperlipidaemia that have received most prominence in the United Kingdom—those of the European Atherosclerosis Study Group[49] and the British Hyperlipidaemia Association[50] (Table 3.2)—offer consistent advice stressing the importance of targeting therapy at patients at highest overall risk, in particular, patients with known CHD and those with inherited disorders of lipoprotein metabolism. Lipid-lowering dietary advice is the recommended initial treatment, although usual dietary advice only results in a mean reduction in total and LDL cholesterol concentration of between one and four per cent[51] (see Chapter 4). To obtain a better dietary response, more intensive intervention than is normally available in primary care is probably necessary.

Table 3.2 British Hyperlipidaemia Association guidelines: Priorities and action limits for lipid-lowering drug therapy in diet-resistant subjects*

Prioritiy	Subject Category	Total cholesterol (mmol/l)	LDL cholesterol (mmol/l)
First	Patients with existing CHD, or post-CABG, angioplasty or cardiac transplant	> 5.2	> 3.4
Second	Patients with multiple risk factors or genetically determined hyperlipidaemia, e.g. familial hypercholesterolaemia	> 6.5	> 5.0
Third	Males with asymptomatic hypercholesterolaemia	> 7.8	> 6.0
Fourth	Postmenopausal females with asymptomatic hypercholesterolaemia	> 7.8 and HDL ratio < 0.2	> 6.0

* Aim of cholesterol lowering should be an LDL cholesterol < 3.4 mmol/l in the presence of CHD and < 4.1 mmol/l in the absence of CHD

Indications for lipid-lowering drug therapy

Patients with established CHD warrant long-term drug therapy since there is convincing clinical trial evidence that treatment substantially reduces total and CHD mortality. Table 3.2 gives the cholesterol concentrations above which drug therapy is recommended, and these are consistent with the evidence that has already been reviewed.

Patients with major inherited disorders of lipoprotein metabolism also warrant drug treatment since there is evidence from angiographic studies in familial hypercholesterolaemia that cholesterol lowering results in regression of coronary atherosclerosis.[52] The effect on total mortality, however, has not been studied, and it would no longer be ethical to do so. The high risk of CHD in familial disorders and the likely benefits of treatment strongly suggest that drug therapy is justified in most patients.

In patients with polygenic hypercholesterolaemia the decision to treat with lipid lowering drugs depends on an assessment of the risks and benefits of therapy. There is limited but persuasive evidence that drug therapy reduces total mortality in patients without pre-existing CHD[23] but caution is needed since the risks of continued drug use for 20 or 30 years are unknown. The high costs of treatment and potential long-term risks of drug therapy are easier to justify in patients with marked multiple cardiovascular risk factors, especially young male patients with a family history of premature CHD, but conclusive evidence of benefit must await the results of current clinical trials which are being undertaken in these groups of patients. There remain uncertainties about the benefit of drug therapy in the elderly and it is rarely justified in pre-menopausal women.

SUMMARY

- Total and LDL cholesterol concentrations are major independent risk factors for CHD.
- There is a continuous, curvilinear, and dose-dependent relationship between cholesterol concentrations and incidence of CHD over the whole cholesterol distribution with no evidence of a threshold effect.
- There is an inverse relationship between HDL cholesterol concentrations and CHD incidence.
- The role of triglycerides as a risk factor for CHD remains poorly defined.
- Cholesterol interacts synergistically with other cardiovascular risk factors to enhance the risk of CHD.
- Levels of cholesterol that characterize polygenic hypercholesterolaemia are relatively poor predictors of individual risk of CHD unless account is taken of other CHD risk factors.
- Major inherited disorders of lipoprotein metabolism that are associated with a high risk of CHD usually warrant treatment with lipid-lowering drugs.

- Patients with CHD and cholesterol concentrations greater than 5.5 mmol/l should be considered for lipid-lowering drug treatment with a statin.
- The limited efficacy of dietary advice and the high costs and potential long-term risks of lipid-lowering drug therapy mean that population-based interventions to lower cholesterol rather than individual medical interventions remain the most appropriate overall strategy for primary prevention.
- Clinical trial evidence of net benefit is the most important determinant when deciding whether drug therapy is appropriate. In the absence of such evidence, only patients at highest risk of CHD should be treated with lipid-lowering drugs.

REFERENCES

1. Keys A. Seven countries: a multivariate analysis of death and coronary heart disease. Cambridge, MA: Harvard University Press, 1980.
2. Kagan A, Harris B, Winkelstein W, *et al.* Epidemiologic studies of coronary heart disease. and stroke in Japanese men living in Japan, Hawaii and California: demographic, physical and biochemical characteristics. J Chron Dis 1974; **27**: 345–64.
3. Kannel WB, Castelli WP, Gordon T, McNamara PM. Serum cholesterol, lipoproteins, and the risk of coronary heart disease. The Framingham Study. Ann Intern Med 1971; **74**: 1–12.
4. Martin JM, Hulley SB, Browner WS, Kuller LH, Wentworth D. Serum cholesterol, blood pressure, and mortality: implications from a cohort of 361 662 men. Lancet 1986; **ii**: 933–6.
5. Pocock SJ, Shaper AG, Phillips AN. Concentrations of high density lipoprotein cholesterol, triglycerides, and total cholesterol in ischaemic heart disease. BMJ 1989; **298**: 998–1002.
6. Gordon DJ. High-density lipoprotein and coronary heart disease: a comparison of recent epidemiologic and clinical trial results. Circulation 1989; **79**: 8–15.
7. Jacobs DR, Mebane IL, Bangdiwala SI, Criqui MH, Tyroler HA. High density lipoprotein cholesterol as a predictor of cardiovascular disease mortality in men and women: The Follow-Up Study of The Lipid Research Clinics Prevalence Study. Am J Epidemiol 1990; **131**: 32–47.
8. Castelli WP, Garrison RJ, Wilson PWF, Abbott RD, Kalousdian S, Kannel WB. Incidence of coronary heart disease and lipoprotein cholesterel levels. The Framingham Study. JAMA 1986; **256**: 2835–8.
9. Brunner D, Weisbort J, Meshulam N, Schwatz S, Gross J, *et al.* Relation of serum total cholesterol and high density lipoprotein cholesterol percentage to the incidence of definite coronary heart events: Twenty year follow-up of the Donolo-Tel Aviv Prospective Coronary Artery Disease Study. Am J Cardiol 1987; **59**: 1271–6.
10. Neil HAW, Mant D, Jones L, Morgan B, Mann JI. Lipid Screening: Is it enough to measure total cholesterol concentration? BMJ 1990; **301**: 584–7.
11. Stampfer MJ, Sacks FM, Salvini S, Willett WC, Hennekens CH. A prospective study of cholesterol, apolipoproteins, and risk of myocardial infarction. N Engl J Med 1991; **325**: 374–81.
12. Schaefer EJ, Lamon-Fava S, Jenner JL, McNamara JR, Ordovas JM, Davis CE, Abolafia JM, Lippel K, Levy R. Lipoprotein (a) levels and risk of coronary heart disease in men: The Lipid Research Clinics Coronary Prevention Primary Trial. JAMA 1994; **13**: 999–1003.

13. Uterman G, Menzel HJ, Kraft H, Duba HC, Kemmler HG, Seitz C. Lp(a) glycoprotein phenotypes. Inheritance and relation to Lp(a) lipoprotein concentrations in plasma. J Clin Invest 1987; **80**: 458–65.
14. Austin MA. Plasma triglycerides as a risk factor for coronary heart disease. Am J Epidemiol 1989; **129**: 249–59.
15. Bottinger LE, Carlson LA. Risk factors for ischaemic vascular death for men in the Stokholm Prospective Study. Atherosclerosis 1980; **36**: 389–408.
16. Bengtsson C, Bjorkelund C, Lapidus L, Lissner L. Association of serum lipid concentrations and obesity with mortality in women: 20 year follow up of participants in prospective population study in Gothenburg, Sweden. BMJ 1993; **307**: 1385–8.
17. Bainton D, Miller NE, Bolton CH, Yarnell JWG, Sweetnam PM, Baker IA, Lewis B, Elwood PC. Plasma triglycerides and high density lipoprotein cholesterol as predictors of ischaemic heart disease in British men. Br Heart J 1992; **68**: 60–6.
18. Barker DJB, Martyn CN, Osmond C, Hales CN, Fall CHD. Growth in utero and serum cholesterol concentrations in adult life. BMJ 1993; **307**: 1524–7.
19. Goldstein JL, Schrott HD, Hazzard WR, Bierman EL, Motulsky G. Hyperlipidaemia in coronary heart disease. J Clin Investigation 1973; **52**: 1544–68.
20. Slack J. Risks of ischaemic heart disease in familial hyerlipidaemic states. Lancet 1969; **ii**: 1380–2.
21. The Simon Broome Register Group. The risk of fatal coronary heart disease in familial hypercholesterolaemia. BMJ 1991; **303**: 893–6.
22. Paterson D, Slack J. Lipid abnormalities in male and female survivors of myocardial infarction and their first-degree relatives. Lancet 1972; **i**: 393–9.
23. Shepherd J, Cobbe SM, Ford I, Isles CG, Lormier AR, Macfarlane PW, *et al.* Prevention of coronary heart disease with pravastatin in men with hypercholesterolemia. N Engl J Med 1995; **333**: 1301–7.
24. Scandanavian Simvastatin Survival Study Group. Randomized trial of cholesterol lowering in 4444 patients with coronary heart disease: the Scandanavian Simvastatin Survival Study (4S). Lancet 1994; **344**: 1383–9.
25. Blankenhorn DH, Nessim SA, Johnson RL, Sanmarco ME, Azen SP, Cashin-Hemphill L. Beneficial effects of combined colestipol-niacin therapy on coronary atherosclerosis and coronary venous bypass grafts. JAMA 1987; **257**: 3233–40.
26. Brown G, Albers JJ, Lloyd D, Schaffer SM, Lin J-T, Kaplan C, *et al.* Regression of coronary artery disease as a result of intensive lipid-lowering therapy in men with high levels of apolipoprotein B. N Engl J Med 1990; **323**: 1289–98.
27. Watts GF, Lewis B, Brunt JNH, Lewis ES, Coltart DJ, Smith LDR, *et al.* Effects on coronary heart disease of lipid-lowering diet plus cholestyamine, in the St Thomas' Atherosclerosis Regression Study (Stars). Lancet 1992; **339**: 563–9.
28. Law MR, Wald NJ, Thompson SG. By how much and how quickly does reduction in serum cholesterol lower risk of ischaemic heart disease? BMJ 1994; **308**: 367–72.
29. Law MR, Wald NJ, Wu T, Hackshaw A, Bailey A. Systematic underestimation of association between serum cholesterol concentration and ischaemic heart disease in observational studies: data from the BUPA study. BMJ 1994; **308**: 363–6.
30. Vartiainen E, Puska P, Pekkanen J, Tuomilehto J, Jousilahti P. Changes in risk factors explain changes in mortality from ischaemic heart disease in Finland. BMJ 1994; **309**: 23–7.
31. Neaton JD, Blackburn H, Jacobs D, Kuller L, Lee D-J, Sherwin R, *et al.* Serum cholesterol level and mortality findings for men screened in the multiple risk factor intervention trial. Arch Intern Med 1992; **152**: 1490–1500.
32. Law MR, Thompson SG, Wald NJ. Assessing possible hazards of reducing cholesterol. BMJ 1994; **303**: 373–9.

33. Henrikson P, Eriksson M, Ericsson S, Rudling M, Stege R, Berglund L, Angelin B. Hypocholesterolaemia and increased elimination of low-density lipoproteins in metastatic cancer of the prostate. Lancet 1989; **ii**: 1178–80

34. Chen Z, Peto R, Collins R, MacMahon S, Lu J, Li W. Serum cholesterol concentration and coronary heart disease in a population with low cholesterol concentrations. BMJ 1991; **303**: 276–82.

35. A co-operative trial in primary prevention of ischaemic heart disease using clofibrate: report from the Committee of Principal Investigators. Br Heart J 1978; **40**: 1069–118.

36. Smith GD, Song F, Sheldon TA. Cholesterol lowering and mortality: the importance of considering initial level of risk. BMJ 1993; **306**: 1367–73.

37. Pekkanen J, Linn S, Heiss G, Suchindran CM, Leon A, Rifkind BM, Tyroler HA. Ten-year mortality from cardiovascular disease in relation to cholesterol level among men with and without preexisting cardiovascular disease. N Engl J Med 1990; **322**: 1700–07.

38. US Department of Health and Human Sciences. The Lipid Research Clinics Population Studies Data Book. Vol 1 The Prevalence Study. NIH Publication No. 80–1527: 1980.

39. Guo S, Beckett L, Chumlea WC, Roche AF, Siervogel RM. Serial analysis of plasma lipids and lipoproteins from individuals 9–21 y of age. Am J Clin Nutr 1993; **58**: 61–7.

40. Cardiovascular Review Group; Committee on Medical Aspects of Food Policy. Nutritional Aspects of Cardiovascular Disease. Department of Health, Report on Health and Social Subjects 46. London: HMSO, 1994.

41. Durrington PN. Hyperlipidaemia, Diagnosis and Management 2nd Ed. Oxford: Butterworth Heinemann 1994.

42. Johansson S, *et al*. Serum lipids and apolipoprotein levels in women with acute myocardial infarction. Arteriosclerosis 1988; **8**: 742–9.

43. Tunstall-Pedoe H, Smith WCS, Tavendale R. How-Often-That-High Graphs of serum cholesterol. Lancet 1989; **i**: 540–2.

44. Grady D, Rubin SM, Petitti DB, Fox CS, Black D, Ettinger B, *et al*. Hormone therapy to prevent disease and prolong life in postmenopausal women. Ann Intern Med 1992; **117**: 1016–37.

45. Stamler J, Wentworth D, Neaton JD. Is the relationship between serum cholesterol and risk of premature cornary heart disease continuous and graded? JAMA 1986; **256**: 2823–7.

46. Kronmal RA, Cain KC, Ye z, Omenn GS. Total serum cholesterol levels and mortality risk as a function of age: a report based on the Framingham data. Arch Intern Med 1993; **153**: 1065–73.

47. Harris T, Kleinman JC, Ettinger WH, Makue DM, Schatzkin AG. The low cholesterol-mortality association in a national cohort. J Clin Epidemiol 1992; **45**: 595–601.

48. Hulley SB, Newman TB. Cholesterol in the Elderly: Is it important? JAMA 1994; **272**: 1372–4.

49. International Task Force for Prevention of Coronary Heart Disease. Prevention of coronary heart disease: scientific background and new clinical guidelines. The recommendations of the European Atherosclerosis Society. Nutrition, Metabolism and Cardiovascular Diseases 1992; **2**: 113–56.

50. Betteridge DJ, Dodson PM, Durrington PN, Hughes EA, Laker MF, Nichols DP, *et al*. Management of hyperlipidaemia: guidelines of the British Hyperlipidaemia Association. Postgrad Med J 1993; **69**: 359–69.

51. Neil HAW, Roe L, Godlee RJP, Moore JW, Clark GMG, Brown J, *et al*. Randomized trial of lipid lowering dietary advice in general practice: the effects on serum lipids, lipoproteins, and antioxidants. BMJ 1995; **310**: 569–73.

52. Kane JP, Malloy MJ, Ports TA, Phillips NR, Diehl JC, Havel RJ. Regression of coronary atherosclerosis during treatment of familial hypercholesterolaemia with combined drug regimens. JAMA 1990; **264**: 3007–12.

4 Nutrition

Margaret Thorogood

INTRODUCTION

Many aspects of diet have been associated with varying the risk of coronary heart disease (CHD), from drinking boiled coffee to eating garlic. This chapter will concentrate principally on the major components of dietary intake which appear to be associated with CHD, that is, fibre, dietary cholesterol, antioxidant containing fruit and vegetables, and, most importantly, both the type and amount of fat. Evidence relating to hypertension and diet is reviewed in Chapter 2.

THE PROBLEM

In Britain, the population is eating a diet which is very high in fat, particularly saturated fat. This is part of a wider European problem, where most of the countries of northern Europe derive more than 40 per cent of energy from fat, as compared with the European Economic Community (EEC) nutrition policy goal that 20 per cent to 30 per cent of energy should be derived from fat.[1] It is generally accepted that a diet with a high proportion of saturated fat, possibly combined with an inadequate supply of foods containing the antioxidants beta carotene and vitamin E, is a major cause of coronary atherosclerosis. In 1992, over 40 per cent of all energy intake in the UK was from fat, with over 15 percent of all energy coming from saturated fat alone.[2] The majority of this fat intake comes from three sources: over one quarter of the intake comes from spreading and cooking fats (butter, margarine, and oil), almost as much from meat and meat products, and a further 10 per cent from milk and milk products. In order to reduce the incidence of CHD, the Department of Health has recommended that proportions of energy from total fat and saturated fat should be reduced to 35 percent and 10 percent respectively.[2]

In reviewing the evidence for the importance of dietary change in relation to coronary heart disease, this chapter will address three questions. These are:

1. **Is there epidemiological evidence of a relationship between diet and CHD?**
2. **Is there epidemiological evidence of a relationship between diet and blood lipid levels?**
3. **What is the evidence concerning the feasibility of intervention to achieve dietary change?**

While many metabolic studies have shown a relationship between diet and blood lipid levels, evidence for the relationship between diet and CHD comes principally from epidemiological studies. One major problem with all epidemiological dietary studies is the difficulty of measuring accurately the nutritional intake of free living individuals. The problems with measuring dietary intake, and the alternative methods of measurement that are available, have been reviewed thoroughly. No method is universally the best.[3,4] Early epidemiological studies relied on recall methods, where subjects were asked to remember what they had eaten over a defined period in the past (typically the last 24 hours). More recently, the problems of faulty remembering and the possible unrepresentativeness of any one day's intake have led epidemiologists to prefer methods based on diet records kept prospectively by the subject over a number of days, or food frequency question-naires in which subjects are asked to estimate their usual intake of listed foods. A seven-day record, in which all food eaten is weighed and recorded, has sometimes been referred to as a 'gold standard' for dietary methodology, but it is certainly not free from problems, particularly relating to biased compliance.[5] None of the methods developed so far are ideal, in that they are all associated with some forms of bias and some inevitable inaccuracies in measurement, and these problems may often dilute the observed relationships between diet and disease. Such a dilution of the evidence, together with the major confounding effect of population change in other coronary risk factors (notably smoking) have made it possible for some authors to attempt to argue that there is no evidence of a relationship between fat intake and coronary disease.[6]

IS THERE EPIDEMIOLOGICAL EVIDENCE OF A RELATIONSHIP BETWEEN DIET AND CHD?

Despite the problems described above, there is considerable epidemiological evidence that nutritional intake is related to the risk of developing CHD and this has been carefully reviewed.[7] Evidence comes from four different types of studies. These are:

- *chronological studies*, concerning data on observed changes over a period of time in food consumption and mortality within a population.
- *comparative studies* of nutrient intake and CHD rates between countries.
- *migrant population studies* providing evidence of the effect on rates of CHD of the change in lifestyle, including diet, as groups settle into new cultures.
- *cohort studies* where information is collected on individuals who eat different diets, and who are followed up for a number of years.

None of the studies by themselves can be said to provide conclusive evidence of a causal relationship between diet and CHD, but considered together they do provide strong suggestive evidence of a relationship between aspects of diet, in particular the quantity and type of fat in the diet, and CHD incidence.

Chronological studies

Two studies have been conducted of changes in food intake in the United States over periods of more than sixty years. One of the studies used government data on food consumption (primarily national food disappearance data) between 1909 and 1980,[8] while the other study collected together data from 171 different research projects which had assessed dietary intake and were conducted between 1920 and 1984.[9] It is notable that although the two studies were based on entirely different sources of nutritional data they both found that the proportion of saturated fat in the diet had been decreasing, and that such a decrease preceded by 10 to 20 years a decrease in mortality from CHD in the United States.

Comparative studies

The *Seven Countries Study* is an important comparative, international study. A number of variables, including dietary intake and blood lipid levels were measured in cohorts of men aged between 40 and 59 years from Japan, Greece, Yugoslavia, Italy, the Netherlands, the United States and Finland. Mean levels of nutrient intake were estimated from seven day weighed diet records kept by a sub-sample of men in most of the cohorts; in two cohorts dietary intake was estimated using a recall method. The 111 579 men were followed up for 15 years, after which time there had been 2288 deaths, with marked variations in death rates between the different cohorts. Death rates were related positively to the proportion of total energy in the diet contributed by saturated fat and negatively to the proportion contributed by monounsaturated fat, while the proportion contributed by poly-unsaturated fat appeared to have no relationship to death rate. Oleic acid accounted for almost all the difference in intake of monounsaturates between cohorts, and CHD death rates were low in cohorts where olive oil was a principle source of dietary fat.[10]

Migrant population studies

The *NI-HO-SAN* migrant study has shown a strong correlation between dietary saturated fatty acids and CHD. Three cohorts of Japanese men were studied: native Japanese living in Japan, Japanese men living in Hawaii and eating a diet richer in fat and dietary cholesterol, and Japanese men living in California and eating a diet even richer in fat and cholesterol. The men who had remained in Japan had the lowest rates of CHD, while those who had moved to Hawaii had twice the rate of those remaining in Japan, and men in California had rates 50 percent higher than men in Hawaii.[11,12]

Cohort studies

Fat

Two cohort studies have found a relationship between the nature of fat consumed and CHD. The *Ireland-Boston* study of 1001 men of Irish descent followed for

20 years found a weak, but statistically significant, relationship between CHD mortality and the Keys dietary score calculated by a dietary recall method.[13] The Keys dietary score has been shown in metabolic studies to be a good predictor of blood cholesterol levels. The formula is based on the amount of saturated and polyunsaturated fat and cholesterol in the diet.

Fish oils

The fat available in fish is rich in eicosapentaenoic acid, and experimental diets rich in fish oils have been shown to change blood lipid levels.[14] In the *Zutphen Study* information on the dietary habits of 852 Dutch men with a wide range of intake of fish was collected by a food frequency method. The men were followed for 20 years, during which time 78 of them died from CHD. Mortality from CHD was more than 50 per cent lower among those men who ate at least 30g of fish a day compared with those who did not eat fish.[15]

Dietary cholesterol

Dietary cholesterol intake was shown to be associated with relative risk of death from cardiovascular disease in the *Western Electric Study*. In this study 1824 male employees of the Western Electric Company in Chicago aged between 40 and 59 were followed for 25 years, after which time 307 of them had died from cardiovascular disease. Dietary information was obtained at recruitment into the study using a recall method for food consumed in the previous 28 days. The relative risk of cardiovascular death for men in the highest quintile of dietary cholesterol intake compared with those in the bottom quintile was 1.5 (95 per cent confidence interval 1.1–1.9).[16]

Fibre

Two cohort studies have shown a relationship between cardiovascular disease and dietary fibre intake. A study of *London bank clerks and bus drivers* involved 337 men who completed seven-day weighed dietary records between 1956 and 1966. By 1976, 45 men had developed clinical CHD. Men who developed CHD had a significantly lower mean daily intake of dietary fibre.[17] In the *Rancho Bernardo Study*, California, 859 men and women aged 50–79 years were followed for 12 years, after which time there had been 65 deaths from ischaemic heart disease. Diet was assessed at entry into the study using a 24 hour recall method. A higher intake of dietary fibre was associated with a lower risk of ischaemic heart disease mortality, in that a 6 gm increment in daily fibre intake was associated with a 25 per cent reduction in such mortality ($p < 0.01$).[18]

Obesity

The relationship between measures of body fatness and risk of death from coronary disease has been examined in several cohort studies. The *Framingham Study* has followed over 5000 men and women living in a community in New England since 1948. After 26 years of follow-up, both men and women aged under 50 years and weighing at least 30 per cent in excess of desirable body weight (this represents a body mass index of around 27 to 29 kg/m^2) were found to be at a significantly increased risk of coronary disease.[19] This relationship was not explained by a relationship between body weight and other risk factors. Similar findings come from the *Northwick Park Heart Study* of 1511 men aged 40–64 years at recruitment. After 12 years, men with a body mass index one standard deviation (about 8 kg) above average were found to have a 44 per cent increase in risk of ischaemic heart disease.[20]

The Gothenburg Study, Sweden has examined the relationship between risk of ischaemic heart disease and several measures of obesity, including body mass index, skinfold thickness and waist to hip ratio, in both 792 men aged 54 years at recruitment and 1462 women aged 38–64 years. The only measure of obesity which showed any relationship with risk of ischaemic heart disease in men was the waist to hip ratio. However, waist to hip ratio was not an independent long-term predictor of ischaemic heart disease once the confounding effects of blood lipid levels and blood pressure were taken into account.[21] By contrast, in the female cohort, waist to hip ratio was found to be positively associated with risk of myocardial infarction even after allowing for the confounding effects of age, body mass index, smoking habit, serum cholesterol, and blood pressure.[22] There is evidence from several studies that the waist to hip ratio, rather than body mass index, is a better predictor of CHD, and may also explain, in part, the sex differences in CHD risk.[23,24]

Calorie restricted diets may, however, not improve the risk unless any weight reduction is maintained long-term. Results from 32 years of follow-up in the *Framingham Study* showed that subjects with highly variable body weights had a significantly increased total and CHD mortality, independent of any risk associated with obesity.[25] Sustained weight loss in obese subjects is very difficult to achieve. The prevention of obesity is therefore particularly important.

Special diets

Studies of Seventh Day Adventist church members provide a good source of data. Adventist members abstain from smoking and alcohol, but are also encouraged to reduce or exclude meat from the diet. About half of Adventist members are lacto-ovo vegetarians, that is, they eat milk and eggs, but not meat or fish. *The Adventist Health Study* involves 24 044 Californian Adventist members aged 35 and over, followed for 20 years. CHD mortality was very low amongst the whole cohort in comparison with the general Californian population. Moreover, within the Adventist population there were significant associations between diet and CHD. Adventist subjects who ate nuts more than four times a week had a lower risk of both fatal CHD (relative risk 0.5, 95 per cent confidence interval 0.4–0.8) and of non-fatal myocardial infarction (relative risk 0.5, 95 per cent confidence interval 0.3–0.9). Those subjects who ate wholewheat bread experienced a small decrease in risk of fatal CHD (relative risk 0.9, 95 per cent confidence interval 0.6–1.3) and a larger, significant, decrease in risk of non-fatal myocardial infarction (relative risk 0.6, 95 per cent confidence interval 0.4–0.9). Men who ate beef regularly had a higher risk of fatal CHD (relative risk 2.3, 95 per cent confidence interval 1.1–4.8), but not of non-fatal disease, and the elevated risk associated with eating beef was not apparent in women. [26]

The British Health Food Shop Users Study of 10 943 people with a particular interest in health foods has provided similar findings. Subjects completed a screening questionnaire relating to the frequency of intake of high fibre foods, and were also asked whether or not they were vegetarian. After 7 years of follow-up 140 subjects had died from ischaemic heart disease. The vegetarians experienced significantly less ischaemic heart disease mortality than the non-vegetarian health food users, and this difference was especially marked amongst the men. [27]

The Oxford Vegetarian Study has followed two cohorts of 6000 non-meat eaters and 5000 meat eaters for 12 years. The death rate from CHD was very low in both these cohorts. The meat eaters had about half the average death rate, but the vegetarians' death rate was even lower at just over a quarter. However, after the data had been adjusted for the differences between the cohorts in body mass index, social class, and smoking history, the CHD death rate in the non-meat eaters was just around 25 per cent lower than in the meat eaters, and the difference was not significant. [28]

Antioxidant intake—The Mediterranean diet

Countries with a high intake of fruit and vegetables, such as France and the Mediterranean countries, appear to have lower than expected rates of coronary disease. The role of a high fruit and vegetable intake in providing an abundance of the antioxidant vitamins C, E and beta carotene, which in turn limit free radical damage to cholesterol, may be an important protective factor in these countries. This issue is discussed at length in Chapter 12.

IS THERE EPIDEMIOLOGICAL EVIDENCE OF A RELATIONSHIP BETWEEN DIET AND BLOOD LIPID LEVELS?

Epidemiological studies of free living subjects within a single population often fail to find a relationship between nutritional intake and blood cholesterol levels. A government sponsored, national survey examined the relationship between nutritional intake of fats and cholesterol and levels of serum total, LDL, and HDL cholesterol in Britain in 860 men and 776 women. The results were disappointing in that few of the correlations were significant, particularly in men, and even the significant coefficients of correlation were very small. [29]

The failure to find relationships between diet and blood lipid levels may be due in part to the problems of accurately measuring dietary intake discussed previously, but such a failure can also be explained by the limited range of levels of intake of fat within most study populations. When subjects within a population who are eating diets that are markedly different in their fat content are compared, a clear relationship can be shown. A study of 208 participants in the *Oxford Vegetarian Study* (including vegans who ate no animal products, lacto-ovo vegetarians, fish eaters who did not eat meat, and meat eaters) found a correlation between plasma total cholesterol and the Keys dietary score of 0.37 (p < 0.001).[30] A similar study of 46 predominantly vegetarian subjects in Boston, Massachusetts found a correlation between the Keys dietary score and plasma total cholesterol of 0.51 (95 per cent confidence interval 0.24–0.70).[31]

Seventh Day Adventist participants in the *Norwegian Cardiovascular Disease Studies* were found to have significantly lower total cholesterol levels than non-adventist participants. This difference was particularly marked for men, where the Adventist men had a mean serum total cholesterol that was 0.9 mmol/l lower (95 per cent confidence interval 0.6–1.1). Amongst the female participants, the Adventist women had a mean serum total cholesterol that was 0.5 mmol/l lower (95 per cent confidence interval 0.3–0.7).[32]

However, a relationship between diet and blood lipid levels may not be as simple as previously thought. The authors of a review of the relationship between diet and CHD have argued that an emphasis solely on the fat content of diet, and in particular on the polyunsaturated to saturated fatty acid ratio, is inappropriate. They discussed the complex relationship between seven dietary factors involved in the development of CHD and put forward a new measure of the propensity of diet to influence the incidence of CHD in terms of two indices of atherogenicity and of thrombogenicity. They argued that total fat consumption and lean meat consumption are not strongly related to either atherogenicity or thrombogenicity, and, indeed, that lean meat is a good source of polyunsaturated fatty acids. They concluded that the best dietary advice is to replace butter and hard margarine with polyunsaturated margarine, replace full-fat with semi-skimmed or skimmed milk, and eat more fish, lean meat, fibre-rich foods, fresh fruit, and vegetables.[33]

Obesity and blood lipid levels

A considerable number of studies have shown a strong positive relationship between body weight and blood lipid levels. While the relationship is strongest for blood triglyceride levels, there is also a positive relationship with levels of total cholesterol and a negative relationship with levels of HDL cholesterol.[34] Data from the *British Regional Heart Study* appear to indicate that the positive relationship between cholesterol and body mass index is only apparent when body mass index is less than 28 kg/m^2, and total cholesterol level less than 7.0 mmol/l. In obese men (that is, men with a body mass index above 30) there was no such relationship.[35]

WHAT IS THE EVIDENCE CONCERNING THE FEASIBILITY OF INTERVENTION TO ACHIEVE DIETARY CHANGE?

It is never easy for individuals to change their diet. In particular, many people find the severely reduced fat diet, that is often recommended, to be unpalatable.

However, there is evidence that the diet of the population is changing, with an increasing consumption of some low-fat products[2.] In the 1980s butter consumption declined to below wartime levels, being replaced in part by a rapidly increasing consumption of low-fat and reduced fat spreads. At the same time consumption of milk and milk products was declining. Skimmed and semi-skimmed milk has replaced some of the whole milk consumption. Changes in intake at a population level, then, are possible, and can happen quite rapidly in some cases.

There has recently been considerable concern expressed about the effects of cholesterol lowering interventions unless patients are at high absolute risk of CHD. This issue is discussed in more detail in Chapter 3. Briefly, there is concern that the use of lipid-lowering drugs does not lead to a lower mortality, and may actually increase mortality. There have been several reviews of this controversial area. A recent review of trials of cholesterol lowering by both diet and drug therapy concluded that dietary change was both more cost effective and probably safer than drug therapy but this remains controversial.[36]

Dietary advice in high risk groups

There have been studies of dietary intervention at an individual level which have shown such intervention to be feasible and to be associated with a positive benefit on cardiovascular outcomes. In the *Life-style Study*, a prospective randomized controlled trial of 48 patients with angiographically documented coronary artery disease, 28 patients were allocated to an experimental group, with a very low-fat vegetarian diet, smoking cessation advice, stress management and exercise, while the remaining 20 patients were allocated to a usual care group. After one year, the fat intake of the experimental group had fallen from 31.5 per cent of total calories to 6.8 per cent, and dietary cholesterol intake had fallen from 213 mg/day to 12 mg/day. There was no significant change in the diet of the usual care group. Serum total cholesterol level had fallen significantly in the experimental group, but not in the usual care group. Coronary angiography showed significant overall regression of coronary atheroma in the experimental group, while atheroma had progressed in the usual care group. The authors concluded that patients with coronary disease can be motivated to make major life-style changes, and that such changes are of benefit.[37]

Trials of fat reducing advice in breast cancer prevention are interesting. In one trial of women with mammographic dysplasia the intervention group reduced their fat intake from an initial level of 37 per cent of energy to 21 per cent at one year[38], while the control group intake had fallen marginally to 35 per cent. In another trial of women at high risk of breast cancer the intervention group had a mean fat intake of 23 per cent of energy at 2 years, while the control group intake remained unchanged at 37 per cent.

The diet recommended in the Life-style study and the breast cancer prevention trials were very low in fat, and would be unlikely to be acceptable in Britain even to patients who have the strong motivation of already suffering from severe coronary disease. A much less restricted diet was used in a British randomized controlled trial of secondary prevention of myocardial infarction (the *DART trial—diet and reinfarction trial*). In this trial, 2033 men who had survived a myocardial infarction were randomized in a four way factorial design to receive or not to receive advice on each of three dietary factors: a reduction in fat intake and an increase in the polyunsaturated to saturated fat ratio (P:S ratio), an increase in fatty fish intake or the use of fish oil capsules, and an increase in cereal fibre intake. After two years, all aspects of the dietary advice had a marked effect on subjects' intake as estimated by an interviewer-administered dietary questionnaire, except for the advice to reduce total fat intake. Total fat intake was only marginally lower in the fat advice group (32 per cent of total energy) than in the no fat advice group (35 per cent of total energy). The **P**:S ratio in the fat advice group was 0.8, compared with 0.4 in the no fat advice group, cereal fibre intake was 17 g/day in the fibre advice group compared with 9 g/day in the no fibre advice group and eicosapentaenoic acid intake was 2.4 g/week in the fish oil advice group compared with 0.6 g/week in the no fish oil advice group.

Although changes in the diet were achieved, advice on fat and fibre intake was not associated with any significant difference in mortality after two years. However, the subjects advised to eat fatty fish had a 29 per cent reduction in two year all cause mortality compared with those not so advised. No information is available on the health effects of these dietary changes over a longer period than two years, so no conclusions about long-term effects can be drawn.[40] The dietary changes achieved in this study were less marked that those achieved in the Life-style study, but probably represent more realistic dietary goals for a British population.

A randomized controlled trial of 90 men with CHD and a total cholesterol concentration between 6.0 and 10.0 mmol/l (the *STARS trial—St Thomas' Atherosclerosis Regression Study*) has provided further evidence of the effectiveness of dietary intervention in the reduction of CHD.[41] The men were randomized to one of three groups. One group received usual care, one group received dietary advice, and one group received dietary advice together with cholesterol lowering drugs. The recommended diet was low in total fat and saturated fat, and was calorie restricted if the men had a body mass index greater than $25 kg/m^2$. The subjects underwent angiography before admission into the trial and again after three years in the trial. Both the intervention groups had significantly less progression of atheroma during the trial period, and the mean absolute width of coronary segments increased in both intervention groups (by 0.003mm in the dietary intervention group and by 0.103mm in the diet and drugs group, compared with a decrease of 0.201mm in the usual care group, $p < 0.05$ for comparison of usual care and diet plus drug groups). Both interventions significantly reduced the frequency of total cardiovascular events. The authors concluded that there was 'growing evidence to support the use of lipid-lowering intervention, first by diet but with drug treatment added if necessary'.

Dietary advice in the groups at mildly elevated risk

Three recent studies have examined the effectiveness of dietary advice in a primary care setting. Two randomized controlled trials have tested the effectiveness of nurse administered health checks in primary care. The *Family Heart Study* randomized patients in a number of practices around the country to either be invited for a health check or to wait one year for their health check. Participants were given advice on all aspects of life-style which affect the risk of CHD, including diet. After one year, cholesterol in the intervention group had fallen by an average of 0.1 mmol/l in comparison with the control groups.[42]

The *OXCHECK Trial* was a longer term trial of nurse administered health checks which randomized patients from five general practices in Bedfordshire. The final results from this trial showed that after three years mean serum cholesterol was three per cent lower in the intervention group than in the controls, and there was a four per cent reduction in the percentage of subjects with a cholesterol greater than 8.0 mmol/l. Self-reported dietary fat intake also changed significantly in the intervention group. These results indicate that a small change in cholesterol levels can be achieved, and maintained for at least three years.[43]

A single factor randomized trial of dietary advice in primary care for patients with mildly elevated cholesterol levels (6.0–8.5 mmol/l) compared personal advice given by a dietitian, personal advice given by a practice nurse, or a leaflet handed to the patient. After six months, only a two percent reduction in total cholesterol was observed. There was no difference in the effectiveness of the three interventions being tested.[44]

Taken together, these three trial results provide strong evidence that dietary advice given to patients at mildly elevated risk is unlikely to achieve more than a small fall in cholesterol. While small downward shifts in mean cholesterol level might be useful at a population level, the clinical value seems more doubtful.

SUMMARY

- Dietary epidemiologic studies are difficult to carry out, and much of the published work is difficult to interpret.
- Eating a diet that is high in saturated fat raises blood lipid levels and increases the risk of premature coronary disease.
- Obesity, particularly central obesity, increases the risk of CHD. Highly variable weight may also increase risk, and weight loss should be sustained long term. This is very difficult to achieve and prevention of obesity is therefore important.
- A diet that is low in saturated fat, but high in monounsaturated and poly-unsaturated fats, with an abundance of fresh fruit and vegetables, a plentiful intake of wholegrain cereals, and a limited intake of dietary cholesterol is likely to provide the best protection against premature coronary disease.
- Changing the diet of individuals is a difficult undertaking, and such studies have shown very limited success, except in patients at very high risk of CHD or with established CHD.

REFERENCES

1. O'Connor M. Europe and nutrition. BMJ 1992; **304**: 178–80.
2. Department of Health and Social Security nutritional aspects of cardiovascular disease report on health and social subjects No 46, London: HO, 1995.
3. Bingham SA. The dietary assessment of individuals; methods, accuracy, new techniques and recommendations. Nutrition Abstracts and Reviews (Series A) 1987; **57**: 705–42.
4. Barret-Connor E. Nutrition epidemiology: how do we know what they ate? Am J Clin Nutr 1991; **54**: 182S-7S.
5. Livingstone MBE, Prentice AM, Strain JJ, Coward WA, Black AE, Barker ME, *et al*. Accuracy of weighed dietary records in studies of diet and health. BMJ 1990; **300**: 708–12.
6. Le Fanu J. Eat your heart out. London: Macmillan, 1987.
7. La Rosa JC, Hunninghake D, Bush D, Criqui MH, Getz GS, Gollo AM, *et al*. The Cholesterol Facts. A summary of the evidence relating dietary fats, serum cholesterol and coronary heart disease. Circulation 1990; **81**: 1721–33.
8. Slattery ML, Randall DE. Trends in coronary heart disease mortality and food consumption in the United States between 1909 and 1980. Am J Clin Nutr 1988; **47**: 1060–7.
9. Stephen AM, Wald NJ. Trends in individual consumption of dietary fat in the United States 1920–1984. Am J Clin Nutr 1990; **52**: 457–69.
10. Keys A (ed.). Coronary heart disease in seven countries. Circulation 1970; **41**: Suppl 1.
11. Kagan A, Harris BR, Winkelstein W, Johnson KG, Kato H, Syme SL, *et al*. Epidemiologic studies of coronary heart disease and stroke in Japanese men living in Japan, Hawaii and California: Demographic, physical, dietary and biochemical characteristics. J Chron Dis 1973; **27**: 345–64.
12. Robertson TL, Kato H, Gordon T, Kagon A, Rhoads GG, Land CE, Worth RM, Belsky JL, Dock DS, Miyanishi, Kavamoto S, *et al* Epidemiologic studies of coronary heart disease and stroke in Japanese men living in Japan, Hawaii, and California. Am J Cardiol 1977; **39**: 239–43.
13. Kushi LH, Lew RA, Stare FJ. Diet and 20-year mortality from coronary heart disease. N Engl J Med 1985; **312**: 811–18.
14. Sanders TAB. Fish and coronary artery disease. Br Heart J 1987; **57**: 214–19.
15. Kromhout D, Bosschieter E, Coulander C. The inverse relation between fish consumption and 20-year mortality from coronary heart disease. N Eng J Med 1985; **312**: 1205–9.
16. Shekelle RB, Stamler J. Dietary cholesterol and ischaemic heart disease. Lancet 1989; **i**: 1177–9.
17. Morris JN, Marr JW, Clayton DG. Diet and heart: a postscript. BMJ 1977; **2**: 1307–14.
18. Khaw KT, Barrett-Connor E. Dietary fibre and reduced ischaemic heart disease mortality rates in men and women: a 12-year prospective study. Am J Epid 1987; **126**: 1093–102.
19. Hubert HB, Feinleib M, McNamara PM, Castelli WP. Obesity as an independent risk factor for cardiovascular disease: A 26-year follow-up of participants in the Framingham Heart study. Circulation 1983; **67**: 968–77.
20. Imeson JD, Haines AP, Meade TW. Skinfold thickness, body mass index, and ischaemic heart disease. J Epidemiol and Community Health 1989; **43**: 223–7.
21. Larsson B, Svardsudd K, Welin L, Wilhelmsen L, Bjorntorp P, Tibblin G. Abdominal adipose tissue distribution, obesity, and risk of cardiovascular disease and death: 13 year follow up of participants in the study of men born in 1913. BMJ 1984; **288**: 1401–4.

22. Lapidus L, Bengtsson C, Larsson B, Pennert K, Rybo E, Sjostrom L. Distribution of adipose tissue and risk of cardiovascular disease and death: a 12 year follow up of participants in the population study of women in Gothenburg, Sweden. BMJ 1984; **289**: 1257–61.
23. Larsson B, Bengtsson C, Bjorntorp P, Lapidus L, Sjostrom L, Svardsudd K, Tibblin G, Wedel H, Welin L, Wilhelmson L. Is abdominal body fat distribution a major explanation for the sex difference in the incidence of myocardial infarction? Am J Epidemiol 1992; **135**: 266–73.
24. Wingard DL. Sex differences and coronary heart disease. A case of comparing apples and pears? Circulation 1990; **81**: 1710–12.
25. Lissner L, Odell PM, D'Agostino RB, Stokes J, Kreger BE, Belanger AJ, Brownwell KD. Variability of body weight and health outcomes in the Framingham population. N Engl J Med 1991; **324**: 1839–44.
26. Fraser GE, Sabate J, Beeson WL, Strahan TM. A possible protective effect of nut consumption on risk of coronary heart disease. Arch Intern Med 1992; **152**: 1416–24.
27. Burr ML, Sweetnam PM. Vegetarianism, dietary fiber and mortality. Am J Clin Nutr 1982; **6**: 873–7.
28. Thorogood M, Mann J, Appleby P, McPherson K. Risk of death from cancer and ischaemic heart disease in meat and non-meat eaters. BMJ 1994; **308**: 1667–71.
29. Gregory J, Foster K, Tyler H, Wiseman M. The dietary and nutritional survey of British adults London: HMSO, 1990.
30. Thorogood M, Roe L, McPherson K, Mann J. Dietary intake and plasma lipid levels: lessons from a study of the diet of health conscious groups. BMJ 1990; **300**: 1297–301.
31. Kushi LH, Samonds KW, Lacey JM, Brown PT, Bergan JG, Sackss FM. The association of dietary fat with serum cholesterol in vegetarians: the effect of dietary assessment on the correlation coefficient. Am J Epidemiol 1988; **128**: 1054–64.
32. Fonnebo V. Coronary risk factors in Norwegian Seventh-day Adventists: A study of 247 Seventh-day Adventists and matched controls. Am J Epidemiol 1992; **135**: 504–8.
33. Ulbricht TLV, Southgate DAT. Coronary heart disease: seven dietary factors. Lancet 1991; **338**: 985–92.
34. Thompson GR. A handbook of hyperlipidaemia. London: Current Science Ltd, 1989
35. Thelle DS, Shaper AG, Whitehead TP, Bullock DG, Ashby D, Patel I. Blood lipids in middle-aged British men. BMJ 1983; **49**: 205–13.
36. Davey-Smith G, Pekkanen J. Should there be a moratorium on the use of cholesterol lowering drugs? BMJ 1992; **304**: 431–4.
37. Ornish D, Brown SE, Scherwitz LW, Bilings JH, Armstrong WT, Ports TA, *et al.* Can life-style changes reverse coronary heart disease? The lifestyle heart trial. Lancet 1990; **336**: 129–33.
38. Boyd NF, Cousins M, Beaton M, *et al.* Quantitative changes in dietary fat intake and serum cholesterol in women: results from a randomized controlled trial. Am J Clin Nutr 1990; **52**: 470–76.
39. Henderson M, Kushi LH, Thompson DJ, *et al.* Feasibility of a randomized trial of a low-fat diet for the prevention of breast cancer: dietary compliance in the women's health trial vanguard study. Preventive Medicine 1990; **19**: 115–133.
40. Burr M, Fehily A, Gilbert JF. Effects of changes in fat, fish, and fibre intakes on death and myocardial reinfarction: diet and reinfarction trial (DART). Lancet 1989; **ii**: 757–61.
41. Watts GF, Lewis B, Brunt JNH, Lewis ES, Coltart DJ, Smith LDR, Mann JI, Swan AV. Effects on coronary artery disease of lipid-lowering diet, or diet plus cholestyramine, in the St Thomas' atherosclerosis regression study (STARS). Lancet 1992; **339**: 563–9.

42. Family Heart Study Group. Randomised controlled trial evaluating cardiovascular screening and intervention in general practice: principal results of British family heart study. BMJ 1994; **308**: 313–20.
43. ICRF OXCHECK Study Group. The effectiveness of health checks conducted by nurses in primary care: Final results form the OXCHECK study. BMJ 1995; **310**: 1099–104.
44. Neil HAW, Roe L, Godlee RJP, Moore JW, Clark GMG, Brown J, Thorogood M, Stratton IM, Lancaster T, Mant D, Fowler GH. Randomised trial of lipid lowering dietary advice in general practice: the effects on serum lipids, lipoproteins and antioxidants. BMJ 1995; **310**: 549–73.

5 Exercise

David Mant and Paul Little

INTRODUCTION

Forty years ago, Morris and his co-workers in London drew attention to the higher cardiovascular morbidity of sedentary workers within similar social groups. They asked why bus drivers should suffer more heart attacks than bus conductors, why clerks more than postmen, and they suggested that one explanation was the degree of exercise taken.[1] This led Morris to set up the *UK Civil Service Study,* concerned with leisure time activity in male civil servants aged 40–64, in which those who reported involvement in vigorous exercise experienced a coronary heart disease (CHD) rate approximately one third lower than that in other men.[2] Importantly, the benefit of vigorous exercise was apparent even within groups of men with cardiovascular risk factors such as smoking, high blood pressure and high serum cholesterol levels.

Exercise was measured in the, now famous, *Framingham Study* at the fourth biennial examination when a 24-hour 'energy output' score was estimated for each participant. A score of more than 35 (achieved by 17 per cent of the population) was associated with a one-third reduction in the annual incidence of CHD.[3] In 1986, Paffenberger reported the relative and attributable risk of death in relation to exercise among 16 936 Harvard alumni. Although a sedentary life-style was less important than smoking, hypertension, or weight gain as an individual risk factor, its high prevalence placed it second only to smoking as a risk factor for the population as a whole (Table 5.1).[4]

A meta-analysis in 1990, of 27 cohort studies examining the effect of physical activity on CHD, reported a relative risk of death for sedentary compared with high activity groups of 1.9 (95 per cent confidence interval 1.6–2.2) for occupational activity and 1.7 (95 per cent confidence interval 1.2–2.3) for leisure time activity.[5] More recently, a further report from the *UK Civil Service Study* has confirmed that it is current rather than past activity which is important.[6] And a 1993 report of the further follow-up of the Havard alumni isolated the effect of beginning moderately vigorous sports activity. During an average follow-up of nine years, those who took up sports activity lowered their subsequent risk of death by 23 per cent (95 per cent confidence interval 4–42 per cent).[7] In comparison, stopping smoking lowered the risk by 41 per cent (95 per cent confidence interval 20–57 per cent).

Not yet convinced

In the light of these findings, and the Royal College of Physicians 1991 Report stating the undisputed benefits to general health which regular exercise confers,[8] we must ask why many general practitioners seem to remain doubtful about the value of promoting exercise as a strategy for the prevention of cardiovascular disease in primary care. The remainder of this chapter will address the specific areas of uncertainty and concern:

1. **How strong is the evidence for a protective effect of exercise?**
2. **Is there a physiologically plausible explanation for a protective effect?**
3. **Is only vigorous exercise beneficial?**
4. **What is the risk of sudden death from exercise?**
5. **Who should exercise, and should people be screened before beginning exercise programmes?**
6. **Is it feasible to give effective advice in primary care?**

Table 5.1 Adjusted relative and attributable risks of death (from all causes) among 16 936 Harvard Alumni, 1962 to 1978. (From Paffenbarger R, Hyde R, Wing A, Hsieh C. Physical activity, all cause mortality and longevity of college alumni. NEJM 1986; **314**: 605–13)

Alumnus characteristic	Prevalence (man-years %)	Relative risk of death (95% CI)	Clinical attributable risk (%)	Community attributable risk (%)
Sedentary life style	62.0	1.31 (1.15–1.49)	23.6	16.1
Hypertension	9.4	1.73 (1.48–1.49)	42.1	6.4
Cigarette smoking	38.2	1.76 (1.56–1.99)	43.2	22.5
Low weight gain	35.1	1.33 (1.17–1.51)	24.6	10.3
Early parental death	33.1	1.15 (1.02–1.30)	13.1	4.8

The clinical attributable risk of death is the risk reduction for persons who do not have the adverse characteristic. The community attributable risk of death is the risk reduction for the community if the adverse characteristics were converted to more favourable characteristics.

The charcteristics were defined as follows: sedentary life style—energy expenditure < 2000 kcal/week in walking, climbing stairs and playing sports; hypertension—doctor diagnosed; low weight gain—less than 3 units BMI since left college (approximately 1 stone); early parental death—parent died < age 65.

HOW STRONG IS THE EVIDENCE FOR A PROTECTIVE EFFECT OF EXERCISE?

Lack of trials

Although there have been a number of multiple intervention trials concerned with both primary and secondary prevention of CHD which have included exercise as a component of the intervention, there have been no trials to assess the effect of exercise alone. In a meta-analysis of cardiac rehabilitation, seven 'exercise predominant' trials were identified, involving more than 2000 patients (Fig. 5.1). The pooled odds ratio for cardiovascular death in these trials was 0.78 (95 per cent confidence interval 0.56–1.08) and for non-fatal re-infarction 1.06 (95 per cent confidence interval 0.75–1.50).[9]

In other words, the trial evidence exists to support the view that a 20 per cent reduction in fatal (but not non-fatal) re-infarction can be achieved by exercise training after a heart attack, but the trials have not been of sufficient size to confirm this with certainty. Trials of primary prevention have not been done.

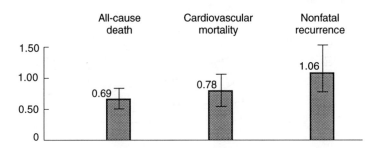

Fig. 5.1 Pooled odds ratios and 95 per cent confidence intervals for all-cause death, cardiovascular mortality, and non-fatal myocardial infarction for exercise predominant trials of cardiac rehabilitation. (From Oldridge N, Guyatt G, Fishe M *et al.* Cardiac rehabilitation after myocardial infarction—combined experiences of randomized trials. JAMA 1988; **260**: 945–50.)

In the absence of evidence from formal trials it is not possible to say with absolute certainty that exercise will protect against heart disease. However, as a formal primary prevention trial is unlikely to be done, decisions on action must be made on the basis of the evidence available from existing research. The strength of this evidence depends upon the extent to which the problems of measurement, selection, and confounding have been met in the cohort studies, and the extent to which a plausible causal mechanism for a protective effect of exercise can be demonstrated.

Was exercise properly measured?

In the early cohort studies the validity of the measurement of activity was often unimpressive: for example, exercise was measured on a single occasion by a simple multiple choice questionnaire allowing only four grades of response. In other studies the ascertainment of cases, particularly non-fatal events, was incomplete. However, in the more recent studies, such as those on Harvard alumni[10] and U.K. Civil Servants,[6] ascertainment was high and measurement of exercise was reasonably precise. Both these carefully conducted studies showed a convincing protective effect.

In three recent American cohort studies, cardiovascular fitness rather than exercise has been measured, in all cases by a treadmill test. Fig. 5.2 shows the results of the *Dallas Study*.[11] The analysis was based on total treadmill test time, which correlates highly with measured maximal oxygen uptake, the most widely accepted index of cardio-respiratory fitness. In the *Lipid Research Clinics Mortality Follow-up Study*[12] and the *US Railroad Study*,[13] the heart rate was used as an indicator of fitness. In all three studies, a clear benefit of cardiovascular fitness was demonstrated which was independent of other risk factors. It is also relevant that in the *Belgian Physical Fitness Study*[14] the main conclusion was that it is the fitness level, but not the physical activity pattern, which is an independent predictor of cardiovascular risk.

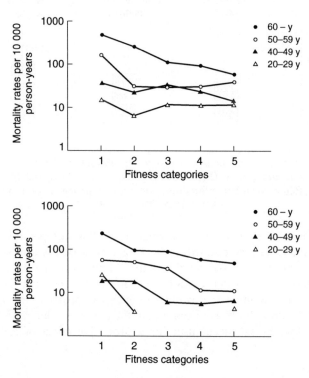

Fig. 5.2   Age specific all-cause death rate per 10 000 person years of follow-up in (a) 10 244 men and (b) 3120 women in the Aerobics Centre Longitudinal Study, by physical fitness quintiles as determined by maximal treadmill exercise tests. (From Blair S, Kohl H, Paffenbarger R *et al.* Physical fitness and all-cause mortality. JAMA 1989; **262**: 2395–401.)

How well was confounding and selection bias avoided?

The authors of the cohort study meta-analysis, using multivariate adjustment regression methods, reported that the protective effect of exercises was not explained in terms of other associated cardiovascular risk factors. In addition, the methodologically stronger studies showed larger benefits than the less well designed studies.[5] However, it must be recognized that in non-randomized studies it is likely that subtle, unmeasured differences between those who do and do not exercise contribute to the observed difference in cardiac death rate. A recent New England Journal of Medicine editorial suggests that this may reduce our estimate of the protective effect of exercise, but is unlikely to eliminate it.[15]

IS THERE A PHYSIOLOGICALLY PLAUSIBLE
EXPLANATION FOR A PROTECTIVE EFFECT?

Blood pressure

In a number of cohort studies, such as the *US Railroad Study*,[13] the beneficial effect of exercise was mediated largely through a reduction in blood pressure. This effect was also demonstrated directly in a group of 33 sedentary men aged 35–50 undertaking a 30 week training programme for their first marathon, whose diastolic blood pressure fell by 10 per cent, probably due to a combination of weight loss and accommodation to measurement.[16]

HDL cholesterol

Exercise has a beneficial effect on HDL cholesterol which is not related to weight loss and may be mediated by an increase in lipoprotein lipase in skeletal muscle tissue. In most studies the extent of increase in HDL cholesterol and fall in LDL cholesterol is small.[17]

Clotting factors

In a recent study from Sweden, fibrinogen concentrations were reported as 3.34, 3.16, and 3.02 g/l in low, medium and high activity groups respectively.[18] (This positive association was not seen in smokers.) Similarly, long term vigorous exercise, but probably not lesser degrees of activity, has been shown to reduce platelet aggregation.[19] Paradoxically, increased platelet aggregation may occur after short-term exercise programmes of high intensity, associated with high levels of catecholamines. However, these bursts of catecholamines, and consequent platelet activation, appear to be less pronounced after exercise training.

Arrythmias

The final common pathway in sudden cardiac deaths is lethal arrythmia, frequently precipitated by myocardial ischaemia. Although exercise increases the immediate risk of ischaemia, training reduces myocardial oxygen demand at a given level of exercise, hence lowering the risk of an individual experiencing the degree of ischaemia necessary to cause fatal arrythmias.[20]

IS ONLY VIGOROUS EXERCISE BENEFICIAL?

The idea that there may be a threshold of activity below which little benefit is to be gained arose from the UK literature. In the first *UK Civil Service Study*, the preventive effect was restricted to those undertaking vigorous exercise. This study was concerned with leisure time activity in male civil servants aged 40–64 (Table 5.2). Total leisure time activity levels did not predict CHD incidence rates, but if the analysis was made in terms of vigorous activity rather than total activity, a strong protective effect was apparent. Vigorous exercise was defined as entailing peaks of energy expenditure of 7.5 kilo calories plus a minute (a standard definition of heavy industrial work) and men who reported vigorous exercise experienced a CHD rate of approximately one third the rate in those not taking vigorous exercise.[2]

Table 5.2   Physical activity and incidence of fatal first episode of CHD in male executive grade Civil Servants, 1968–77. (Adapted from Morris JN, Everitt MG, Semmence AM. Coronary heart disease and exercise. Health Trends 1987; **19**: 13–16.)

Reported activity	Number	Age standardized CHD rates (%)
Vigorous exercise	646	0.9
No vigorous exercise		
– High activity*	641	2.2
– Medium activity	518	3.1
– Low activity	433	2.7

* Total leisure time activity levels (tertiles)

The second report from the UK Civil Service Study clarified the 'threshold'. The nine per cent of men who reported that they often participated in vigorous sports or cycling or that the pace of their regular walking was fast (over four miles per hour) experienced less than half the non-fatal and fatal CHD of the other men. Older men aged 55–64 men who reported the next lower degree of vigorous aerobic exercise (taking part in sport once a week, walking 'briskly', or cycling occasionally), experienced a rate two thirds that of men participating in sport once a month or claiming to walk 'fairly briskly', whose overall rate was similar to those taking no vigorous exercise at all. In the younger men aged 45–54, the event rates were similar irrespective of the amount of non-vigorous exercise taken. A history of vigorous sports in the past were not protective.[6]

Most recently, the *British Regional Heart Study* has reported the effect of exercise on cardiovascular morbidity in its cohort of nearly 8000 men recruited from 24 UK general practices. Overall, an inverse relationship between physical activity and heart attacks was seen, which does not suggest a threshold effect (Fig. 5.3). Interestingly, benefit was not so apparent in men with existing ischaemic heart disease, and no protective effect was shown for regular walking.[21]

North American data are generally unsupportive of the existence of a vigorous exercise threshold.[4,13,22] For example, the Harvard alumni[4] showed CHD incidence rates, after indirect standardisation for cigarette habit and diagnosed hypertension, of 16.4, 21.2 and 25.7/1000 for vigorous, moderate, and inactive groups. In line with the Civil Service studies, alumni who were active but subsequently adopted a sedentary life-style experienced disease rates consistent with that life-style.

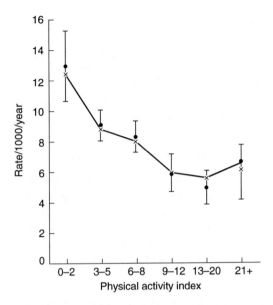

Fig. 5.3 Heart attack rates according to the physical activity index of middle aged men in the British Regional Heart Study. Crude rates (*circles*) with 95 per cent confidence intervals and age adjusted rates (X). (From Shaper A, Wannamethe G. Physical activity and IHD in middle aged British men. Br Heart J 1991; **66**: 384–94.)

Fitness studies

No threshold is seen in the cohort studies which measured 'fitness'. *The Dallas Study*[11] involved eight year follow-up of 10 200 men and 3100 women and the age-adjusted cardiovascular disease death rates per ten thousand person years in the first, second plus third, and fourth plus fifth quintiles of fitness score were 3.1, 7.8 and 24.6 in men and 0.8, 2.9, and 7.4 in women. This significant trend remained after statistical adjustment for age, smoking habit, cholesterol level, systolic blood pressure, fasting blood glucose level, history of CHD, and follow-up intervals. A similar relationship was also seen for total mortality. The *Lipid Research Clinic Study*[12] followed 4276 men aged 30–69 years for an average of 8.5 years. A three-fold increase in relative risk of cardiovascular disease was associated with each increment of 35 beats per minute in the heart rate during stage two of the exercise test. Once again, the benefit of physical fitness appeared to be independent of conventional coronary risk factors.

Minimum exercise to achieve fitness

Wenger has analysed the success of exercise programmes in achieving different degrees of fitness.[23] His review characterises exercise training programmes according to four dimensions: intensity, frequency, duration, and length. The intensity of exercise can be assessed without a treadmill machine in terms of heart rate as described below. His data suggest a steadily increasing benefit over the following ranges: frequency 2–4 times per week, duration 15–45 minutes, and programme length 5–11 weeks. He was not able to address the existence of a lower threshold, nor duration greater than 45 minutes as few studies had reported in these ranges. However, it appears that low intensity exercise of longer duration is equivalent to more intense exercise of short duration; low intensity activity was helpful particularly for those with low baseline fitness.

Why an exercise threshold in the Civil Service studies?

One explanation for the threshold seen in the UK Civil Service studies is that the participants were healthy workers with a relatively high baseline fitness. The study by Wenger, reported in the last paragraph showed that to achieve a training effect from aerobic exercise the individual must exercise at a threshold intensity of at least 50 per cent of maximum capacity: less than vigorous exercise may not have achieved this in the Civil Servants, and so may not have achieved a training effect.

WHAT IS THE RISK OF SUDDEN DEATH FROM EXERCISE?

There is no doubt that exercise is associated with sudden cardiac death. In 1986 the British Heart Journal reported the circumstances surrounding 60 sudden deaths associated with squash playing—the certified cause of death was coronary artery disease in 51 cases.[24] An American review of sudden cardiac deaths among athletes showed that at least 80 per cent in the over 35 age group were due to coronary artery disease.[25] The important practical questions relate to the magnitude of this risk of sudden death from CHD as a result of exercise in relation to the benefit gained, and the extent to which the risk can be avoided.

Gibbons, *et al*[26] studied nearly 3000 volunteer exercisers for 375 000 person hours of exercise. These were healthy volunteers who were habitual runners. Only two cardiac events were seen, with no deaths. In cardiac rehabilitation, sudden cardiac death rates have been estimated as 0.13 to 0.61 per 100 000 person-hours of exercise.[27]

A case control approach has the benefit of allowing a comparison of risk and benefit, and such a study of married men aged 25–75 years was carried out in Seattle, Washington and reported in 1984.[28] This study found that men were fifty times more likely to die during vigorous exercise if they were habitually sedentary (95 per cent confidence interval 23–151) but only five times more likely to die during vigorous exercise if habitually active (95 per cent confidence interval 2–14). As it is possible to increase cardiac fitness and probably achieve a two-fold reduction in overall risk by exercising for about three hours per week, on this estimate the benefits of this degree of vigorous exercise outweigh the risks by about twenty-fold. However, it is also clear from these data that the risks of occasional vigorous exercise may be greater than the benefit and great care must be taken at the initiation of an exercise programme.

WHO SHOULD EXERCISE, AND SHOULD PEOPLE BE SCREENED BEFORE BEGINNING EXERCISE PROGRAMMES?

Screening

The fact that vigorous exercise is not risk free has led to suggestions in the US that patients should be screened before being accepted into an exercise programme. However, if we believe that exercise is protective, then the benefit outweighs the risk even for those with coronary artery disease. The only clear benefit of identifying pre-existing coronary artery disease is to stress the need for gradual initiation of exercise programmes. Although structural cardiac abnormalities probably account for at least 80 per cent of sudden cardiac deaths in athletes aged under 35 years (mainly hypertrophic cardiomyopathies) and 15 per cent in older athletes (mainly valvular disease),[25] sudden cardiac death is extremely rare in the young and it seems unlikely that the benefits of screening for valvular disease in asymptomatic older patients will outweigh the costs.

As we have already discussed, there is a considerable body of evidence that rehabilitation programmes after myocardial infarction reduce overall risk of cardiac death.[9,29] Although it has already been noted that it is impossible to reach a definitive conclusion about the role of physical exercise alone from these trials, advice to exercise is an important part of an effective rehabilitation package aimed at reducing overall risk. It is therefore reasonable to surmise, on both theoretical and empirical grounds, that the benefits of exercise in patients with proven coronary artery disease outweighs the risk as long as a graduated programme of slowly increasing exercise is taken.

There is no indication of an age threshold in benefit from physical activity. As the relative protection of exercise appears to be comparatively constant, and the risk of cardiovascular disease increases markedly with age, the absolute benefit should be greater for older people. The UK Civil Service Study suggests that benefit can be obtained from less vigorous exercise in older people,[6] and this result is also consistent with data from the US.[30] However, the proportion of individuals over the age of 50 with pre-existent cardiovascular disease is high and the risk of sudden death at the commencement of regular exercise must also be high. The issue of 'safe' training and gradual increase in exercise is very important in this group.

IS IT FEASIBLE TO GIVE EFFECTIVE ADVICE IN PRIMARY CARE?

Lack of trials

There seems to be only one reported UK trial of exercise promotion through primary care.[31] This was a doctor-led community campaign, rather than a trial of individual advice, and it concerned two villages in a rural area of Hampshire. The doctor in question literally led from the front by running daily through the intervention village and participating in a number of marathon events. Although the increase in exercise in the intervention village was significantly greater than in the control village, the absolute difference was rather small—the increase in the proportion of respondents taking vigorous exercise more than three times each week in the intervention village was four per cent. There is also one primary care based study from the US which reports a small positive effect on exercise activity as a result of doctor given advice.[32] Of the various descriptive reports, the most interesting is a letter recently published in the British Medical Journal reporting a system of direct referral from 20 GPs to a leisure centre for fitness training—it was claimed that more than 90 per cent of those referred attended, about 80 per cent completed the course, and about 50 per cent continued to attend after the formal programme was completed.[33]

Indirect evidence of the effectiveness of advice and the extent of patient compliance can be gleaned from other settings, such as cardiac rehabilitation units, workplace and community programmes, and from exercise clinics. Most reports are from the US and suggest high dropout rates of at least 50 per cent, although in the US Task Force report, Harris points out that the non-compliance problem is similar to that seen for programmes related to smoking, substance abuse, and diet.[34] Not surprisingly, programmes showing the best compliance and greatest effect have concentrated on spontaneous, health conscious volunteers, but the potential problem of 'inverse care' is obvious.

Practical guidance

The evidence presented to the US and Canadian Task Forces on Prevention,[34] and the results of the recently reported *UK Civil Service Study*,[6] suggest that advice to undertake regular brisk walking is likely to be both effective and acceptable to sedentary patients. This should probably be the focus of advice given in general practice. However, it is important to tailor advice to the patient's needs and expectations, to make the advice practical, and to provide follow-up support. Exercise targets, and brief questionnaires to assess patients' activity, are provided in Chapter 19.5.

It is also important that the patient recognizes that the objective of taking exercise is to improve fitness, and that this can be measured and monitored as an 'outcome'. As with diet, there is distressingly little evidence about how to achieve this 'minimum effective intervention' in primary care, but certain important elements can be identified:

1. Patients take very different amounts of activity and will have very different ideas about terms like 'brisk'. It is probably not necessary to try to asses fitness formally but it is necessary to characterise and to counsel about exercise in terms of intensity, frequency, and duration and to take account of the patients age and baseline fitness.
2. Although frequency (per week) and duration (in minutes) are easy to describe, intensity is difficult. The best subjective target for intensity is breathlessness.

The only feasible objective measure for setting a target in general practice is pulse rate. GPs can use the following simple formulae to recommend a target pulse rate (taking account of the patients age) in order to achieve a target level of intensity of exercise.

Common methods of calculating a target heart rate to improve aerobic fitness are

Karvonen method:
1. Calculate predicted 'maximum' heart rate (MHR) = 220 − age.
2. Take resting heart rate (RHR)
3. Calculate difference between resting and maximal heart rates (DHR) = MHR − RHR
4. Recommend target heart rate = RHR + 0.6DHR

70% method:
1. Calculate predicted 'maximum' heart rate (MHR) = 220 − age.
2. Recommended target heart rate = 0.7 MHR.

These formulae are based on physiological considerations of the minimum intensity of exercise necessary to achieve improvement in cardio-respiratory fitness. There is no clear evidence about the opimal pace at which sedentary patients should be advised to achieve these target rates—for the reasons outlined above a gradual attainment of these targets, subject to previous activity and health, is necessary. Patients should be advised that exceeding the target heart rate is unnecessary and, certainly at the onset of an exercise programme, should be avoided.

3. Formal testing of fitness is unlikely to be part of routine care in many general practices. It is however valuable in judging how rapidly to increase the intensity of an exercise programme, and in monitoring improvement. Methods are described in Chapter 19.5. Patients can also be instructed on monitoring fitness by the time taken for the pulse to return to the resting rate.

Resources, cost and opportunity cost

The prevalence of physical inactivity in the United Kingdom is high. The *Allied Dunbar National Fitness Survey* compared activity with national target levels of at least three 20 minute periods of exercise a week which have to be 'vigorous' for the under 35s, 'moderately vigorous' for those aged 35–54, and 'moderate' for those aged over 55 years. The survey showed that 81 per cent of middle aged men did not reach the target, and that walking up a slight incline would be too much for nearly a third of men and two thirds of women.[35] In the *Heartbeat Wales* survey, only 22 per cent of men and 3 per cent of women considered themselves very active and 34 per cent and 73 per cent respectively considered themselves minimally active or sedentary.[36]

In primary care, there is an urgent need to establish the necessary intensity of counselling to effect change—is advice enough or is intensive support and referral necessary? In secondary prevention, existing cardiac rehabilitation programmes have been proven to be effective—but again, there is a lack of evidence about their practical implementation. It is unlikely that primary care teams will assign high priority to exercise promotion until there is better guidance on the effective interventions and a better estimate of resulting workload.

SUMMARY

- There is good circumstantial evidence that people who exercise adequately have a reduced risk of CHD.
- The minimum exercise which affords some protection is the minimum exercise which will improve individual fitness, and the intensity of exercise should be at least 50 per cent of maximum capacity.
- The minimum exercise required to improve fitness in the averagely fit middle aged person is brisk walking (four miles per hour) for at least 20 minutes twice a week. People who are less fit or elderly may benefit most from sustained low intensity exercise (for example walking at ordinary pace).
- There is a trade-off between intensity, duration, and frequency of exercise in achieving and maintaining fitness, and primary care workers must understand how to assess and to advise about intensity of exercise.
- There is a marked (x50) increased risk of sudden cardiac death associated with too vigorous commencement of an exercise programme in sedentary individuals with pre-existing cardiovascular disease (both detected and undetected) so a graduated programme of slowly increasing exercise is essential.
- Except for people with acute, current illness or structural heart defects, the benefit of an exercise regime outweighs the risks. The value of pre-exercise screening is not proven.
- There is little evidence, as yet, that advice to exercise from primary care workers is effective. An effective programme may well involve considerable expenditure of time in explanation, guidance, follow-up and support.
- When the opportunity cost of exercise promotion in primary care is considered, the benefits of exercise to general health and well-being, as well as to CHD prevention, must be taken into account.

REFERENCES

1. Morris JN, Heady JA, Raffle PAB. Coronary heart disease and physical activity of work. Lancet 1953, ii; 1057–1054: 1111–20.
2. Morris J N, Chave S P W, Adam C, Sirey C, Epstein L, Sheehan D. VigorousExercise in Leisure Time and the Incidence of Coronary Heart Disease. Lancet 1973; i: 333–9.
3. Dawber T R, The Framingham Study: the epidemiology of atherosclerotic disease. Cambridge, Mass: Harvard University Press, 1980; pp. 157–67.
4. Paffenbarger R S, Hyde R T, Wing A L, Hsieh C C. Physical activity, all cause mortality and longevity of college alumni. N Eng J Med 1986; **314**: 605–13.

5. Berlin JA, Colditz GA. A meta-analysis of physical activity in the prevention of coronary heart disease. Am J Epidemiol 1990; **132**: 612–28

6. Morris J N, Clayton D G, Everitt M G, Semens A N, Burgess E H. Exercise in leisure time: coronary attack and death rates. British Heart Journal 1990; **63**: 325–34.

7. Paffenbarger RS, Hyde PH, Wing AL, Lee IN, Jungh DL, Klampet JB, *et al*. The association of changes in physical activity level and other lifestyle characteristics with mortality in men. N Engl J Med 1993; 328 (8): 538–45.

8. Royal College of Physicians Working Party Report. Medical aspects of exercise: benefits and risks. London: RCP, May 1991.

9. Oldridge NB, Guyatt GH, Fischer ME, Rimm AA. Cardiac rehabilitation after myocardial infarction. JAMA 1988; 260 (7): 945–50.

10. Paffenbarger R S, Hyde R T, Wing A L, Steinmetz C H. A natural history of athleticism and cardiovascular health. JAMA 1984; **252**: 491–95.

11. Blair S N, Kohl H W, Paffenbarger R S, Clarke D G, Cooper K H, Gibbons L W. Physical fitness and all-cause mortality: a prospective study of healthy men and women. JAMA 1989; **262**: 2395–401.

12. Ekelund L G, Haskell W L, Johnson J L, Whaley F S, Criqui M H, Sheps D S, Physical fitness as a fredictor of cardiovascular mortality in asymptomatic north American men: the Lipid Research Clinic's mortality follow-up study. N Engl J Med 1988; **319**: 1379–84.

13. Slattery M L, Jacobs D R. Physical fitness and cardiovascular disease mortality: the US railroad study. Am J of Epidemiol 1988; **127**: 571–80.

14. Sobolski J, Kornitzer M, De-Backer G, Dramaix M, Abramowicz M, Degre S, Denolin H. Protection against ischaemic heart disease in the Belgian physical fitness study: physical fitness rather than physical activity? Am J Epidemiol 1987; **125**: 601–10.

15. Curfman GD. The health benefits of exercise. N Engl J Med 1993; 328(8): 574–6.

16. Findlay F I, Taylor R, Dargieh, Grant S, Pettigrew A, Wolfson J, *et al*. Cardiovascular effects of training for a marathon run in unfit middle-aged men. BMJ 1987; **295**: 521–4.

17. Correspondence. Brisk walking and high density lipoprotein cholesterol. BMJ 1990; **300**: 195–6.

18. Rosengren A, Wilhelmsen L, Welin L Tsipogiannia, Teger-Nilsson A C, Wedel H. The relationship between social factors and fibrinogen concentration in a general population sample of middle-aged men. BMJ 1990; **300**: 634–8.

19. Correspondence. Reduced platelet aggregation in long-distance runners. Lancet 1989; **1**: 1398–9.

20. Kohl HW, Powell KE, Gordon NF, Blair SN, Paffenburger RS. Physical activity, physical fitness and sudden cardiac death. Epidemiologic Reviews 1992; **14**: 37–58.

21. Shaper AG, Wannamethee G. Physical activity and ischaemic heart disease in middle aged British men. Br Heart J 1991; **66**: 384–94.

22. Leon AS, Conneet J, Jacobs DR, Rauramaa R. Leisure time physical activity levels and risk ofcoronary heart disease and death: the Multiple Risk Factor International Trial (MRFIT). JAMA 1987; **258**: 2388–95.

23. Wenger HA, Bell GJ. The interaction of intensity, frequency, and duration of exercise training in altering cardiovascular fitness. Sports Medicine 1986; **3**: 346–56.

24. Northcote R J, Flanagan C, Ballantyne D. Sudden death and vigorous exercise: a study of 60 deaths associated with squash. Br Heart J 1986; **55**: 198–03.

25. Maron BJ, Epstein SE, Roberts WC. Causes of sudden death in competitive athletes. Am Coll Cardiol 1986; **7**: 204–14

26. Gibbons L W, Cooper K H, Mayer B M, Ellison R L. The acute cardiac risk of strenuous exercise. JAMA 1980; **244**: 1799–801.

27. Thompson PD. Benefits and risks of exercise training in patients with coronary artery disease. JAMA 1988; **259**: 1537–40.

28. Siscovick D S, Yseissns, Fetcher R H, Laski T. The incidence of primary cardiac arrest during vigorous exercise. N Eng J Med 1984; **311**: 874–7.

29. O'Connor G T, Buring J E, Yusuf S, Goldharber S, Olmstead E, Paffenbarger R S, Hennekens C H. An overview of randomised trials and rehabilitation with exercise after myocardial infarction. Circulation 1989; **80**: 234–44.

30. Devries HA. Exercise intensity threshold for improvement of cardiovascular-respiratory function in older men. Geriatrics 1971; **26**: 94–101.

31. Campbell MJ, Browne D, Waters WE. Can general practitioners influence exercise habits? A controlled trial. BMJ 1985; **290**: 1043–6.

32. Mulder JA. Prescription home exercise therapy for cardiovascular fitness. J Family Practice 1981; **13**: 345–8.

33. Osbourne M. Exercising for health (letter). BMJ 1992; **305**: 891.

34. Harris S, Caspersen C, De Friese G, Estes E. Physical activity for healthy adults. In Goldbloom R, Lawrence R Preventing Disease: beyond the rhetoric. New York: Springer-Verlag, 1990.

35. Gloag G. The lazy English. BMJ 1992; **304**: 1591.

36. Welsh Heart Programme Report No7 Pulse of Wales: social survey supplement, 24 Park Place, Cardiff: Heartbeat Wales, 1987

6 Alcohol

Peter Anderson

INTRODUCTION

There is evidence for a dose–response relationship between alcohol consumption and risk of liver cirrhosis, cancers of the oropharynx, larynx, oesophagus, rectum (beer only), liver, and female breast, and violent death, but the relationship between alcohol consumption and cardiovascular disease is more complex.[1-4] It is now recognized that alcohol may reduce the risk of coronary heart disease (CHD), despite its adverse effect on blood pressure and the association with an increased risk of stroke.

This review considers six questions:

1. **What is the relationship between alcohol consumption and CHD?**
2. **What is the relationship between alcohol consumption and stroke?**
3. **What is the relationship between alcohol consumption and total mortality?**
4. **What is the explanation of the reduced risk for CHD?**
5. **What are the individual and public health implications of the reduced risk for CHD?**
6. **What is the evidence for the effectiveness of brief interventions for hazardous alcohol consumption in primary health care?**

WHAT IS THE RELATIONSHIP BETWEEN ALCOHOL CONSUMPTION AND CHD?

Reviews of the relationship between alcohol consumption and CHD have concluded that alcohol consumption in the range of less than one drink a day to up to five drinks a day reduces the risk of CHD by about 40–60 per cent,[3,5-8] (Fig. 6.1). Of seventeen studies in men published between 1978 and 1994, eleven showed a significant negative association[9-19] and six no significant relationship[20-25] between alcohol consumption and risk of CHD. Of four reports in women, three demonstrated a significant negative association[11,13,26] and one no relationship between alcohol consumption and risk of CHD.[24] The negative relationship between alcohol consumption and risk of CHD is present across all age ranges for both men and women, although it appears stronger for older people. The reduction in risk appears to be achieved at consumption levels of less than 10 g a day and is not strongly dose-related. Some studies have shown an increased risk of CHD at consumption levels of over six drinks a day. Although the relationship is present amongst populations from many different countries, most studies have been undertaken in populations in economically developed countries and the effect in lesser developed countries is not known.

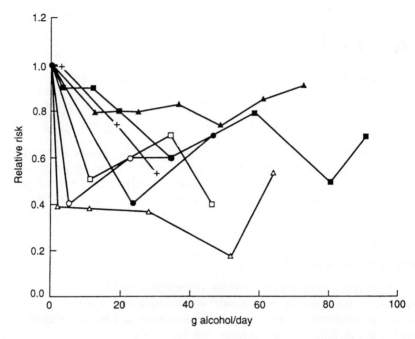

Fig. 6.1 Coronary heart disease mortality among men: alcohol consumption and relative risk. Results from seven studies; Hennekens CH, *et al*. Am J Epidemiol 1978; **107**: 196–200 (*closed circle*); Rimm EB, *et al*. Lancet 1991; **338**: 464–8 (*cross*); Gordon T, Kannel WB. Am Heart J 1983; **105**: 667–73 (*closed square*); Gordon T, Doyle J. Am J Epidemiol 1987; **125**: 263–70 (*open square*); Boffeta P, Garfinkel L. Epidemiology 1990: **1**: 342–8 (*closed triangle*); Scragg R, *et al*. Am J Epidemiol 1987; **126**: 77–85 (*open circle*); Jackson R, *et al*. BMJ 1991; **303**: 211–6 (*open triangle*).

The negative relationship between alcohol consumption and risk of CHD is greater when alcohol consumption is spread throughout the week on a regular basis than when consumption is concentrated and consumed on one occasion during the week. It is not clear if the relationship is both long-term and short-term or only of a short-term nature. Nor is it clear if the relationship is equally strong for all beverage types, although there is some evidence that wine is more beneficial than beer or spirits.[27]

In summary, there is evidence that light to moderate consumption of alcohol consumption can lead to a reduced risk for CHD in both men and women. The effect does not appear to be strongly dose-related and it appears that much of the reduced risk can be achieved by low doses of alcohol consumption.

WHAT IS THE RELATIONSHIP BETWEEN ALCOHOL CONSUMPTION AND STROKE?

Reviews of the relationship between alcohol consumption and stroke have concluded that alcohol consumption increases the risk of stroke, particularly haemorrhagic stroke.[1,4,28] It has been suggested that low doses of alcohol may reduce the risk of non-haemorrgahic stroke although not all reviews agree on this.[4]

Of seven studies in men, published between 1986 and 1992, four demonstrated a dose-response relationship,[9,20,29,30] one a J-shaped curve[31] and two no relationship[32,33] between alcohol consumption and risk of stroke, (Fig. 6.2). Of three studies in women, one showed a positive relationship between heavy drinking and stroke mortality,[30] another showed a J-shaped relationship[26] and the third no relationship between alcohol consumption and risk of stroke.[31] Of two studies of men and women, one found a non-significant dose-response relationship[34] and the other a significant reduced risk between alcohol consumption and risk of stroke.[35]

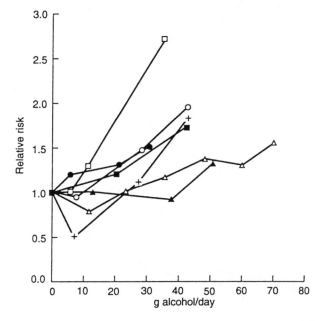

Fig. 6.2 Mortality from stroke among men: alcohol consumption and relative risk. Results from seven studies; Donahue RP, *et al.* JAMA 1986; **255**: 2311–14 (*closed circle*); Gill JS, *et al.* N Engl J Med 1986; **315**: 1041–6 (*cross*); Kone S, *et al.* Int J Epidemiol 1986; **15**: 527–32 (*closed square*); Semenciw RM, *et al.* Int J Epidemiol 1988; **17**: 317–24 (*open square*); Shaper AG, *et al.* BMJ 1991; **302**: 1111–15 (*closed triangle*); Ben-Shlomo Y, *et al.* Stroke 1992; **23**; 1093–8 (*open circle*); Boffeta P, Garfinkel L. Epidemiology 1990; **1**: 342-8 (*open triangle*). The Kono *et al* report subsumed incidence of stroke as well as mortality.

Because there is a dose-response relationship between alcohol consumption and blood pressure, controlling for blood pressure removes some of the alcohol effect for risk of stroke.[32,36] Three of the above studies subdivided stroke into non-haemorrahigic and haemorrhagic.[20,26,29] All three studies found a significant dose response relationship between alcohol consumption and risk of haemorrhagic stroke. For non-haemorrhagic stroke, a dose relationship was found in one study,[20] no association in another[29] and an inverse U-shaped relationship in the third.[26]

In summary, there is evidence for a dose-response relationship between level of alcohol consumption and all strokes in men. There is some evidence of a positive relationship for women, which may be J-shaped. The evidence suggests that drinking alcohol increases the chance of haemorrhagic, more than other types of stroke.

WHAT IS THE RELATIONSHIP BETWEEN ALCOHOL CONSUMPTION AND TOTAL MORTALITY?

Reviews of the relationship between alcohol consumption and total mortality have concluded that for most industrialized countries, the overall relationship between alcohol consumption and all cause mortality is J-shaped for both sexes,[1,3,4,37] (Fig. 6.3).

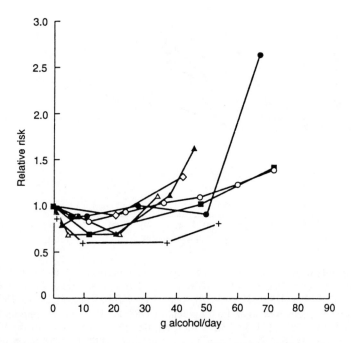

Fig. 6.3 All-cause mortality among men. Alcohol consumption (g/day) and relative risk. Eight prospective studies; Dyer AR, *et al.* Preventive Medicine 1980; **9**: 78–90 (*closed circle*); Shaper AG, *et al* Lancet 1988; **ii**: 1267–73 (*cross*); Kagan A, *et al.* Circulation 1981; **64**: 27–31 (*closed triangle*); Klatsky AL, *et al.* Circulation 1981; **64**: 32–41 (*closed square*); Kono S, *et al.* Int J Epidemiol 1986; **15**: 527–32 (*open diamond*); Marmot M, *et al* 1982 (*open triangle*); Boffeta P, Garfinkle L Epidemiology 1990; **1**: 342–8 (*open circle*).

Of sixteen studies published between 1978 and 1995, 13 showed a significant positive association[9,16,17,19,21,25,36–42] and three no significant relationship between alcohol consumption and all cause mortality.[11,12,23]

When taking different age groups into consideration, the relationship between alcohol consumption and all cause mortality is linear in the younger age groups, with a steeper gradient for women than men, and J-shaped in the older age groups. The reason for the age specific pattern is due to the different causes of death for the different age groups. In younger age groups, accidents and poisoning are a more common cause of death, whilst in older age groups, cardiovascular diseases become the major causes of death. In industrialized countries, the age when the relationship between alcohol and mortality changes from linear to J-shaped is about 50 years. The lowest part of the J corresponds to a consumption of 5–15 g of alcohol a day and the cross-over is at about 30–40 g (three to four units) a day.

In summary, in industrialized countries, for men and women under the age of 50, there is a linear relationship between alcohol consumption and total mortality. For men and women aged 50 and over, the relationship is J-shaped, due to a reduced risk of CHD at lower levels of alcohol consumption.

WHAT IS THE EXPLANATION OF THE REDUCED RISK FOR CHD?

At least four arguments have been made to suggest that the lower risk of CHD amongst moderate drinkers might be an artefact.[5]

First, it has been suggested that non-drinkers include people who have given up drinking because they were unwell. Such people would be expected to have an increased rate of disease. Although both former drinkers and never-drinkers, have been shown to have a higher incidence of CHD than light to moderate drinkers,[13,20,21,22,43] former drinkers have a greater risk of death from CHD than lifetime non-drinkers.[21,21,44]

Second, it has been suggested that abstainers have a greater burden of ill health than moderate drinkers, regardless of their previous drinking status.[36,45] However, the reduced risk of CHD from light to moderate alcohol remains when those with cardiovascular illness or risk factors at enrollment are removed from the analysis,[9,46] although not all studies have demonstrated this.[18] Furthermore, the reduction in risk persists throughout the total length of follow-up periods.[9,47]

Third, it has been suggested that non-drinkers are an unusual group in a society in which alcohol intake is the norm.[48–49] Both former drinkers and lifetime abstainers have charateristics which might account for the excess mortality over light to moderate drinkers.[50]

Fourth, although many studies have controlled for the effect of cigarette smoking, it is clear that smoking is very much involved in the relationship between alcohol and total mortality.[48] The J-shaped function is most pronounced for current cigarette smokers and the greatest mortality is found amongst non-drinkers who smoke.[39,40,47,48,51,52]

So, if the protective effect is real, what is the biological mechanism? The protective effect may be mediated through atherosclerotic processes, including an increase in blood high density lipoprotein levels[53-55] as well as antithrombotic effects, including a reduction in plasma fibrinogen levels and decreased platelet aggregation.[56-58] It may be that the antithrombotic effects are more important,[59] and could be an explanation as to why the protective effect can be achieved with small doses of alcohol and for the presence of the protective effect amongst older people.

In conclusion, although the role of social and psychological factors have not yet been sufficiently explored, there is a consistent epidemiological finding that alcohol, in light to moderate doses, reduces the risk of CHD. Because the incidence of CHD is low in early adulthood this is not an important effect for men and women under the age of 50.

WHAT ARE THE INDIVIDUAL AND PUBLIC HEALTH IMPLICATIONS OF THE REDUCED RISK FOR CHD?

What are the implications for individuals?

The following advice for individuals should probably hold:[60]

1. Except for CHD, across all ranges of alcohol consumption, the less the consumption of alcohol, the better with respect to health.
2. Taking CHD into account (and for industrialized countries) age must be considered. For men and women up to the age of 50 years, across all ranges of alcohol consumption, the less the consumption of alcohol, the better with respect to health. For older men and women, there appears to be an optimum level of alcohol consumption, with regard to reducing total mortality, at one or two drinks a day; most of the health benefit is achieved by drinking as little as one drink every other day.
3. In view of the implications for the population (see below), individual advice to abstainers with high risk of CHD should be concentrated on alternative ways of reducing CHD risk, other than consuming alcohol.

What are the implications for populations?

There are two important characteristics in relation to the distribution of alcohol consumption in populations. First, in most populations, the distribution of alcohol consumption is strongly skewed with a long tail towards high consumption levels.[61] Second, there is a strong relationship between the average consumption level in the population and the percentage of heavy drinkers. Studies have demonstrated that the proportion of heavy drinkers in the population increases as the overall population consumption of alcohol increase.[61] Collective movements of populations up and down the consumption scale suggests that normal drinking represents the cultural foundation of heavy drinking, and that the consumption level, and thus the risk of drinking problems, for an individual drinker is directly related to the amount of alcohol to which he or she is exposed in the cultural environment.

The alcohol-related mortality rate in the population depends on how many people are at risk, the numerical size of the risk, and on the shape of the risk relation.[61] A J-shaped function, as might relate to total mortality, implies that there might be an average consumption level in the population, where the risk for mortality is at a minimum level. If those who consume less than this average level increase their intake and those who consume more than the average level decrease their intake, total mortality in the population should decrease. However, this is an unlikely outcome, since those who are drinking at a level which is a risk to their health are unlikely to reduce their consumption in the knowledge that light to moderate drinking will reduce their chance of death. On the contrary, if lighter drinkers, who form a substantial proportion of the population started to drink more frequently, then even those who already drank above the level might be induced to drink more, since they would find themselves in a heavier drinking culture with more pressure to drink.

In setting public health policies in the presence of a J-shaped risk function, it is necessary to make a distinction between the level of intake for an individual that minimizes risk and the average level for the population that minimizes risk. Because of the skewed distribution of alcohol consumption, and the fact that individuals tend to change their drinking by roughly the same percentage when population changes occur, the average level of consumption with minimal risk for a population will be considerably lower (perhaps more than twice as low) than the level of consumption with minimal risk for an individual.[61] For most populations in industrialized countries, it remains appropriate to advocate for overall decreases in alcohol consumption, since this will result in better health

WHAT IS THE EVIDENCE FOR EFFECTIVENESS OF BRIEF INTERVENTIONS FOR HAZARDOUS ALCOHOL CONSUMPTION IN PRIMARY HEALTH CARE?

Reviews of the effectiveness of brief interventions in general practice settings have concluded that brief advice is effective in reducing alcohol consumption by over 20 per cent in the large group of people with raised alcohol consumption.[62,63]

In the *MRC Study* on life-styles and health in the United Kingdom, 907 male and female heavy drinkers (defined as men consuming over 350 g per week and women 210 g per week) were recruited, on the basis of a health screening questionnaire, and were allocated randomly to a control group which received an assessment interview or a treatment group which received 15 minutes of advice from their general practitioner to reduce alcohol consumption.[64] Men in the control group reduced their alcohol consumption from an average of 640 g per week to 560 g per week at one year follow-up. Men in the treatment group reduced their consumption from 620 g per week to 440 g per week. This was a highly significant difference (p < 0.001) which was corroborated by significant differences in GGT (gamma-glutamyl transferase) level (p < 0.01). For the women a treatment effect was also observed, although the magnitude was less and there was no significant difference in GGT levels at follow-up between the treatment and control groups. The *MRC study* also demonstrated that the proportion of excessive drinkers was decreased in relation to the number of general practitioner advice sessions attended. For those men who only received one advice session, at one year follow up 79 per cent remained excessive drinkers whereas for those men who received five advice sessions 41 per cent remained as excessive drinkers. Similar figures for the women were 67 per cent and 31 per cent.

In the *Oxford Study* in England, 154 men and 72 women were recruited using a screening questionnaire.[65,66] Heavy drinkers (defined as men consuming over 350 g per week and women consuming over 210 g per week) were randomly allocated to a control group which received an assessment interview and a treatment group which received 10 minutes of advice from their general practitioner to cut down on their drinking. At one year follow-up, men in the control group reduced their consumption from 530 g per week to 440 g per week and men in the treatment group from 520 g per week to 360 g per week. The difference between the two groups was significant (p < 0.05). For the women, both the treatment and the control groups reduced their consumption by the same proportion from 360 g per week to 250 g per week.

In conclusion, studies on the effectiveness of general practitioner interventions for individuals with hazardous alcohol consumption suggest that brief advice can lead to reductions of alcohol consumption of over 20 per cent at one years follow-up. There is greater evidence for an intervention effect for men than women and inconclusive evidence for a superior effect of more intensive intervention.

CONCLUSIONS

- There is evidence that alcohol consumption in the range of 5–50 g of alcohol a day reduces the risk of CHD.
- Alcohol consumption leads to an increased risk of haemorrhagic stroke, but may reduce the risk of non-haemorrhagic stroke.
- All cause mortality rises linearly with consumption in people under the age of 50, but shows a J-shaped relationship in older people, with the minimum mortality corresponding to 5–15 g (0.5–1.5 units) a day.
- Although the role of psychosocial variables has not been adequately explored, the relationship between alcohol consumption and risk of CHD remains when controlling for other relevant variables. The effect may be mediated through both atherosclerotic and antithrombotic mechanisms, with the latter possibly being more important.
- The number of heavy drinkers in any society is related to the average consumption. For this reason it is not advisable to encourage abstainers to drink alcohol in order to improve their health.

- Except for CHD, the less the consumption of alcohol the better, with respect to health.
- Ten to fifteen minutes of advice is effective in reducing heavy drinking by over 20 per cent.

REFERENCES

1. Duffy JC (ed.). Alcohol and illness. Edinburgh University Press. 1992.
2. Verschuren PM (ed.). Health issues related to alcohol consumption. Brussels: International Life Sciences Institute, Europe, 1993.
3. Anderson P. Alcohol and risk of physical harm. In Holder HD, and Edwards G. Alcohol and public policy: evidence and issues. Oxford University Press. 1995.
4. Holman D'A J, Armstrong BK. The quantification of drug caused morbidity and mortality in Australia 1992. Canberra, Government Printing House. 1995.
5. Marmot M and Brunner E. Alcohol and cardiovascular disease: the status of the U-shaped curve. BMJ, 1991; **303**: 565–8.
6. Jackson R, Beaglehole R. The relationship between alcohol and coronary heart disease: is there a protective effect? Current Opinion in Lipidology 1993; **4**: 21–6.
7. Maclure M. Demonstration of deductive meta-analysis: ethanol intake and risk of myocardial infarction. Epidemiologic reviews 1993; **15**: 328–51.
8. Renaud S, Criqui MH, Farchi G and Veenstra J. Alcohol drinking and coronary heart disease. In Health issues related to alcohol consumption, (ed. PM Verschuren), Brussels, International Life Sciences Institute, Europe, 1993, pp. 81–123.
9. Boffetta P, Garfinkel L. Alcohol drinking and mortality among men enrolled in an American Cancer Society prospective study. Epidemiology 1990; **1**: 342–8.
10. Hennekens CH, Rosner B & Cole DS. Daily alcohol consumption and fatal coronary heart disease. Am J Epidemiol 1978; **107**: 196–200.
11. Gordon T, Kannel WB. Drinking habits and cardiovascular disease: The Framingham Study. Am Heart J 1983; **105**: 667–3.
12. Gordon T, Doyle J. Drinking and mortality. Am J Epidemiol 1987; **125**: 263–70.
13. Jackson R, Scragg R, Beaglehole R. Alcohol consumption and risk of coronary heart disease. BMJ 1991; **303**: 211–16.
14. Rimm EB, Giovannucci EL, Willett WC, Colditz EA, Ascherio A, Rosner B, *et al.* Prospective study of alcohol consumption and risk of coronary disease in men. Lancet 1991; **338**: 464–8.
15. Scragg R, Stewart A, Jackson R, Beaglehole R. Alcohol and exercise in myocardial infarction and sudden coronary death in men and women. Am J Epidemiol 1987; **126**: 77–85.
16. Farchi G, Fidanza F, Mariotti S, Menotti A. Alcohol and mortality in the Italian rural cohorts of the seven countries study. Int J Epidemiol 1992; **21**: 74–82.
17. Gronbaek M, Deis A, Sorensen TIA, Beckel U, Borch-Johnsen K, Muller C. Influence of age, gender, body mass index and smoking on alcohol intake and mortality. BMJ 1994; **308**: 302–6.
18. Shaper A G, Wannamethee G, Walker M. Alcohol and coronary heart disease: a perspective from the British regional heart study. Int J Epidemiol 1994; **23**: 482–94.
19. Doll R, Peto R, Hall E, Wheatley K, Gray R. Mortality in relation to consumption of alcohol: 13 years' observations on male doctors. BMJ 1994; **309**: 911–18.

20. Kono S, Ikeda M, Tokudome S, Nishizumi M, Kuratsune M. Alcohol and mortality: a cohort study of male Japanese physicians. Int J Epidemiol 1986; **15**: 527–32.
21. Dyer AR, Stamler J, Paul O, *et al.* Alcohol consumption and 17-year mortality in the Chicago Western Electric Company study. Preventive Medicine 1980; **9**: 78–90.
22. Yano K, Rhoads GG, Kagan A. Coffee, alcohol and risk of coronary heart disease among Japanese men living in Hawaii. N Engl J Med 1977; **297**: 405–9.
23. Suhonen O, Aromaa A, Reunanen A & Knekt P. Alcohol consumption and sudden coronary death in middle-aged Finnish men. Acta Medica Scandinavica 1987; **221**: 335–41.
24. Camacho TC, Kaplan GA, Cohen RD. Alcohol consumption and mortality in Alameda County. J Chron Dis 1987; **40**: 229–36.
25. Kittner SJ, Garcia-Palmieri MR, Costas R, *et al.* Alcohol and coronary heart disease in Puerto Rico. Am J Epidemiol 1983; **117**: 50.
26. Stampfer MJ, Colditz GA, Willett WC, *et al.* A prospective study of moderate alcohol consumption and the risk of coronary disease and stroke in women. N Engl J Med 1988; **319**: 267–73.
27. Gronbaek M, Deis A, Soresen TIA, Becker U, Schnohr P, Jensen G. Mortality associated with moderate intakes of wine, beer or spirits. BMJ 1995; **310**: 1165–1168.
28. Van Gn J, Stampfer MJ, Wolfe C, Algra A. The association between alcohol and stroke. In Verschuren, PM. (ed.) Health issues related to alcohol consumption. Brussels: International Life Sciences Institute, Europe, 1993.
29. Donahue RP, Abbott RD, Reed DM & Yano K. Alcohol and haemorrhagic stroke. The Honolulu heart program. JAMA 1986; **255**: 2311–14.
30. Semenciw RM, Morrison HI, Mao Y, *et al.* Major risk factors for cardiovascular disease mortality in adults: results from the nutrition Canada cohort. Int J Epidemiol, 1988; **17**: 317–24.
31. Gill JS, Zezulka AV, Shipley MJ, Beevers DG. Stroke and alcohol consumption. N Engl J Med 1986; **315**: 1041–6.
32. Shaper AG, Phillips AN, Pocock SJ, Walker M, Macfarlane PW. Risk factors for stroke in middle aged British men. BMJ 1991; **302**: 1111–15.
33. Ben-Shlomo Y, Markowe H, Shipley M, Marmot MG. Stroke risk from alcohol consumption using different control groups. Stroke 1992; **23**: 1093–8.
34. Klatsky AL, Friedman GD. Siegelaub AB. Alcohol use and cardiovascular disease: the Kaiser-Permanente experience. Circulation 1981; 64 (suppl III): 32–41.
35. Von Arbin M, Britton M, De Faire U, Tisell A. Circulatory manifestations and risk factors in patients with acute cerebrovascular disease and in matched controls. Act Med Scand 1985; **218**: 373–80.
36. Shaper AG, Wannamethee G, Walker M. Alcohol and mortality in British men: explaining the U-shaped curve. Lancet 1988; **ii**: 1267–73.
37. Poikplainen K. Alcohol and mortality: a review. J Clin Epidemiol 1995; **48**: 455–65.
38. Kagan A, Yano K, Rhoads G, McGee DL. Alcohol and cardiovascular disease: The Hawaiian experience. Circulation 1981; 64 (suppl.III): 27–31.
39. Marmot MG, Rose G, Shipley MJ, Thomas BJ. Alcohol and mortality: a U-shaped curve. Lancet, 1991; **i**: 580–3.
40. Klatsky AL, Friedman GD, Siegelaub AB. Alcohol and mortality. A ten-year Kaiser Permanente experience. Ann Int Med 1981; **95**: 139–45.
41. Andreasson S, Allbeck P, Romelsjö A. Alcohol and mortality among young men: longitudinal study of Swedish conscripts. BMJ 1988; **296**: 1021–5.
42. Rehm J, Sempos CT. Alcohol and mortality. Br J Addict 1995; **90**: 471–80.
43. Klatsky AL, Armstrong MA, Friedman GD. Mortality in ex-drinkers. Circulation 1990; 81, 720.

44. Lazarus NB, Kaplan GA, Cohen RD, Leu D-J. Change in alcohol consumption and risk of death from all causes and from ichaemic heart disease. BMJ 1991; **303**: 553–6.
45. Wannamethee G, Shaper AG. Men who do not drink: a report from the British Regional Heart Study. Int J Epidemiol 1988; **17**: 201–10.
46. Klatsky AL, Armstrong MA, Friedman GD. Alcohol and cardiovascular deaths. Circulation 1989; **80**: 611–14.
47. Friedman LA, Kimball AW. Coronary heart disease mortality and alcohol consumption in Framingham. Am J Epidemiol 1986; **24**: 481–489.
48. Kozlowski LT, Ferrence RG. Statistical control in research on alcohol and tobacco: an example from research on alcohol and mortality. Br J Addict 1990; **85**: 271–8.
49. Knupfer G. Drinking for health: the daily light drinker fiction. Br J Addict 1987; **82**: 547–55.
50. Fillmore KM, Golding JM, Graves KL, Kniep S, Leino EV, Romelsjö A, Shoemaker C, Ager CR, Allebeck P, Ferrer HP. Alcohol use and mortality risk in multiple follow-up studies; characteristics of groups at risk. Addiction. In Press.
51. Dyer AR, Stamler J, Paul O. Alcohol consumption, cardiovascular risk factors, and mortality in two Chicago epidemiologic studies. Circulation 1977; **56**: 1067–74.
52. Razay G, Heaton KW, Bolton CH, Hoghes AO. Alcohol consumption and its relation to cardiovascular risk factors in British women. BMJ 1992; **304**: 80–3.
53. Gaziano JM, Buring JE, Breslow JL, Goldhaber SZ, Rosner B, VanCenburgh M, Willet W, Henneckens CH. Moderate alcohol intake, increased levels of high-density lipoprotein and its subfractions, and decreased risk of myocardial infraction. N Engl J Med 1993; **329**: 1829–34.
54. Criqui MH, Cowan LD, Tyroler HA, Bangdiwala S, Heiss G, Wallace RB, *et al.* Lipoproteins as mediators for the effects of alcohol consumption and cigarette smoking on cardiovascular mortality: results from the lipid research clinics follow-up study. Am J Epidemiol 1987; **126**: 629–37.
55. Criqui MH. The reduction of coronary heart disease with light to moderate alcohol consumption: effect or artefact. Br J Addict 1990; **85**: 837–47.
56. Meade TW, Chakrabarti R, Haines AP. Characteristics affecting fibrinolytic activity and plasma fibrinogen concentrations. BMJ 1979; **1**: 153–6.
57. Hendriks JFJ, Veenstra J, Wierik W, Schaafsma G, Kluft C. Effect of moderate dose of alcohol with evening meal on fibrinolytic factors. BMJ 1994; **308**: 1003–6.
58. Rankin JG. Biological mechanisms at moderate levels of alcohol consumption that may affect the development, course and/or outcome or coronary heart disease. Contemporary Drug Problems 1994; **21**: 45–57.
59. World Health Organization. Cardiovascular disease risk factors: new areas for research. WHO Technical report Series 841. Geneva: World Health Organization, 1994.
60. World Health Organization Working Group on Population levels of Alcohol Consumption. Copenhagen: World Health Organization Regional Office for Europe, 1994.
61. Skog O-J. Epidemiological and biostatistical aspects of alcohol use, alcoholism and their complications. In Erickson PG, Kalant H. (ed.) Windows on Science. Toronto, Addiction Research Foundation, 1992; pp. 3–35.
62. Nuffield Institute of Health. Brief interventions and alcohol use. Effective Health care No 7. University of Leeds: Nuffield Institute of Health, 1993.
63. Bien TH, Miller WR, Scott Tonnigan J. Brief interventions for alcohol problems: a review. Br J Addict 1993; **88**: 315–36.
64. Wallace PG, Cutler S, Brennan PJ, Haines A. Randomised controlled trial of general practitioner intervention in patients with excessive alcohol consumption. BMJ 1988; **297**: 663–8.

65. Scott E, Anderson P. Randomised controlled trial of general practitioner intervention in women with excessive alcohol consumption. Drug and Alcohol Review. 1990; **10**: 313–21.
66. Anderson P, Scott E. The effect of general practitioners' advice to heavy drinking men. Br J Addict 1992; **87**: 891–900.

7 Personality and psychological environment

John Muir

INTRODUCTION

Physiology links stress to the fight and flight reaction, whilst in psychology increasing stress is related to improving performance on a curve which peaks at an optimum level and then deteriorates. Pathophysiology relates extreme stress to sudden death—the fate of John Hunter when flatly contradicted at a hospital board meeting. With this background to heighten curiosity and fervour, researchers in the last 40 years have addressed the task of searching for a relationship between stress, personality, environment, and disease. The results provide intriguing conflicts in findings and have led to swings in consensus.

This chapter addresses the following areas of uncertainty:

1. **Are there coronary prone personality types?**
2. **Is there a relationship between workplace, environment, and the development of coronary heart disease (CHD).**
3. **Is there a relationship between stressful psychosocial factors and the development of CHD?**
4. **Are there mechanisms whereby stress may induce CHD?**
5. **Can modification of psychological stresses reduce CHD risk?**

ARE THERE CORONARY PRONE PERSONALITY TYPES?

The type A personality concept was developed in the 1950s in the USA by Friedman and Rosenman, and others.[1] It describes a hard driving, aggressive, competitive person who experiences time urgency, hostility, and has difficulty relaxing. Those not showing this cluster of characteristics are designated type B. Early studies were convincing and in 1981 sufficient data had accumulated in North America for The Review Panel on Coronary-Prone Behaviour and Coronary Heart Disease to pronounce type A behaviour an independent risk factor for CHD.[2] A key report in the Review Panel's judgement was the 8.5 year follow-up of the 3524 men in the *Western Collaborative Group Study*.[3] These 39–59 year olds were prospectively assessed for personality type in 1960/61 using a structured interview method. The 257 individuals developing clinical CHD had, on average, higher levels of each of the other principal risk factors, but after adjustment an approximate doubling of CHD risk in type A personalities remained (P < 0.003).

Subsequent studies have not confirmed the strength of these early conclusions.

In 1987, workers from the University of California published a quantitative review of psychological predictors of heart disease risk.[4] They examined 150 reports relating to type A behaviour published between 1945 and 1984. The analysis was based on 83 reports meeting appropriate selection criteria, and the results are shown in Table 7.1, which summarizes both cross-sectional and prospective studies. The data indicate a very small, but highly significant association of CHD with type A personality. This applies for both of the principal methods of its assessment (JAS; Jenkins Activity Score and SI; Structured Interview).

Table 7.1   Relationship between type A behaviour and all CHD outcomes (myocardial infarction, angina, cardiac death) from Booth-Kewley S, Friedman HS. Psychological Bulletin 1986; **101**; 343–62.

Personality variable	No. of publications	Effect size (r)	P
Type A: all measures	36	0.112	< 0.0000
– JAS type A	18	0.065	< 0.0000
– SI type A	11	0.197	< 0.0000
Sub-groups			
Speed: impatience:			
time urgency	9	0.061	0.0001
Job involvement	6	0.033	NS
Competitive: hard			
driving: aggressive	11	0.207	< 0.0000
Anger	7	0.042	0.001
Hostility	9	0.171	< 0.0000
Aggresion	5	0.059	NS
Depression	13	0.225	< 0.0000
Anxiety	14	0.136	< 0.0000

JAS: Jenkins activity score.   SI: structured interview.

The meta-analysis also indicates that the relationship is weaker in the prospective studies, which are less prone to bias, and in studies published since 1977. However, in almost all analyses the sub-components of hostility, competitive hard driving with aggression, and particularly, depression, have the strongest association with disease outcomes. The relationship between type A personality and CHD did not appear to be explained by effects of age, smoking, serum cholesterol, blood pressure, or years of education, but the authors admit that not enough data were available for a firm conclusion.

It is suggested that the apparent weakening of the type A–CHD relationship since the mid 1970s could be explained by changing patterns in the method of assessing type A personality, changing population personality (there has been an apparent increase from 50 per cent to over 70 per cent of the USA population being categorised as type A between the 1960s and 1980s), greater scientific stringency of investigators, or publication bias.[5] The latter would operate if there was a tendency for studies indicating positive associations to be accepted initially, followed by a bias to selective publication of the contrary findings.

There is a possible alternative explanation which does not appear in the literature. During the 1970's and 1980s life-style changes in western populations have been paralleled by significant reductions the incidence of CHD (see Chapter 4), a reversal of the social class relationship of CHD (see Chapter 9), and reductions in risk factor levels, particularly smoking, all with the lead occurring in the higher socio-economic groups. It would seem possible that the go-getting, type A personalities would be more likely to adapt their life-styles and indeed be more likely to be in the higher socio-economic groups. Resultant changes in more strongly predictive risk factors might then overcome the deleterious effect of having the 'wrong' personality.

This hypothesis is supported by an interesting quirk in the follow-up of the *Western Collaborative Study Group* cohort cited above.[3] Whereas type A was initially associated with a doubling of CHD mortality in 1975, an analysis reported in 1988 indicated a startling change.[6] After 22 years of follow-up the mortality rate of those developing CHD during the first 8.5 years was one third lower if labelled type A in 1960/61, than if type B (p = 0.04). An accompanying editorial commented that 'This is a topsy turvy career for a risk factor'.[5]

Most of the data in the meta-analysis refer to middle aged US white males.[4] Type A personality has, however, been associated with coronary proneness in both sexes and various cultures.[7] The two community based British reports come from *The British Regional Heart* and *Caerphilly* studies.[8,9] The former found no relationship between type A characteristics, assessed using a shortened rating scale (Bortner questionnaire), and CHD events. In both studies there was a significant association between type A and diagnosis of angina, based on the WHO chest pain questionnaire, but there was no relationship with ECG change, CHD morbidity, or CHD mortality.

These two studies imply that type A personalities report angina more than type B personalities, without necessarily having more disease. An earlier British report of 99 patients undergoing coronary angiography suggested the same phenomenon; patients with normal or minimally diseased arteries had significantly higher type A scores.[10] Again, in patients with stable angina both personality types A and B had similar ECG changes, but type A personalities reported one in two ECG documented episodes of ischaemia as angina in their symptom diaries whereas type Bs only reported one in four.[11]

Depression

The association of depression and acute myocardial infarction has recently been separately reviewed.[12] The evidence suggests that, although depression may be a potential sequel to CHD and hospitalisation, it is also more common in subjects destined to suffer acute myocardial infarction in the future. In particular, it is suggested that a chronic maladaptive depressive coping style is the adverse state, rather than frank clinical depression or bipolar/manic disorders.[12]

IS THERE A RELATIONSHIP BETWEEN WORKPLACE, ENVIRONMENT, AND THE DEVELOPMENT OF CHD?

The inverse association between socio-economic status and CHD in western societies (see Chapter 9) is only partly explained by the established physical risk factors and personality attributes. Other possibilities include variations and quality of medical resources, genetic factors, fetal growth and effects related to the environment.[13] The psychosocial aspects of the latter have been extensively studied in the workplace with particular emphasis on psychological stress and job characteristics.

Attempts to measure work stress directly have failed to predict CHD events, but examination of particular job characteristics have proved more fruitful. Studies done in the 1960s and 1970s suggested that role conflicts at work, high work load, job dissatisfaction, and poor social support at work were linked to increases in recognised CHD risk factors and related to increased CHD morbidity and mortality.[13,14] Further, chronic socio-emotional distress has been linked to increases in blood pressure, atherogenic lipids and thrombogenic risk and is more prominent in lower socio-economic groups.[15]

Decision latitude hypothesis

In 1981, Karasek, *et al* reported on a random sample of 1461 employed Swedish males aged 18–60 years surveyed in 1968 and again in 1974.[16] Working environment characteristics were assessed in a case-control study of 22 cases of cerebrovascular or cardiovascular death and 66 matched controls. A 'hectic and psychologically demanding job' were associated with increased risk of developing overt CHD (odds ratio 1.25 $p < 0.025$), and vascular death (odds ratio 4.1 $p < 0.01$). 'Low intellectual discretion' (i.e. little decision making ability or choice) was associated with CHD (odds ratio 1.44, $p < 0.01$) and 'low personal schedule freedom', in workers with relatively few education years, with increased vascular death (odds ratio 6.6, $p < 0.001$). Analyses were adjusted for age, education years, smoking and weight but not blood pressure, blood cholesterol levels, nor personality type.

The factors 'low intellectual discretion' and 'low personal schedule freedom' together constitute 'low decision latitude'. The latter has been combined with job demands in a 'job strain' model which the authors have proposed. This is summarised in Fig. 7.1. According to the model, where work demands were high but control of work was low (example in production line workers) there were raised vascular disease risks. But high job demands when there was control over decisions and the environment did not predict increased risk (example professionals and managers). Where demands were relatively low and decision latitude high (example administrators) work related CHD risk was lowest.

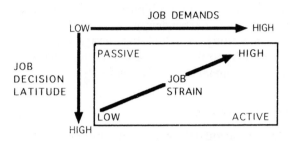

Fig. 7.1 Karasek workplace hypothesis.

This hypothesis from Karasek and co-workers[16] has been widely accepted[13, 14], but the data on which it is based include few fatal events (n = 22) and no data were collected on blood pressure or lipid levels, which tend to be higher in those having the greatest job stress.[15]

In 1989 Piper, La Croix, and Karasek published an analysis of five studies conducted in the USA between 1949 and 1980 which included 12 500 working males.[17] Using a separate national labour survey, the authors attached measures of job characteristics, psychological demands, and decision latitude to each subject by occupation. The hypothesis was that these job characteristics might be related to blood cholesterol, blood pressure, and smoking status. The analysis was controlled for age, years of education, body mass index, and type A behaviour pattern and showed a significant relationship between low decision latitude and both smoking and systolic blood pressure (p < 0.05).

A second analysis of nearly 5000 employed US males, and using logistic regression, enabled comparison of stress between the 69 cases having a history of myocardial infarction and the rest of the population, after adjustment for age, race, education, systolic blood pressure, serum cholesterol levels, smoking status (half the population only), and physical exertion.[18] A low decision latitude in association with a highly psychologically demanding job occurred in 20 per cent of the working population and had a significant (p < 0.01), independent association with the prevalence of past myocardial infarction. The estimated strength of the association was of similar or greater magnitude than that for the effects of cholesterol and smoking. The analysis on low decision latitude alone also yielded similar results. The occupations having high job strain were mostly classified in social classes four and five, and had a strong time pressure element (example production line workers, waiters, freight handlers).

Attributing the same level of stress, as reported by job characteristics, to all individuals in a particular type of work (imputation strategy) is a blunt methodology since individuals are so disparate. The analysis is also based on past history of myocardial infarction, which might have influenced selection of less stressful jobs before the studies were performed. These factors would dilute the estimated associations between work stress and CHD events.

Overall, Karasek's studies suggest (albeit with few numbers of cardiac events for analysis) that high psychological job demands, associated with low decision latitude, may be associated with both higher than average levels of conventional physical risk factors and, independently, with CHD directly by some other mechanisms. It is interesting to reflect that though the work strain hypothesis is largely attributed to Karasek, *et al*, research in the 1960s had indicated almost the same conclusions (summarized by Groen in 1974).[19]

German blue collar worker studies

One small study has adequately controlled for all of the relevant variables including type A personality and was specifically designed to examine prospectively the relationship of workplace characteristics and the incidence of new CHD events.[14] Four hundred and sixty blue collar workers aged 25–55 years, and without previous ischaemic heart disease at first examination, were sampled from three German steel industry plants. A structured interview determined a range of work related variables. Follow-up covered 85 per cent of the sample over the first 6.5 years during which there were 21 CHD events.

In multivariate regression analysis, cases not only had significantly raised levels of conventional risk factors (odds ratios for age, systolic blood pressure, low density lipoprotein cholesterol were 3.0, 8.2, and 11.6 respectively) but four psychological indicators also contributed to the coronary risk in a substantial way—status inconsistency, which defines people holding occupational grades with either unusually high or low educational background related to the work demands (odds ratio 4.4); job insecurity (odds ratio 3.4); work pressure, an evaluation of frequency and intensity of self-perceived time pressure (odds ratio 3.5); and immersion, a state of exhaustive coping, reflecting frustrated but continued efforts, without control (odds ratio 4.5). Further analyses indicated a particularly adverse risk state in which conventional physical risk factors combined synergistically with low perceived reward and high work effort. This comparison was found in 38 per cent of cases and only seven per cent of controls ($p < 0.0001$). This work also identified a new psychosocial risk factor 'need for control'. This is an indicator of coping in response to the work environment and is of adverse effect particularly if combined with status inconsistency. Though the number of events in the studies by Siegrist, *et al*[14] are few, the findings are important because they used a prospective study design and appropriately controlled for effects of all known influencing variables, they also support the theory of Karasek, *et al* that high psychological stress combined with reduced control over the working environment (decision latitude) is independently predictive of CHD events.[15]

Recommendations concerning conditions of employment

The implications of research in this area have been summarised by Michael Argyle in The social psychology of work.[20] The proposals made to reduce stress and disease associated with the work environment are divided between work situations where stress is inevitable and non-stressful work situations. Where stress cannot be entirely avoided (example police, firemen) employee selection can seek out persons with past experience of successfully coping with stress or use appropriate personality tests; training in stress management may be considered; job rotation can avoid extended periods of very high stress levels and short shift duration is advised in certain occupations (e.g. radar plotters). Also, regular medical check ups can be conducted and counselling made available.

Where the problem is continuous work pressure, Argyle recommends planned examination of the structure of the working environment to reduce repetition, physical overload, time pressures and avoidance of unnerving factors such as high noise levels or dangerous moving equipment. He also suggests that organisational changes should allow all workers to have some autonomy and to feel a cohesive identity, having some decision making ability about the way their work is run. This should be coupled with consultation procedures with supervisors and managers who have had appropriate training, and surveys of job satisfaction.

Though these recommendations are based on observational research and seem pragmatically to make good sense, evidence is lacking from intervention studies that introducing these changes will reduce the likelihood of CHD events.

IS THERE A RELATIONSHIP BETWEEN STRESSFUL PSYCHO-SOCIAL FACTORS AND THE DEVELOPMENT OF CHD?

The literature on psychosocial stress has recently been reviewed in a Handbook of life, stress, cognition and health.[21] This cites research indicating a wide variety of states which have been linked to subsequent CHD events. These vary from conflicts at work to being shown too little affection by a spouse. Included are upward and downward changes in social class, migration, lack of social ties and social support, bereavement, marital breakdown, major stresses such as air raids, as well as other factors covered in this chapter. Unfortunately, much of this literature does not include appropriate statistical analysis and is based on retro-spective data. But there are a number of reports of prospective studies appro-priately controlled for accepted risk factors.

The effects of social isolation and poor social relationships have been recently investigated in a Swedish study of nearly 1000 men in their 50s and 60s, followed for nine years.[22] Results were adjusted in multiple regression analysis for age, smoking status, blood pressure, blood total cholesterol levels, and alcohol consumption. The investigators observed a 2.5 times lower CHD event rate in participants who were most active whether at home (e.g. hobbies, reading, DIY) or outside the home (e.g. travelling, fishing, theatre going). In those having most social activities (e.g. parties, meetings, visiting friends and relatives) a three–four fold lower event rate was noted than in the most socially isolated. The possibility that reduced social activity was the result of prior disease, rather than habit, was considered and it was found the relationships were independent of initial health status.

Another Swedish study of nearly 7000 men in middle age employed a ques-tionnaire to assess personal feelings of tension, irritability, anxiety, and sleeping difficulties related to problems at home or work.[23] After 11.8 years of observation, the 1070 having 'permanent' stress from these factors, compared to all the others, had an odds ratio of 1.7 for CHD death (95 per cent confidence interval 1.2–2.4), and 1.4 for all cause mortality (95 per cent confidence interval 1.1–1.7). These differences are impressive since analyses were controlled for 11 possible confounding factors including the important physical ones, as well as family history of CHD, employment class, leisure time activity, and alcohol abuse.

The 20 year follow-up of women in the *Framingham Study* also reported data fully controlled for usual physical risk factors.[24] The data implicate low educational level, tension, and lack of vacations as having independent association with CHD ($p < 0.05$).

A recent study of 10 000 male and female British Civil Servants provides new insights, indicating that lack of social support, social activity, and emotional support are encountered progressively more frequently from the upper to lower socio-economic groups.[25] This study has also reported an association with CHD risk in relation to the work characteristics of low levels of control; lack of variety and use of skills; pace of work; and lack of support at work.

A British prospective study of phobic anxiety has indicated a three to four-fold increase in CHD event risk in the most anxious.[26] Results were adjusted for the effects of established risk factors and the investigation included about 1500 middle aged males who were followed for 13 years.

A prospective investigation by Dutch workers followed 4000 male Civil Servants over 4.2 years and controlled for major risk factors. They found a condition termed 'vital exhaustion' (i.e. symptoms such as unusual fatigue, dejection, and irritability) was twice as common in subjects developing subsequent angina or experiencing non-fatal myocardial infarction.[27] Previous reports have suggested similar conclusions, but most involved relatively few subjects, were retrospective, or failed to control for effects of accepted risk factors.[27] Since the association was not found in relation to fatal myocardial infarction (though numbers were few) the possibility remains that dejected subjects, like type A personalities[11], may perceive and report their symptoms more than the less morose.

ARE THERE MECHANISMS WHEREBY STRESS MAY INDUCE CHD?

There is a large literature on the effect of stress on CHD risk factors which has been assessed in recent reviews.[28] In the majority of 60 short-term studies, increases in blood pressure and blood lipid levels occurred in response to a variety of stressful stimuli (including emotional arousal, serial addition tests, cold immersion, confrontational interviews, and video games[28]). In 70 per cent of 37 studies, type A personalities demonstrated greater reactivity of risk factors in response to such stresses than type B personalities. Risk factor changes were made more extreme by nicotine, caffeine, and high salt intake and less pronounced by alcohol, increased exercise, low salt and high potassium diets, and beta blockade.[28]

The possibility of increased platelet reactivity as a response to psychological stress has also been investigated. A recent review supports this hypothesis, which could be important in the context of both acute CHD events and the development of atheroma.[29]

It is proposed that acute stress, working primarily through the limbic system, hypothalamus, and adrenal medulla, results in increased catecholamine release. This leads to increased blood pressure, heart rate, and mobilization of cholesterol as well as lowering the threshold to ventricular fibrillation and increasing platelet stickiness.[29,30] Chronic stress has effects through central influences on the pituitary/adrenocortical axis with concomitant increase in cortisol release. Long-term effects of stimulating cortisol release are sodium retention, increased blood volume, decreased ventricular ectopic threshold, and increased sensitivity of arterioles to catecholamines.[28,30]

CAN MODIFICATION OF PSYCHOLOGICAL STRESSES REDUCE CHD RISK?

A number of studies have explored the possibility that stress management may lower blood pressure. Techniques used include relaxation, breathing exercises, meditation, and biofeedback. These can be taught in groups of eight to ten people, with treatment sessions lasting 1–1.5 hours for eight to ten weeks; follow-up is required. A recent review concluded that many patients do indeed have significant benefit, compared to controls, and this may be sustained over some years.[31]

One study has explored the role of type A behaviour modification in CHD. Meyer Friedman, still working in the Harold Brunn Institute in San Francisco and over a quarter of a century after his first communications in the field, studied 1013 subjects who had survived myocardial infarction by six months or more.[32] The intervention group (n = 592) was randomized to receive both post-coronary and type A behaviour modification counselling; controls (n = 270) received post-coronary counselling alone. A further observation group (n = 151) received no counselling. During 4.5 years of follow-up, the controls were offered 33 group sessions of 90 minutes each (attending 25 on average). The intervention group were offered 62 sessions (attending 38 on average). Type A counselling comprised instruction on techniques of relaxation, behaviour modification, and environmental restructuring, combined with efforts to change beliefs, learning abilities, and instructions in specific drills.

Results indicated a significant reduction in markers of type A behaviour in the intervention (-35 per cent) compared to the control (-10 per cent) groups (p < 0.001). There were also fewer recurrent myocardial infarctions in the intervention group than in the controls (13 per cent versus 21 per cent p < 0.005), with a total of 119 events. The observation only group had similar results to the controls. The inter-group differences could not be explained by changes in blood pressure, blood lipid levels, or smoking status.

If these results could be confirmed, and if simple and less intensive techniques (e.g. audio or video cassette) are also effective, this form of risk reduction 'therapy' could become widely applicable. However this single report must be interpreted with appropriate caution.

SUMMARY

Type A personality

- This personality type appeared to be associated with a doubling of CHD risk in early studies.
- There was only a weak association with increased CHD risk in a comprehensive meta-analysis, including more recent studies.
- It is too broad a construct and should be divided into:
  - positive aspects including job involvement, hardworking drive, and time urgency which appear to have little or no association with CHD risk
  - negative aspects of hard driving, aggressiveness, and hostility, which relate to increased CHD risk.
- Type A personality appears to be associated with reporting more symptoms than type B with similar CHD pathology.

Working environment and CHD

- Evidence is emerging to support a hypothesis which suggests that high work pressure in association with lack of decision making ability, and little or no control over the working environment, is independently associated with:
  - raised levels of conventional physical risk factors.
  - raised CHD rates.
- This state is commoner in:
  - low socio-economic groups
  - production line workers and others who have to cope with a continuous demand.
- This state has greatest effect on:
  - subjects with a high personal need for control.
- There is a dearth of research on the effects of modifying work stress.

Stressful psychosocial factors and CHD risk

- There is evidence indicating an independent effect of at least a doubling of CHD event risk in association with:
  - social isolation and inactivity
  - phobic anxiety.
- Depression and chronic anxiety have a minor, but statistically significant, association with increased CHD event risk.

Mechanisms whereby stress may induce CHD

- There is a body of evidence suggesting that levels of blood pressure and blood cholesterol may increase in response to a variety of physical, mental, and psychological stimuli.
- Type A individuals appear to demonstrate greater reactivity of adverse risk factors to stress.

Studies of stress reduction and life management

- These interventions have led to sustained reduction in blood pressure in compliant individuals.
- The studies provide inadequate data to evaluate the possibility that stress reduction advice given by GPs will reduce the incidence of either primary or recurrent vascular events.

REFERENCES

1. Friedman M, Rosenman R.H. Type a behaviour and your heart. New York: Alfred A Knopf 1974.
2. The Review Panel on Coronary-Prone Behaviour and Coronary Heart Disease. Coronary prone behaviour and coronary heart disease: a critical review. Circulation 1981; **63**: 1199–215.
3. Rosenman RH, Brand RJ, Jenkins D, Friedman M, Straus R, Wurm M. Coronary heart disease in the Western Collaborative Group study. JAMA 1975; **233**: 872–7.
4. Booth-Kewley S, Friedman HS. Psychological predictors of heart disease: a quantitative review. Psychological Bulletin 1987; **101**: 343–62.
5. Dimsdale JE. (Editorial) A perspective on type A behaviour and coronary disease. New Eng J Med 1988; **318**: 110–12.
6. Ragland DR, Brand RJ. Type A behaviour and mortality from coronary heart disease. New Eng J Med 1988; **318**: 65–9.
7. Sensky T. (Editorial) Refining thinking on type A behaviour and coronary heart disease. BMJ 1987; **295**: 69–70.
8. Johnson DW, Cook DG, Shaper AG. Type A behaviour and ischaemic heart disease in middle aged British men. BMJ 1987; **295**: 86–9.
9. Gallacher JEJ, Yarnell JWG, Elwood PC, Phillips KM. Type A behaviour and heart disease prevalent in men in the Caerphilly study. BMJ 1984; **289**: 732–3.
10. Bass C, Wade C. Type A Behaviour: not specifically pathogenic? Lancet 1982; **ii**: 1147–50.
11. Freeman LJ. Type A behaviour and ischaemic heart disease. BMJ 1987; **295**: 501.
12. Fielding R. Depression and acute myocardial infarction: a review and reinterpretation. Soc Sci Med 1991; **32**: 1017–27.
13. Marmot M. Look after your heart: stress and cardiovascular disease—a studiable case? Health Trends 1987; **19**: 21–2.
14. Sigrist J, Peter R, Junge A, Cremer P, Seidel D. Low status control, high effort at work and ischaemic heart disease: prospective evidence from blue-collar men. Soc Sci Med 1990; **31**: 1127–34.

15. Sigrist J.Contributions of sociology to the prediction of heart disease and their implications for public health. Eur J Publ Health 1991; **1**: 10–21.

16. Karasek R, Baker D, Marxer F, Ahlbom A, Theorell T. Job Decision Latitude, Job demands, and cardiovascular disease: a arospective study of Swedish men. Am J Public Health 1981; **71**: 694–705.

17. Pieper C, LaCroix AZ, Karasek RA.The relation of psychosocial dimensions of work with coronary heart disease risk factors: a meta-analysis of five United States data bases. Am J Epidemiol 1989; **129**: 483–94.

18. Karasek RA, Theorell T, Schwartz JE, Schnall PL, Pieper CF, Michela JL. Job characteristics in relation to the prevalence of myocardial infarction in the US Health Examination Survey (HES) and the Health and Nutrition Examination Survey (HANES). Am J Public Health, 1988; **78**: 910–18.

19. Groen JJ. Psychosomatic aspects of ischaemic (coronary) heart disease. In Modern trends in psychosomatic medicine (ed. Hill OW) London: Butterworth, 1974: 288–29.

20. Argyle M. Stress health and mental health at work. In The social psychology of work. (2nd edn.) London: Penguin Books, 1989: pp. 260–84.

21. Boman B. Stress and heart disease. In Handbook of life stress, cognition and health (ed. Fisher S and Reason J) New York : John Wiley & Sons Ltd., 1988: pp. 301–35.

22. Welin L, Tibblin G, Svardsudd K, Tibblin B, Ander-Peciva S, Larsson B, and Wilhelmsen L. Prospective study of social influences on mortality. Lancet 1985, **i**: 915–18.

23. Rosengren A, Tibblin G, Wilhelmsen L. Self-perceived psychological stress and incidence of coronary artery disease in middle-aged men. Am J Cardiol 1991; **68**: 1171–75.

24. Eaker ED, Pinsky J, Castelli WP. Myocardial infarction and coronary death among women: psychosocial predictors from a 20-year follow up of women in the Framingham study. Am J Epidemiol 1992; **135**: 854–64.

25. Marmot MG, Davey Smith G, Stansfeld S, Patel C, North F, Head J, White I, Brunner E, Feeney A. Health inequalities among British civil servants: the Whitehall II study. Lancet 1991; **337**: 1387–93.

26. Haines AP, Imeson JD, Meade TW. Phobic anxiety and ischaemic heart disease. BMJ 1987; **295**: 297–9.

27. Apels A and Mulder P. Fatigue and heart disease. The association between 'vital exhaustion' and past, present and future coronary heart disease. J Psychosomat Res 1989; **33**: 727–38.

28. Dembroski TM, Matthews KA. In Handbook of stress, reactivity and cardiovascular disease (ed. Matthews KA, Weiss SM, Detre T, Dembroski TM, *et al.*) New York: John Wiley and Sons 1986: pp. 275–89 461–73.

29. Markovitz JH, Matthews KA. Platelets and coronary heart disease: potential psycho-physiologic mechanisms. Psychosomatic Medicine 1991; **53**: 643–68.

30. Frank C, Smith S. Stress and the heart: biobehavioural aspects of sudden cardiac death. Psychosomatics 1990; **31**: 255–64.

31. Anon. Relaxation therapy for hypertensive patients. Drug and Therapeutics Bulletin 1989; **27**: 77–9.

32. Friedman M, Thoresen CE, Gill JJ, Ulmer D, Powell LH, Price VA, Brown B, Thompson L, Rabin DD, Breall WS, Bourg E, Levey R, Dixon T. Alteration of type A behaviour and its effect on cardiac recurrences in post myocardial infarction patients: summary results of the recurrent coronary prevention project. Am Heart J 1986; **112**: 653–66.

8 Diabetes

Jim Mann

INTRODUCTION

Coronary heart disease (CHD) is a major cause of serious morbidity and the commonest cause of mortality among people with diabetes. It accounts for much of the excess morbidity and mortality associated with both insulin dependent (IDDM) and non insulin dependent diabetes (NIDDM). There are four major issues which are considered in this chapter:

1. **The frequency of CHD in diabetes**
2. **The determinants of CHD in diabetes**
3. **Approaches to CHD risk reduction in diabetes and the evidence of benefit**
4. **CHD in impaired glucose tolerance and the insulin resistance syndrome (syndrome 'X').**

THE FREQUENCY OF CORONARY HEART DISEASE IN DIABETES

Over many decades, autopsy studies have suggested that people with diabetes have more extensive coronary atherosclerosis than non-diabetic people of the same age. The early studies were potentially biased since patients with diabetes may be more likely to come to autopsy than people without diabetes. However, most of the recent autopsy studies, which have used control groups and standardized techniques, have confirmed and extended these observations. People with diabetes appear to have an excess of complicated atherosclerotic lesions (haemorrhage, ulceration, thrombosis, calcification, and stenosis) and the frequency of myocardial infarction in men and women is double that in non-diabetics.[1,2]

Epidemiological studies in the past have generally underestimated the risk of clinical CHD in diabetes for two reasons. First, people with diabetes may experience silent myocardial infarctions which will not be detected unless the research methodology includes the routine use of electrocardiography. Second, studies which are based on death certificates may underestimate CHD risk because diabetes is frequently not mentioned on the death certificate when diabetic patients die from CHD. More recent studies, however, permit reliable estimates. The *World Health Organisation (WHO) Multinational Study*[3] of vascular disease in diabetes provides an indication of the extent to which circulatory diseases contribute to total mortality in diabetic patients in different countries (Fig. 8.1). The striking geographic variation in the percentage of deaths attributable to circulatory disease, evident in this study, may be explained by potentially modifiable environmental risk factors.

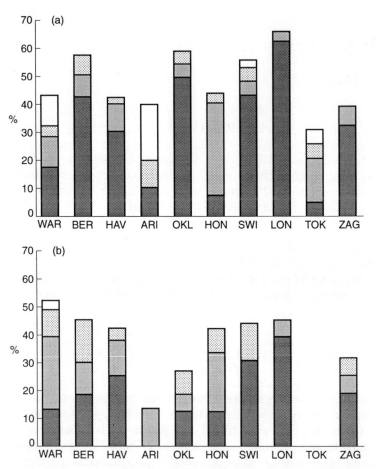

Fig. 8.1 Percentage of deaths attributable to circulatory disease; ischaemic heart disease (black), stroke (hatched), other circulatory disease (stippled), sudden death (white), for (a) males and (b) females. WAR = Warsaw; BER = Berlin; HAV = Havana; ARI = Arizona; OKL = Oklahoma; HON = Hong Kong; SWI = Switzerland; LON = London; TOK = Tokyo; ZAG = Zagreb. (From Head J, Fuller J. Diabetologia 1990; **33**: 477–81.)

Large within-population prospective studies provide the best estimate of the increased risk of CHD associated with diabetes. Not surprisingly, the results differ slightly from one study to another, but in general it appears that diabetes is associated with a two to three-fold greater risk of CHD. Some studies suggest that the effect is even more marked in women than men, so that among people with diabetes the CHD gender difference is less marked than in those who do not have the disease. The *Framingham Study* [4] has provided one of the longest periods of follow-up of diabetic patients. During a 20-year period of follow-up, the age adjusted incidence for all CHD was 24.8/1000 for diabetic men, 14.9/1000 for non-diabetic men, 17.8/1000 diabetic women and 16.9/1000 for non-diabetic women. This increase in risk applies to people with both IDDM and NIDDM.

DETERMINANTS OF CORONARY HEART DISEASE IN DIABETES

When attempting to explain increased risk of CHD in diabetes it is necessary to consider the extent to which diabetes is associated with increased levels of cardiovascular risk factors, and whether these factors have a greater impact in people with diabetes. It is also necessary to establish whether the duration and degree of hyperglycaemia, and other metabolic abnormalities associated with diabetes, or even treatment of diabetes might increase the risk of CHD.

Plasma lipids and lipoproteins

Total cholesterol concentrations in patients with NIDDM and IDDM tend to be slightly higher than in non diabetic subjects. Total cholesterol appears to have the same impact as a CHD risk determinant as in non-diabetics. For example, in a Swedish prospective study, diabetic men with a total cholesterol concentration above 7.3 mmol/l had a significantly higher incidence of CHD during follow-up than those with concentrations less than 5.5 mmol/l (28 per cent vs. 5 per cent); corresponding figures for non-diabetic men were nine per cent and two per cent respectively. Most prospective studies have involved, principally, patients with NIDDM but total cholesterol also appears to predict CHD in patients with IDDM.[5,6]

Prospective studies have often measured only the total cholesterol concentration and, much less frequently, total triglyceride and high density lipoprotein (HDL) cholesterol concentrations. Several case control studies using more sophisticated laboratory methods suggest that the dyslipidaemia of diabetes is complex, and that it differs in NIDDM and IDDM. It may therefore be important to consider the composition of the various lipoprotein fractions as well as their concentrations when determining CHD risk.

The predominant lipid abnormalities in IDDM are raised concentrations of total triglyceride, reflecting an increase in very low density lipoprotein (VLDL), together with reduced HDL cholesterol concentrations. These abnormalities are associated with inadequate glycaemic control. When control is satisfactory, the major difference between people with IDDM and controls is that the HDL cholesterol concentrations are higher among the diabetics.[7] In IDDM, total cholesterol and low density lipoprotein (LDL) cholesterol appear to be the most important lipoprotein mediated determinants of risk of CHD, a finding which is similar to that observed in the population at large.[6]

The situation differs considerably in NIDDM where the predominant features of the dyslipidaemia are reduced concentrations of HDL cholesterol (in particular HDL_2) and elevated concentrations of triglyceride, again reflecting an increase in VLDL. However, these features are present even in individuals with satisfactory glycaemic control.[8] Furthermore, in NIDDM, triglyceride and HDL cholesterol levels appear to be more important risk determinants for CHD than total and LDL cholesterol concentrations.[9]

Recent studies involving sophisticated laboratory techniques suggest that the composition of lipoproteins may be markedly different in both IDDM and NIDDM compared with people who do not have diabetes.[10] These features of the diabetic dyslipidaemia may be of equal or greater importance than the concentrations of total cholesterol, LDL, VLDL, and HDL cholesterol in determining the lipoprotein mediated risk of CHD, but there are at present no definitive data.

The recently identified lipoprotein(a), Lp(a), may also be relevant in this respect. In a group of patients with NIDDM, higher concentrations of Lp(a) was an important distinguishing characteristic of the group who suffered myocardial infarction.[11] The extent to which lipoproteins, and LDL in particular, are oxidized and the intake of dietary antioxidants have also been shown in both experimental studies and in prospective studies in non-diabetics to be important predictors of CHD. High intakes of food with antioxidant properties may reduce the athero-genic potential of elevated LDL cholesterol concentrations (see Chapter 12). However, while it seems likely that the extent to which LDL cholesterol is oxidized also influences CHD risk in people with diabetes, there are as yet no published data. For this reason, and because the observations regarding Lp(a) and lipoprotein composition have not been tested in prospective studies, it seems practically appropriate, for the present, to emphasise the role of total and LDL cholesterol, triglyceride, and HDL cholesterol. Finally, it should be noted that case control studies from Finland suggest that lipid risk factors may differ in men and women.[12] Hopefully, future prospective studies will be able to confirm or refute these various findings.

Smoking

There have been few systematic studies of smoking habits in representative groups of people with diabetes. However, in prospective studies in the United States and Sweden, smoking appears to have a similar effect in those who do and do not have diabetes. For example, in the *Gothenburg Study* current cigarette smoking was associated with an approximately three-fold increase in risk of CHD and all cause mortality.[5]

Blood pressure

People with diabetes tend to have higher levels of blood pressure than non-diabetics. While this may in part be due to the presence of early or overt nephropathy, there is some evidence from studies such as the *Framingham Study* that higher than average blood pressures may be detected even before the diagnosis of diabetes. This is discussed further in a later section of this chapter. There is no doubt that increased levels of blood pressure are associated with increasing risk of cardiovascular disease (see Chapter 2) and debate centres around whether this risk is more marked in people with diabetes than in those who do not have the disease. Several studies suggest that this is likely to be the case in IDDM but not in

NIDDM. For example, in the London cohort of the *WHO Multinational Study*, hypertension in patients with IDDM was found to be associated with a nearly twenty-fold increase in CHD risk.[13] The findings are less consistent in people with NIDDM, among whom an approximately two-fold increase in risk has been observed in several studies: this is of the same order of magnitude which has been observed in the general population. The association between systolic hypertension and CHD in diabetics is more consistent than that which has been observed for diastolic hypertension.[13,14,15]

Obesity and physical inactivity

Increasing levels of body mass index are strongly associated with an increased risk of NIDDM, especially when the obesity is centrally distributed.[16] Several important CHD risk factors, most notably hypertension and dyslipidaemia, are associated with obesity in people with diabetes, as is the case in non-diabetics. However, epidemiological studies to date have not shown a consistent association between any measure of obesity and cardiovascular risk in diabetes. Although increasing physical activity can favourably influence several risk determinants, no study has examined the association between physical inactivity and risk.

An independent effect of diabetes

There has been considerable debate as to whether the presence of diabetes makes an independent contribution to CHD risk. Several prospective studies have examined this issue. In most studies multivariate analyses suggest that even after adjusting for age and other important risk factors, a strong independent effect of diabetes remains. In the *Framingham Study* adjusting for other risk factors reduces the relative risk of CHD associated with diabetes from 1.70 to 1.66 in men and from 2.66 to 2.06 in women.[17] It is of interest to consider the mechanisms by which diabetes may exert an effect independent of other risk factors. There is as yet no evidence that, in people who already have diabetes, hyperglycaemia *per se* influences CHD risk although the *United Kingdom Prospective Diabetes Study*[18] (UKPDS) should soon provide definitive data about this. However, elevated plasma insulin concentrations may be an important risk determinant. In the *Paris Prospective Study*[19], among those with NIDDM and impaired glucose tolerance insulin concentrations greater than 108 pmol/l (or 2 hour insulin more than 40 pmol/l) were associated with an approximately two-fold increased risk in CHD. No data are available concerning the effect of exogenous insulin in IDDM or insulin-treated NIDDM.

A wide range of haemorrheological disturbances associated with diabetes may contribute to increased CHD risk. Compared with non-diabetics, people with diabetes have been shown to have an enhanced platelet aggregation in vitro, increased concentrations of β thromboglobulin, fibrinogen, factor VII, and reduced fibrinolytic activity.[20,21] Several of these indicators of thrombogenesis have been shown to be related to CHD in non-diabetics (see Chapter 11) but they have yet to be examined in prospective studies of people with diabetes, although the *Paris Prospective Study* found that raised mean corpuscular volume levels were associated with a two-fold increase in total mortality.[20]

The findings of the *University Group Diabetes Program*[22] (UGDP) trial suggested that some forms of treatment might be associated with an increased cardiovascular risk. In this large randomized trial, those treated with tolbutamide and phenformin had an increased risk of cardiovascular disease. While this observation has not been confirmed by other studies, uncertainties have lingered because of the large size of the trial and the prominence given to the results. Several studies have shown that insulin treated NIDDM patients have a two to four-fold greater CHD risk than those treated with oral hypoglycaemic agents or diet alone. However, the nature of most of the studies was such that it is not possible to disentangle the effects of treatment from diabetes severity, since insulin treatment was more likely to have been initiated in those with more marked metabolic derangements or associated risk factors. The question of whether any form of diabetes therapy is likely to increase or reduce the risk of cardiovascular disease in NIDDM will hopefully be answered by the *United Kingdom Prospective Diabetes Study*.[18]

In summary, the excessive occurrence of CHD in diabetes may be partly explained by the increased level of general cardiovascular risk factors associated with diabetes. Apart possibly from the effects of hypertension in IDDM, it is probable that the impact of these risk factors is similar in diabetics and non-diabetics. An appreciable proportion of the excess CHD risk appears, however, to be due to an effect of diabetes which is independent of the major general cardiovascular risk factors. Some of this effect might be explained by the effect of diabetes on components of the lipoprotein mediated risk, or factors influencing thrombogenesis which were not measured and therefore could not be examined in the published prospective studies. Equally, it is conceivable that there may be other mechanisms which remain to be identified.

APPROACHES TO CORONARY HEART DISEASE RISK REDUCTION IN DIABETES AND THE EVIDENCE OF BENEFIT

For many decades therapy in both IDDM and NIDDM aimed at reducing blood glucose levels to a range where patients were free of symptoms associated with hyperglycaemia. More recently there has been a change in attitudes and the goal is now to try to achieve levels approaching normoglycaemia. This has been justified by the recent publication of the *Diabetes Control and Complications Trial*[23] which showed a dramatic reduction in the microvascular complications of IDDM in association with successful attempts to achieve near optimal glycaemic control.

Evidence suggesting that careful control of blood pressure levels reduces the risk of diabetic renal disease has also resulted in recommendations for regular monitoring of blood pressure and early treatment of elevated levels.[24] It is of interest to note that while clinical trial evidence now provides justification for both these recommendations there was strong circumstantial evidence before trial data were available. Treatment of hypertension may also reduce the risk of cerebrovascular disease as is the case in people without diabetes (see Chapter 2).

The strength of evidence favouring identification and treatment of other potentially modifiable cardiovascular risk factors should also be considered. For smoking there is as strong a case for action as there is in those without diabetes and, given the high risk of CHD amongst diabetics, it is imperative to identify smokers and then to offer them appropriate support. A major debate has centred around the approach which should be taken towards modifying the dyslipidaemia of diabetes. There are several strands of evidence which suggest that it is worth paying considerable attention to this component of risk. The geographic epidemiology of CHD in people with diabetes is remarkably similar to that in non-diabetics. CHD in diabetics is more common in those countries where there is a high prevalence of CHD in the background population and where blood cholesterol concentrations also appear to be the principal determinants of the population risk of CHD. Case control, and more importantly prospective studies, confirm the importance of lipid and lipoprotein mediated risk in people with diabetes. Dietary and drug treatments which modify diabetic dyslipidaemia are available, and clinical trials in the non-diabetic population (see Chapter 3) provide convincing evidence that it is possible to reduce clinical CHD by favourably altering blood lipid levels especially in the context of multiple risk factor intervention.

A conservative approach is to argue that in the absence of clinical trial data, since the components of the lipoprotein mediated risk are not identical in diabetics and non-diabetics, there is no justification for special attention to the lipid abnormalities of diabetes. The alternative approach is to suggest that in view of the magnitude of the problem of CHD in diabetes and the strong body of circumstantial evidence it is negligent not to try to influence all modifiable components of CHD risk. The *The United Kingdom Prospective Diabetes Study*[18] may provide evidence as to whether one of several oral hypoglycaemic agents or insulin confers cardioprotective effects in NIDDM and whether optimal glycaemic control reduces the risk of macrovascular disease in diabetics. Several trials of lipid lowering drugs have been proposed and further trials of antihypertensive agents may be expected. Nevertheless, it seems unlikely that further definitive information will be available in the near future and it is therefore necessary to decide on what, if any, preventive action should be taken on the basis of current evidence. From a practical point of view, it is important to point out that all diabetic patients should be regularly reviewed as this provides the only means of ensuring that adequate glycaemic control is achieved. This provides opportunities to assess and treat cardiovascular risk. Possible therapies are reviewed briefly below.

Life-style measures

There is now general agreement about the most appropriate dietary prescription for people with diabetes. Most national recommendations follow those suggested by the European Association for the Study of Diabetes or the American Diabetes Association.[25,26] Advice to achieve ideal body mass, to reduce saturated fat intake to 10 per cent or less of the energy intake, and to reduce all extrinsic or 'free' sugars (i.e. those which are not an integral part of plant foods and which are not rapidly absorbed) form the cornerstone of these recommendations. Such measures will help to reduce blood glucose levels, but the expert committees have all regarded the reduction of cardiovascular risk that is likely to accrue from reducing obesity and saturated fat as being of equal importance in justifying the recommendations. Weight loss in the obese reduces blood glucose, blood pressure, total and LDL cholesterol, and triglycerides, and is associated with an appreciable increase in HDL cholesterol. Substantial reductions in saturated fat intake will reduce total and LDL cholesterol, and favourably influence levels of factor VIII, which is known to be associated with CHD risk in non-diabetics. Increased physical activity is an important aspect of the life-style prescription both because weight loss may be facilitated and because regular exercise is associated with an increase in levels of HDL cholesterol. All expert committees have regarded the evidence summarized here as being sufficient to make these recommendations, even in the absence of data from clinical trials. While these general principles are recommended for all people with diabetes, there is agreement that lipid levels should be regularly measured and more restrictive advice offered to those with marked dyslipidae-mia. In particular, those with elevated total or LDL cholesterol levels should be advised to restrict saturated fatty acids to eight per cent or less of total energy.

There are several other dietary measures which may reduce cardiovascular risk, but which have not been universally incorporated into dietary recommendations. Increased intake of fruit and vegetables may increase blood levels of dietary antioxidants and so reduce the tendency towards oxidation of lipoproteins[27] (see Chapter 12). While this seems to be a generally sensible recommendation, there is as yet no clear evidence concerning the quantities which may be clinically useful. This reservation applies equally to the use of various dietary antioxidants taken as nutritional supplements. Monounsaturated fatty acids derived from vegetable oils provide useful substitutes for saturated fatty acids since they facilitate the maintenance or increase levels of HDL cholesterol. When saturated fatty acids are replaced by carbohydrate, LDL cholesterol levels tend to fall. Furthermore, increased intakes of monounsaturated fatty acids from olive oil have been shown to be associated with reduced LDL cholesterol oxidation.[28] Earlier research suggested that soluble forms of non-starch polysaccharide (dietary fibre) derived from lentils, various cooked dried beans, oats, and pasta helped to decrease blood glucose and LDL cholesterol levels. However, it is now clear that this effect is seen with only very high levels of intake and the effects are relatively small by comparison with those resulting from the other changes described above. It is, nevertheless, extremely important to emphasise that if energy lost by reducing saturated fat is replaced by carbohydrate it is essential that the carbohydrate be rich in soluble non-starch polysaccharides. Failure to comply with this aspect of dietary advice may result in the beneficial effects of LDL cholesterol reduction being offset by a parallel decrease in HDL cholesterol and an increase in triglycerides.[29]

It must be emphasised that translating these nutritional principles into practice involves substantial dietary manipulation for those accustomed to a western diet. Few patients succeed in achieving the degree of change required without the support of a dietitian or other trained nutritional counsellor and this applies particularly to those with more marked dyslipidaemia who need to make even greater changes. Failure to achieve appreciably improved lipid levels usually reflects unwillingness or inability to comply with dietary advice rather than physiological unresponsiveness.

Another dietary modification which might appreciably reduce cardiovascular risk is restriction of dietary sodium which might in turn be expected to reduce blood pressure levels. Meta-analyses of epidemiological studies and clinical trials in non-diabetic populations have suggested that an appreciable reduction in sodium could markedly reduce mortality from cerebrovascular and cardiovascular disease (see Chapter 2). There have been no comparable, large, epidemiological studies in diabetics, but the importance of hypertension as a cardiovascular risk factor and the fact that salt restriction has been shown to reduce blood pressure levels in people with diabetes suggests that it may be a worthwhile measure, and should be part of routine dietetic advice.

Lipid lowering drug therapy

It is important to stress that no trials of lipid-lowering drugy therapy with clinical end points have been conducted in diabetic patients. Decisions concerning drug therapy are based on extrapolating from the experience of trials in non-diabetics, and knowledge of the effects of drugs on metabolic end points. The common lipid abnormalities in NIDDM are raised triglycerides and reduced HDL cholesterol. Fibrate derivatives are the most effective agents for reversing these abnormalities and are often prescribed if diet alone has not effectively reduced unacceptably high levels of triglycerides. The HMG CoA reductase group of drugs (statins) may be tried if fibrate treatment is unsuccessful or if elevated LDL or total cholesterol are the predominant abnormalities. Ion exchange resins are also used occasionally in instances when raised LDL occurs without elevation of triglycerides.

There is no universal agreement on the indication for lipid lowering drug therapy in diabetes. It has been argued that the existence of dyslipidaemia in an individual with diabetes warrants even more energetic management than in a person with no cardiovascular risk factors, and drug therapy should be recommended for those with even modest elevation of lipid levels who do not respond to diet alone. This argument is even stronger in those who are hypertensive, since the multiplicity of risk factors compounds the degree of risk.[30] Lipid levels should be monitored regularly and drugs considered if, after intensive dietary advice, the patient fails to achieve satisfactory levels (see Table 3.2, Chapter 3). Controversies regarding the role of drug therapy are unlikely to be resolved until clinical trials which are currently proposed provide information concerning morbidity and mortality. The known side effects of lipid lowering drugs do not differ between people with diabetes and those without, although it should be noted that ion exchange resins may result in elevated triglyceride levels, despite producing marked reductions in LDL. The importance of triglycerides in the aetiology of CHD in diabetes suggests that resins should therefore be used with caution.

Oral hypoglycaemic and antihypertensive drugs

In the light of current data, it is not possible to recommend with any degree of certainty that one oral hypoglycaemic agent should be used in preference to another in order to reduce cardiovascular risk. Several agents have some beneficial effects on plasma lipids and the haemorrheological disturbances associated with diabetes and hopefully the *United Kingdom Prospective Diabetes Study* [18] will provide information as to whether these have sufficient clinical effect to influence prescribing practices. Similarly, it has been suggested that certain antihypertensive agents, especially ACE inhibitors, are particularly appropriate for use by people with diabetes. It seems appropriate to recommend that those diuretics and beta blockers which have been associated with increase in blood glucose and triglyceride should be used with caution but less clear whether others with relatively small beneficial effects on lipids should be preferentially prescribed.

IMPAIRED GLUCOSE TOLERANCE AND INSULIN RESISTANCE SYNDROME (SYNDROME 'X')

It has long been known that individuals with impaired glucose tolerance are at increased risk of CHD, as is shown (Fig. 8.2) by the data from the prospective *Bedford Study*.[31] It is well recognized that in some individuals there is a tendency towards clustering of several inter-related metabolic and clinical cardiovascular risk factors: hyperglycaemia, hyperuricaemia, hyperinsulinaemia, hypertriglycer-idaemia, low HDL levels, and hypertension. This constellation of abnormalities has been described as 'Syndrome X' and attention has been drawn to its strong association with CHD.[32] It has been suggested that insulin resistance with consequent hyperinsulinaemia is the underlying defect of this syndrome and, on this basis, it has also been described as the insulin resistance syndrome.

An important limitation of most studies linking insulin resistance and hyper-insulinaemia to other metabolic variables and hypertension is that they have all been cross sectional. As a result, insulin resistance could conceivably be a consequence rather than a cause of other disturbances. Hyperinsulaemia and insulin resistance have been shown to predict NIDDM and CHD. Data from the *Paris Prospective Study*[19] are shown in Fig. 8.3. More recently, two prospective studies have shown that raised insulin levels precede the development of hypertension, hyperglycaemia and low levels of HDL providing further evidence that insulin resistance may indeed be the common aetiological factor.[32] Insulin resistance is associated with central obesity, and the high frequency of the insulin resistance syndrome in association with central obesity has been suggested as an important explanation for the high mortality from CHD in certain population groups, including the South Asians settled in Britain.

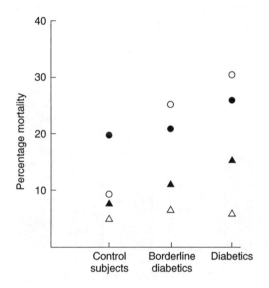

Fig. 8.2   All-causes age adjusted mortality by sex for the years 0–5 and 6–10 of the prospective study. Percentage mortality for the years 6–10 is calculated from the number of survivors at 5 years. Years 6–10 males (*closed circle*); females (*open circle*); years 0–5 males (*closed triangle*); females (*open triangle*). (From Bonanome A, *et al.* Arteriosclerosis and Thrombosis 1992; **12**: 529–33.)

The precise mechanisms by which hyperinsulinaemia causes these various consequences has not been firmly established. Release of non-esterified fatty acids from intra-abdominal fat cells into the portal circulation may affect hepatic insulin metabolism and peripheral glucose intake. Failure of insulin to suppress release of non-esterified fatty acids from intra-abdominal fat cells, which are less sensitive than subcutaneous fat cells to the antilipolytic action of insulin, could lead to increased hepatic synthesis of VLDL triglyceride. Proposed mechanisms for the effect of insulin on blood pressure include effects on the sympathetic nervous system, proliferation of vascular smooth muscle cells, cation transport, and renal sodium reabsorption.

If the insulin resistance hypothesis is correct, it is possible to consider means by which this might be reversed both in individuals in whom the syndrome has been diagnosed and in high risk populations such as South Asians living overseas. Thus far, the only known human environmental influences on insulin resistance are dietary energy intake and physical activity. Reducing the former and increasing the latter will not be an easy task but may provide the best hope of decreasing CHD in this group. In NIDDM it may be appropriate to avoid the use of thiazide diuretics and beta blockers which aggravate insulin resistance, when antihypertensive medication is required for those with the insulin resistance syndrome. ACE inhibitors and alpha blockers on the other hand, may improve insulin sensitivity and it has been argued that these are the drugs of choice in this situation. The evidence for such a recommendation is not conclusive, but circumstantial evidence is strong and the major argument against its adoption is the cost of the drugs involved.

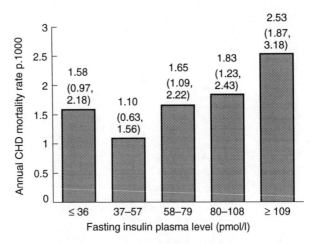

Fig. 8.3 Annual mortality rates for coronary heart disease (CHD) along quintiles of fasting plasma insulin levels at entry to 15 year follow-up. Number of subjects with complete information: 6937. Number of CHD deaths: 178. On top of the bars the annual mortality rates are shown with 95 percent confidence intervals in parenthesis. (From Bonanome A *et al.* Arteriosclerosis and Thrombosis 1992; **12**: 529–33.)

It will be apparent from much of the above discussion that most recommendations concerning CHD risk reduction in diabetics are based on powerful circumstantial evidence. However, in the absence of clinical trials with morbidity and mortality from CHD as end points there is little alternative since the immensely high rates of CHD in people with diabetes demand action. It may well be that surveillance of CHD rates in those with diabetes in conjunction with changing therapeutic practices will provide an indication of the benefits of life-style modification and drug therapy before the results of further clinical trials are available. One conclusion which may be offered, without fear of contradiction, is that ignoring the issue of cardiovascular risk in diabetes will mean that premature mortality and serious morbidity in people with this condition is unlikely to improve.

SUMMARY

- The incidence of CHD is appreciably greater amongst people with diabetes than in the general population.
- The increased risk of CHD in those with diabetes is greater among women than men so that the gender difference in CHD is less marked in those with diabetes than in the general population.
- Rates of CHD in diabetes show geographic variation similar to those in non-diabetics suggesting that environmental (potentially modifiable) factors may be important in the aetiology.
- Increased levels of general CHD risk factors (raised cholesterol and blood pressure, smoking) account for a proportion of the increased CHD risk, but diabetes itself is associated with an increase in risk which is independent of these factors.
- Despite the lack of clinical trials involving coronary events or death as end points there is strong circumstantial evidence that modifying general risk factors will produce clinically useful results.
- Patients with IDDM and NIDDM need regular surveillance, and individualized dietary and drug therapy.

REFERENCES

1. Waller B, Palumbo P, Lie J, Roberts W. Status of the coronary arteries at necropsy in diabetes mellitus with onset after age 30 years: analysis of 229 diabetic patients with and without clinical evidence of coronary heart disease and comparison to 183 control subjects. Am J Med 1980; **69**: 498–506.
2. Vigorita V, Moore G, Hutchins G. Absence of correlation between coronary arterial atherosclerosis and severity or duration of diabetes mellitus of adult onset. Am J Cardiol 1980; **46**: 535–42.
3. Head J, Fuller J. International variations in mortality among diabetic patients: the WHO multinational study of vascular diseases in diabetics. Diabetologia 1990; **33**: 477–81.
4. Garcia M, McNamara P, Gordon T, Kannel W. Morbidity and mortality in diabetics in the Framingham population: sixteen year follow-up. Diabetes 1974; **23**: 105–11.
5. Rosengren A, Welin L, Tsipogianni A, Wilhelmsen L. Impact of cardiovascular risk factors on coronary heart disease and mortality among middle aged diabetic men: a general population study. BMJ 1989; **299**: 1127–31.
6. De Leeus I. Atherogenic profiles in insulin-dependent diabetic patients and their treatment. Europ J Epidemiol 1992; **8**: 125–8.
7. Nikkila E. High density lipoproteins in diabetes. Diabetes 1981; **30**: 82–7.
8. Taskinen MR, Nikkila E, Kuusi T, Harno K. Lipoprotein lipase activity and serum lipoproteins in untreated Type 2 (insulin-independent) diabetes associated with obesity. Diabetologia 1982; **22**: 46–50.
9. Laakso M, Lehto S, Penttila I, Pyorala K. Lipids and lipoproteins predicting coronary heart disease mortality and morbidity in patients with non-insulin-dependent diabetes. Circulation 1993; **88**: 1421–30.

10. Winocour P, Durrington P, Bhatnagar D, Ishola M, Arrol S, Mackness M. Abnormalities of VLDL, IDL, and LDL characterise insulin-dependent diabetes mellitus. Arteriosclerosis and Thrombosis 1992; **12**: 920–8.

11. Velho G, Erlich D, Turpin E, Nell D, Cohen D, Forguel P, *et al.* Lipoprotein(a) in diabetic patients and normoglycemic relatives in familial NIDDM. Diabetes Care 1993; **16**: 742–7.

12. Lehto S, Palomaki P, Miettinen H, Penttila I, Salomaa V, Tuolmilehto J, *et al.* Serum cholesterol and high density lipoprotein cholesterol distributions in patients with acute myocardial infarction and in the general population of Kuopio Province, Eastern Finland. J Int Med 1993; **233**: 179–85.

13. Morrish N, Stevens L, Head J, Fuller J, Jarrett R, Keen H. A prospective study of mortality among middle-aged diabetic patients (the London cohort of the WHO Multinational Study of Vascular Disease in Diabetics) II: associated risk factors. Diabetologia 1990; **33**: 542–8.

14. Dupree E, Meyer M. Role of risk factors in complications of diabetes mellitus. Am J Epidemiol 1980; 112(1): 100–12.

15. Pell S, D'Alonzo CA. Some aspects of hypertension in diabetes mellitus. JAMA 1967; 202(1): 104–10.

16. McKeigue P, Shah B, Marmot M. Relation of central obesity and insulin resistance with high diabetes prevalence and cardiovascular risk in South Asians. Lancet 1991; **337**: 382–6.

17. Kannel W, McGee D. Diabetes and cardiovascular disease: the Framingham Study. JAMA 1979; **337**: 382–6.

18. UK Prospective Diabetes Study Group. UK prospective diabetes study (UKPDS). VIII. Study design, progress and performance. Diabetologia 1991; **34**: 877–90.

19. Fontbonne A, Charles M, Thibult N, Richard JL, Claude JR, Warnet JM, Rosselin GE, Eschwege E, *et al.* Hyperinsulinaemia as a predictor of coronary heart disease mortality in a healthy population: the Paris prospective study, 15-year follow-up. Diabetologia 1991; **34**: 356–61.

20. El-Khawand C, Jamart J, Donckier J, Chatelain B, Lavenne E, Moriau M, Buysschaert M, *et al.* Hemostasis variables in type 1 diabetic patients without demonstrable vascular complications. Diabetes Care 1993; **16**: 1137–45.

21. Balkau B, Eschwege E, Papoz L, Richard JL, Claude JR, Warnet JM, Ducimetiere P, *et al.* Risk factors for early death in non-insulin dependent diabetes and men with known glucose tolerance status. BMJ 1993; **307**: 295–9.

22. UGDP. A study of the effects of hypoglycemic agents on vascular complications in patients with adult-onset diabetes: V. Evaluation of Phenformin therapy. Diabetes 1975; 24: 65–184.

23. The Diabetes Control and Complications Trial Research Group. The effect of intensive treatment of diabetes on the development and progression of long-term complications in insulin-dependent diabetes mellitus. N Engl J Med 1993; **329**: 977–86.

24. Working Group on Hypertension in Diabetes. Statement on hypertension in diabetes. Diabetes Care 1987; **10**: 764–76.

25. Diabetes and Nutrition Study Group of the European Association for the Study of Diabetes—1988. Nutritional recommendations for individuals with diabetes mellitus. Diabetes, Nutrition and Metabolism 1988; **1**: 145–9.

26. Nutritional Recommendations and principles for individuals with diabetes mellitus. Diabetes Care 1991; **14**: 20–7.

27. Steinberg D. Summary of the Proceedings of an NHLBI workshop: antioxidants in the prevention of human atherosclerosis. Circulation 1992; **85**: 2237–44.

28. Bonanome A, Pagnan A, Biffanti S. Effect of dietary monounsaturated and polyunsa-

turated fatty acids on the susceptibility of plasma low density lipoproteins to oxidative modification. Arteriosclerosis and Thrombosis 1992; **12(4)**: 529–33.

29. Riccardi G, Rivallese A. Effects of dietary fibre and carbohydrate on glucose and lipoprotein metabolism in diabetic patients. Diabetes Care 1991; **14**: 1115–25.

30. Mann J, Crooke M, Fear H, *et al.* Guidelines for detection and management of dyslipidaemia. Scientific Committee of the National Heart Foundation of New Zealand. NZ Med J 1993; **106**: 133–41.

31. Jarrett R, McCartney P, Keen H. The Bedford Survey: ten year mortality rates in newly diagnosed diabetics, borderline diabetics and normoglycaemic controls and risk indices for coronary heart disease in borderline diabetics. Diabetologia 1982; **22**: 79–84.

32. Haffner S, Valdez R, Hazuda H, Mitchell B, Morales P, Stern M. Prospective analysis of the insulin-resistance syndrome (syndrome X). Diabetes 1992; **41**: 715–22.

9 Social deprivation

Angela Coulter and David Mant

INTRODUCTION

Socio-economic differences in life expectancy in Britain have been reported since 1921, when the first official statistics linking mortality to social class were published. Figure 9.1 shows standardized mortality ratios (SMRs) for diseases of the circulatory system by social class for the years 1979–83. There is a two-fold mortality gradient in men and almost a four-fold gradient in women between social classes I and V.

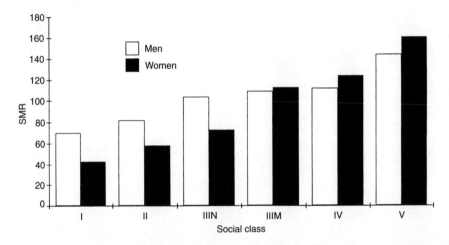

Fig. 9.1 Standardized mortality ratios for CHD by social class in Great Britain 1979–83, men aged 20–64, women aged 20–59. (From British Heart Foundation coronary heart disease statistics 1993; British Heart Foundation, London, 1994. Data from OPCS Occupational mortality decennial supplement, 1986.)

The social class gradient was not apparent earlier this century. Between 1931 and 1951, men in social classes IV and V had slightly lower mortality rates from coronary heart disease than those in social classes I and II. However, mortality rates from coronary heart disease were rising in all social groups, particularly in working class men, and by 1961 men in social classes IV and V had overtaken those in classes I and II. Among women, deaths due to coronary heart disease were more common among those in social classes IV and V during the whole of the time period.[2] Since 1961, the relative disadvantage of those in manual groups appears to have increased in both men and women.[3]

Just as socio-economic status is a powerful predictor of mortality in individual people, census variables also predict geographical variations in cardiovascular mortality in the UK. Figure 9.2 shows standardised mortality ratios for men and women according to the relative deprivation of electoral wards in five representative health regions. The deprivation gradient is apparent for all regions from the most to the least affluent and is greater for men than for women.[4]

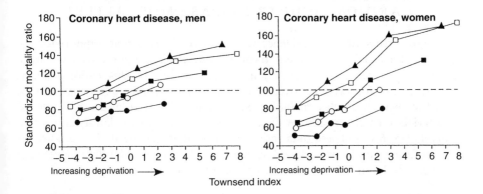

Fig. 9.2 Premature mortality from CHD in relation to degree of social depravation in five regions of England. (From Eames M, Ben-Shlomo Y, Marmot M. Social depravation and premature mortality: regional comparison across England. BMJ 1993; **307**: 1097–107.)

These social inequalities in health arouse considerable political controversy. Wilkinson has shown that trends in the size of socio-economic differentials in mortality over time mimic those of inequalities in income: between 1921 and 1981 widening disparities in the distribution of income were accompanied by increasing mortality differentials and vice-versa.[5] Mortality differentials from 1991 will not be available until the publication of the decennial census supplement in about 1996 but a recent editorial in the British Medical Journal argues that evidence is already emerging that increasing mortality differentials have accompanied the social polarization of the Thatcher years.[6]

This chapter reviews the evidence for the existence of a social gradient in cardiovascular mortality rates and the possible causes of such inequality in health. These issues are important because of what they can reveal about the impact of health service interventions and about policies for prevention. In particular, this chapter reviews:

1. **The strength of the evidence for an association between social class and cardiovascular disease mortality**
2. **The likelihood that this association is artefactual**
3. **The extent to which the association is mediated by identified risk factors including smoking, diet and stress**

4. **The extent to which the association can be explained by factors acting before birth (*in utero*) and in early childhood**
5. **The most appropriate intervention strategy to reduce the social class gradient.**

WHAT IS THE STRENGTH OF THE EVIDENCE FOR AN ASSOCIATION BETWEEN SOCIAL CLASS AND CARDIOVASCULAR DISEASE MORTALITY?

There are three sources of evidence which provide very strong support for the existence of a social class gradient in cardiovascular disease in the UK. The most recent data source is the OPCS longitudinal study.[7] In this national study, individuals are followed up over time and their mortality experience can be related to their social class at initial recruitment rather than at death. Table 9.1 gives SMRs for ischaemic heart disease by social class for the latest time period available (1976–81). These data indicate clearly that the social class gradient is greatest for men and women aged less than 65 and the two-fold difference between social classes I and V is not due to artefact or selection.

Table 9.1   Standardized mortality ratios for ischaemic heart disease 1976–81, according to social class at recruitment to the OPCS longitudinal survey in 1971. Data source: Goldblatt P (ed): OPCS Longitudinal Survey 1971–81—mortality and social organisation. (OPCS; LS6) HMSO, London 1990.

Social class	15–64 years	65–74 years	75+ years
I	67	78	84
II	80	88	87
IIIN	116	89	106
IIIM	95	103	102
IV	109	100	106
V	123	95	99

Another principle source of data on the relationship between socio-economic position and coronary heart disease mortality in Britain are two major cohort studies—the *Whitehall Study* and the *British Regional Heart Study*. In the *Whitehall Study*, 17 530 male Civil Servants working in London were recruited in 1967–9 when a number of baseline measurements were taken. After seven-and-a-half years of follow-up, men in the lowest employment grade had 3.6 times the mortality from coronary heart disease of men in the highest grade.[8] At entry to the study, men in the lower grades were shorter, heavier for their height, had higher blood pressure, higher plasma glucose, smoked more, and reported less leisure time physical activity than men in the higher grades. The only measure of risk factor which exhibited the opposite pattern was plasma cholesterol, which was positively associated with employment grade. Yet after allowance had been made for the influence on mortality of all these factors, the inverse association between employment grade and coronary heart disease mortality was still strong (Fig. 9.3). After ten years follow-up and adjustment for these measured risk factors, the relative risk of death for those in the lowest grade to those in the highest was still 2.1.[9] Since the men in this study were all Civil Servants, the employment grade classification results in more homogeneous groupings than the Registrar General's social class classification used in other studies.

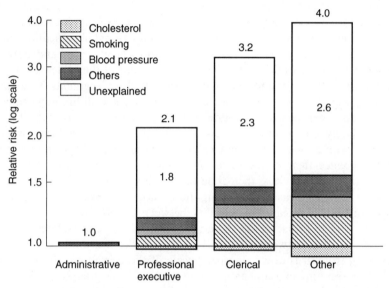

Fig. 9.3 Relative risk of death from CHD according to Civil Service employment grade, and proportions of differences that can be explained statistically by various risk factors. (From Marmot MG, Rose G, Shipley M, Hamilton P. Employment grade and CHD in British Civil Servants. J Epid Comm Health 1978; **32**: 244–9.)

Similar inequalities in ischaemic heart disease incidents were revealed in the *British Regional Heart Study*.[10] In this study the sample was divided into only two groups for social class analysis—manual (working class) and non-manual (middle class). After six years of follow-up of the 7735 middle aged men in this study, the prevalence of ischaemic heart disease at screening was higher among manual workers than among men in middle class occupation; the manual to non-manual ratio was 1.44 unadjusted and 1.24 after adjustment for blood pressure, body mass index, leisure time exercise, and smoking.

The third source of data is from military records—the army, like the Civil Service, is easily stratified into relatively homogeneous groups with regard to income and social position. A study of coronary heart disease mortality in the British army found SMRs of 33 for direct entry officers and 205 for junior soldiers.[11] The death rates among soldiers under 40 were significantly higher than their civilian counterparts, and this may be accounted for by high smoking rates due to the availability of cheap cigarettes at that time, despite the fact there is fairly rigorous health surveillance at entry to the forces and during military service, and all ranks are required to keep fit and to participate in regular exercise programmes.

IS THE SOCIAL GRADIENT ARTEFACTUAL?

Social class is a complex concept. Although it is a commonly used term, there are disagreements about its meaning and about the best way to measure it. The usual method is to use occupation as an indicator, but the concept is broader than simply the skill level or job status implied by an occupational classification. Social class embraces income, wealth, housing, education, social origin and networks, life-style, and cultural outlook. The best known review of the evidence on inequalities and health adopted the following definition of class: 'segments of the population sharing broadly similar types and levels of resources, with broadly similar styles of living and some shared perception of their collective condition'.[12] It is clear that there is likely to be a complex inter-relationship between social class and the risk of disease: people's social class may reflect their genetic predisposition to disease and may influence their exposure to risk factors, their preventive behaviour, their access to health services, their time to recovery, and their likelihood of survival.

Social class as measured by occupation is not static: occupational change results in a considerable degree of mobility between the Registrar General's six social classes. An additional factor, therefore, which has to be considered when assessing the relationship between class and disease, is the possibility of selection effects resulting from drift down the social scale of those in ill health as well as genetic selection resulting in a concentration of those with the greatest predisposition to ill health in the lowest classes. There may also be statistical problems inherent in the official figures on social class differences in mortality rates. There is the possibility of a numerator–denominator bias arising from differential recording of social class at the census and on death certificates; the data may be inaccurately recorded; the definitions and classification systems may change over time; and, because the occupational groupings are so heterogeneous, they may mask a stronger effect which would be apparent when comparing more homogeneous groups.

However there is no evidence from the studies cited of a strong selection effect. The *OPCS Longitudinal Study* excludes the possibility of downward social mobility due to ill health during the duration of the study. The authors of the *Whitehall Study* considered the possibility of selection at entry to the study since it was known that some men had entered the lowest Civil Service grade following a period of ill health: separate analyses of the data for those who were symptom free and for those with disease at entry to the study revealed the same social class trend, leading the authors to discount health selection as an important factor. The differences in height between the grades might point to an effect of genetic selection or childhood nutrition, but the association between grade and mortality was largely independent of the differences in height. This issue is explored in more detail later in this chapter.

TO WHAT EXTENT CAN THE GRADIENT BE
EXPLAINED BY THE TRADITIONAL RISK FACTORS?

Aspects of individual life-style, such as smoking, lack of exercise, and unhealthy dietary habits, clearly make a considerable contribution to the social class inequality. All of these risk factors are more common among those in lower social classes.[13] However, researchers disagree on the extent to which the traditional risk factors for coronary heart disease can account for all of the class difference in risk. The *Whitehall Study* group's finding that the known risk factors could account for only 40 per cent of the difference between the highest and lowest grades led the authors to conclude that there may be other important risk factors for coronary heart disease, as yet undefined and measured, which are associated with socio-economic position. In addition, further analysis of the *Whitehall Study* using a combination of socio-economic indicators (employment grade and car ownership) found a much greater excess risk of cardiovascular disease death among the lower group which could not be explained by risk factor prevalence, including smoking.[14]

In contrast, the *British Regional Heart Study* found only 24 per cent excess risk among the manual classes as against those in non-manual occupations after adjustment for blood pressure, obesity, leisure time exercise, and smoking. This difference was only marginally significant and the authors concluded that cigarette smoking is by far the most important risk factor when considering social differences in ischaemic heart disease. They considered it unlikely that there could be undiscovered risk factors associated with social class, arguing that a single measurement of risk factors at screening is inadequate for assessing the effect of unhealthy behaviours over a lifetime. The weakness in this argument is that the *British Regional Heart Study* divided the population into only two broad manual and non-manual groups and it is likely that the social class effect would have been more apparent if the sample had been stratified into a larger number of socio-economic groups.

Recent studies have attempted to resolve this debate by attempting to identify other intervening variables, including psycho social factors such as stress, associated with type of occupation, unemployment, or lack of social support (see Chapter 7).[15–17] Markowe, *et al.* in 1985 reported a relationship between social status and fibrinogen concentration which was independent of smoking status but was related to a measure of job stress.[18] A positive relationship between social class and haemostatic factors (fibrinogen, viscosity, and clotting time) was also reported from the *Caerphilly and Speedwell Studies* but this effect was lost after adjustment for smoking.[19]

IS CARDIOVASCULAR MORTALITY DETERMINED BY
EVENTS IN UTERO OR EARLY CHILDHOOD?

The most exciting recent research into the aetiology of cardiovascular disease has come from Professor David Barker's group in Southampton. They have reported the results of follow-up studies of people identified from maternity records which indicate that low growth rates *in utero* and during infancy are associated with high death rates from cardiovascular disease. Follow-up of 1586 men born in a maternity hospital in Sheffield during 1907–25 show that death rates from cardiovascular disease fell progressively with increase in weight, head circumference and ponderal index (weight/length^2) at birth.[20] Similarly, follow-up of 5654 men born in Hertfordshire during 1911–30 show death rates from coronary heart disease almost three times higher among those who weighed 8 kg. or less at age one year than among those who weighed 12 kg. or more.[21]

This specific relationship between cardiovascular mortality and growth rates *in utero* and early infancy has now been documented consistently in a number of different populations both within and outside the UK. Moreover, the relationships show a consistent gradient and hold not just for cardiovascular disease mortality but also for established risk factors including blood pressure, and plasma concentrations of glucose, insulin, fibrinogen, factor VII, and apolipoprotein B.[22]

The long-term consequences of altered nutrition during foetal life and infancy appear to depend on its timing and its duration. Different patterns of early growth are associated with different adult abnormalities. Babies who are thin at birth (low ponderal index) have a higher incidence of syndrome X—insulin resistance, hypertension, non-insulin dependent diabetes, and lipid disorders.[23] Those who are short in relation to head size exhibit higher plasma fibrinogen concentrations and higher blood pressure.[24]

Critics of the programming hypothesis argue that people whose growth has been impaired *in utero* and during infancy will continue to experience an adverse environment in childhood and adult life. The relationship between infant mortality and subsequent ischaemic heart disease is markedly attenuated after adequate control for socio-economic variables.[25] There is certainly an interaction between early experience and events in later life. The risk of non-insulin dependent diabetes is highest in people who have low weight at birth and during infancy and become obese as adults.[26] However, the relationship between low birth weight and impaired glucose tolerance occurs in each social class and at each level of cigarette smoking, alcohol consumption, and obesity.[27] A study from Eastern Finland found an association between socio-economic conditions during childhood and the presence of ischaemic heart disease in middle age after adjustment for smoking, cholesterol levels, fibrinogen, and serum selenium concentrations. The authors suggested that ischaemic heart disease may develop earlier in those men who experienced adverse conditions in childhood.[28]

Overall, the consistency of the 'programming' evidence and the specificity of the links with cardiovascular risk factors are extremely convincing. Evidence from other countries, such as the Dutch famine in 1944–45, confirm the long-term effect of deprivation of nutrients during gestation. There is also emerging evidence that early nutritional experience sets homeostatic mechanisms which regulate levels of insulin and growth hormone, both of which are closely linked to subsequent cardiovascular mortality. However, recent results from a trial of different nutritional programmes for pre-term babies seem to indicate that levels of major nutrients are in themselves an insufficient explanation for the relationship between birth weight and subsequent blood pressure,[29] and elucidation of the underlying biological mechanism requires further research.

In political terms, it is unproductive to speculate further on the relative contribution of poor nutrition *in utero* and in infancy and of other aspects of social deprivation in later life. The political importance of recognizing the influence of programming in the uterus and in early childhood is that it inconsistent with victim blaming. The fetus and child are not responsible for their own environment. As Barker and his colleagues continue to work to elucidate the biological mechanisms whereby early life experiences affect later life morbidity and mortality, there is already sufficient evidence to show the importance of addressing the social issues of inequality and deprivation at all stages of life as part of an effective prevention strategy.

THE EFFECT OF SOCIAL CLASS—WHAT ARE APPROPRIATE STRATEGIES FOR PREVENTION?

The authors of the Black Report on inequalities in health emphasised the importance of material inequality and pressed the government to provide income support in order to promote the health of mothers and young children, in particular.[12] In recent years, the British Government has preferred to emphasize the importance of individual lifestyle choices and general practitioners have been enlisted to provide life-style advice to adults. The evidence presented in this chapter suggests that the latter approach is unlikely to diminish cardiovascular disease due to socio-economic deprivation. Individuals make few personal choices *in utero* and during early childhood. Life-style behaviour is rooted in cultural values and the ability to deviate from cultural norms is related to educational achievement and social status.

There is direct evidence that an approach to health promotion which ignores socio-economic and psychosocial influences on health, and focuses only on individual life-style choice, widens social inequalities.[30] Smoking rates have declined faster among those in the higher social classes, who appear to be more receptive to health education messages. There is also accumulating evidence that the model of prevention currently embraced in general practice is failing to reach many of those in high risk groups. Three published reports of attendance at preventive health checks from practices in West Lothian, inner city Cardiff, and Oxford[31–33] have all found that people in working class groups are less likely to attend. It is true that a concerted effort by a primary health care team in Stockton-on-Tees resulted in an increased uptake of preventive care services among a deprived population but this was achieved only by intensive intervention involving the entire practice team (see Chapter 18).[34]

Overall, the evidence suggests that interventions focussed on individual patients in primary care are unlikely to succeed in reducing the social class differentials in cardiovascular disease risk. The interaction between socio-economic conditions and individual life-styles may make it harder for those in relatively deprived circumstances to modify their behaviour. A healthy diet can be relatively expensive for those on low income; smoking and alcohol consumption may compensate for stresses of living in a poor environment; and recreational facilities may not be so accessible for those without transport or those who have small children. Even within the individual behaviour change model, successful programmes will need to work towards creating conditions which make it easier for people in all social classes to adopt a health life-style. Such an approach has implications for the whole spectrum of socio-economic policies and cannot be left to health care professionals alone.

SUMMARY

- There is a distinct social gradient in ischaemic heart disease mortality rates which is probably widening. The relationship between low income, social deprivation, and cardiovascular disease is seen consistently between countries, within countries, and over time. Selection of less healthy people into the lower social classes does not account for these differences.
- Unhealthy behaviours, such as smoking, lack of exercise, and unhealthy diet are more prevalent among those in working class groups. There is debate about the extent to which these risk factors, especially smoking, can explain the social class gradient. Most commentators feel that they cannot explain more than 50 per cent of the social inequality in cardiovascular disease.
- Although it is difficult to unravel the effect of deprivation in earlier and later life, there is accumulating evidence that maternal nutrition and growth rates *in utero* and early childhood have a major effect in determining subsequent cardiovascular mortality.
- Although helping patients in lower social classes to stop smoking and ensuring equal access to early diagnosis and treatment of ischaemic heart are laudable objectives, preventive strategies aimed at changing individual behaviour through general practice advice are likely to increase rather than to decrease social inequality. Uptake of preventive procedures can be increased by intensive effort and careful targeting, but those in the lower social classes remain the least likely to attend and to comply.
- The general practitioner's main role in preventing the social gradient in cardiovascular disease is to treat recognized disease effectively (thereby reducing mortality) and to ensure that politicians remain aware of the social inequalities they meet in their practice.

REFERENCES

1. Office of Population Censuses and Surveys. Occupational mortality 1979–80 and 1982–3, Series DS6. London: HMSO, 1986.

2. Marmot MG, Adelstein AM, Robinson N, Rose GA. Changing social class distribution of heart disease. BMJ 1978; **2**: 1109–12.
3. Marmot MG, McDowall ME. Mortality decline and widening social inequalities. Lancet 1986; **2**: 274–6.
4. Eames M, Ben-Shlomo Y, Marmot MG. Social deprivation and premature mortality: regional comparison across England. BMJ 1993; **307**: 1097–102.
5. Wilkinson RG. Class mortality differentials, income distribution and trends in poverty 1921–81. Journal of Social Policy 1989; **18**: 307–35.
6. Davey-Smith G, Egger M. Socio-economic differentials in wealth and health. BMJ 1993; **307**: 1085–6.
7. Goldblatt P (ed). 1971–81 longitudinal study: mortality and social organisation OPCS, LS6. London: HMSO, 1990.
8. Marmot MG, Rose G, Shipley M, Hamilton PJS. Employment grade and coronary heart disease in British civil servants. Journal of Epidemiology and Community Health 1978; **32**: 244–9.
9. Marmot MG, Shipley MJ, Rose G. Inequalities in death—specific explanations of a general pattern? Lancet 1984; **1**: 1003–6.
10. Pocock S, Shaper A, Cook D, Phillip S, Walker M. Social class differences in ischaemic heart disease in British men. Lancet 1987; **ii**: 197–201.
11. Lynch P, Oelman BJ. Mortality from coronary heart disease in the British army compared with the civil population. BMJ 1981; **283**: 405–7.
12. Townsend P, Davidson N, Whitehead M. Inequalities in health: the Black Report and the health divide. London: Penguin, 1988.
13. Blaxter M. Health and lifestyles. London: Tavistock-Routledge, 1990.
14. Davey-Smith G, Shipley MJ, Rose G. Magnitude and causes of socio-economic differentials in mortality: further evidence from the Whitehall Study. J Epidemiol Community Health 1990; **44**: 265–70.
15. Alfredsson L, Spetz CL, Theorell T. Type of occupation and near future hospitalisation for myocardial infarction and some other diagnoses. Int J Epidemiol 1985; **14**: 378–88.
16. Mattiasson I, Lingarde F, Nielsson JA, Theorell T. Threat of unemployment and cardiovascular risk factors: longitudinal study of quality of sleep and serum cholesterol concentrations in men threatened with redundancy. BMJ 1990; **301**: 461–6.
17. Welin L, Tibblin G, Spardsudd K, Tibblin B, Ander-Peciba S, Larsson B, Wilhelmsen L. Prospective study of social influences on mortality. Lancet 1985; **1**: 915–18.
18. Markowe HLJ, Marmot MG, Shipley MJ, Bulpitt CJ, Meade TW, Stirling Y, Vickers MV, Semmence A. Fibrinogen: A possible link between social class and coronary heart disease. BMJ 1985; **291**: 1312–14.
19. Baker IA, Sweetnam PM, Yarnell JWG, Bainton D, Ellwood PC. Haemostatic and other risk factors for ischaemic heart disease and social class: evidence from the Caerphilly and Speedwell studies. Int J Epidemiol 1988; **17**: 759–65.
20. Barker DJP, Osmond C, Simmonds SJ, Wield GA. The relation of head size and thinness at birth to death from cardiovascular disease in adult life. BMJ 1993; **306**: 422–6.
21. Barker DJP, Winter PD, Osmond C, Margetts B, Simmonds SJ. Weight in infancy and death from ischaemic heart disease. Lancet 1989; **2**: 577–80.
22. Barker DJP, Gluckman PD, Godfrey KM, Harding JE, Owens JA, Robinson JS. Foetal nutrition and cardiovascular disease in adult life. Lancet 1993; **341**: 938–41.
23. Barker DJP, Hales CM, Fall CH, Osmond C, Phipps K, Clark PMS. Type 2 diabetes mellitus, hypertension and hyperlipidaemia (syndrome X): relation to reduced foetal growth. Diabetologia 1993; **36**: 62–7.

24. Barker DJP, Meade TW, Fall CHD, *et al.* Relation of foetal and infant growth to plasma fibrinogen and factor 7 concentrations in adult life. BMJ 1992; **304**: 148–52.
25. Ben-Schlomo Y, Davey-Smith G. Deprivation in infancy or in adult life: which is more important for mortality risk? Lancet 1991; **337**: 530–4.
26. Hales CN, Barker DJP, Clarke PMS, Cox LJ, Fall C, Osmond C, *et al.* Foetal and infant growth and impaired glucose tolerance at age 64. BMJ 1991; **303**: 1019–22.
27. Phipps K, Barker DJP, Hales CN, Fall CHD, Osmond C, Clarke PMS. Foetal growth and impaired glucose tolerance in men and women. Diabetologia 1993; **36**: 225–8.
28. Kaplan GA, Salonen JT. Socio-economic conditions in childhood and ischaemic heart disease during middle age. BMJ 1990; **301**: 121–3.
29. Lucas A, Morley R. Does early nutrition in infants born before term programme later blood pressure? BMJ 1994: 309; 304–8.
30. Coulter A. Lifestyles and social class: implications for primary care. J R Coll Gen Pract 1987; **37**: 533–6.
31. Waller D, Agass M, Mant D, Coulter A, Fuller A, Jones L. Health checks in general practice: Another example of inverse care? BMJ 1990; **300**: 1115–18.
32. Pill R, French J, Harding K, Stott NCH. Invitation to attend a health check in a general practice setting: comparison of attenders and non-attenders. J R Coll Gen Pract 1988; **38**: 53–6.
33. Wrench J, Irvine R. Coronary heart disease: account of a preventive clinic in general practice. J R Coll Gen Pract 1984; **34**: 477–81.
34. Marsh GN, Channing. Narrowing of the health gap between a deprived and an endowed community. BMJ 1988; **296**: 173–6.

10 Hormone Replacement Therapy

Edel Daly and Martin Vessey

INTRODUCTION

Diseases of the circulatory system are the leading causes of death and serious illness among post-menopausal women in most developed countries. Epidemiological evidence suggests that endogenous oestrogen plays a role in protecting younger women from coronary heart disease (CHD). First, incidence rates of CHD are substantially higher in men than in women before the menopause, at which point the sex differential begins to diminish.[1] Secondly, among women with premature ovarian failure, higher rates of CHD are seen compared with pre-menopausal women of the same age.[2] The most compelling evidence comes from studies of the effects of replacement oestrogen on cardiovascular disease risk in post-menopausal women. The great majority of studies suggest that treatment is protective against CHD;[3] however, evidence of a protective effect against stroke is less conclusive.

This chapter will consider five main issues concerning the effects of hormone replacement therapy (HRT) on cardiovascular disease:

1. **What are the major shortcomings of studies on HRT and cardiovascular disease?**
2. **What are the possible mechanisms of cardioprotection?**
3. **What is the evidence for a reduction in coronary heart disease risk associated with HRT use?**
4. **What is the evidence supporting a reduction in stroke risk among HRT users?**
5. **Other effects of HRT, including those on breast cancer and osteoporosis.**

WHAT ARE THE MAJOR SHORTCOMINGS OF STUDIES ON HRT AND CARDIOVASCULAR DISEASE?

Numerous qualitative reviews of the epidemiological literature on this topic have been published recently.[4-6] On the basis of the evidence reviewed, many conclude that the use of HRT confers a substantial reduction of up to 50 per cent in the risk of cardiovascular disease. Behind this summary estimate, which has been extensively quoted in the general HRT literature, lies an array of epidemiological observations from over 30 studies measuring a variety of end-points in different populations.

Most of the larger studies have been carried out in the United States and relate to the use of unopposed oestrogen therapy (ORT), which in the United Kingdom is generally only prescribed for women who have undergone hysterectomy. The majority of women who have intact uteri use combined (oestrogen and progestogen) replacement therapy (CRT) and the magnitude of cardioprotection associated with the use of CRT remains a major unresolved issue. Since it is believed that cardioprotection is mediated partially through favourable changes in blood lipid levels, and since many progestogens are capable of diminishing or negating beneficial changes induced by oestrogen, it has been suggested that adding a progestogen may attenuate any cardioprotective effect of oestrogen. Only a handful of studies, however, have examined cardiovascular disease end-points in CRT users, and results have been conflicting.[7-11]

Guidelines published recently by the *American College of Physicians* state that women at increased risk of CHD and those with CHD are likely to benefit from HRT, whether opposed or unopposed oestrogen is used.[12] The validity of the epidemiological data on which these guidelines are based has been challenged by some who argue that results from observational studies may overestimate the cardioprotective effect of oestrogen.[13] With one exception[7] all studies which have looked at cardiovascular disease end-points in relation to HRT use, have been observational in design. Unlike randomized controlled trials, observational studies may not control adequately for biases in selecting women for treatment. It has been suggested that HRT users may be inherently healthier than those who choose to forgo treatment. In view of the evidence relating oral contraceptive use to an increased risk of cardiovascular disease, menopausal women considered to be at high risk may not have been selected for oestrogen treatment in the past.

Despite these shortcomings, case-control and cohort studies provide strong evidence of a cardioprotective effect of treatment. It is the size of this effect which is currently being debated. Those who argue that selection bias may be contributing to the cardioprotection seen in oestrogen users,[13] have estimated a reduction in risk of 15–20 per cent rather than the 50 per cent reduction which is frequently quoted in literature reviews of this topic. Given the prominence of cardiovascular disease in causing death among post-menopausal women, even a 20 per cent reduction in risk would have a major impact on health in this age group.

WHAT ARE THE POSSIBLE MECHANISMS OF CARDIOPROTECTION?

While the mechanism by which oestrogen replacement therapy confers cardioprotection is not fully understood, the effects of treatment on serum lipid and lipoprotein levels provide the most plausible explanation. In general, oestrogens lower total and low-density lipoprotein (LDL) cholesterol, and increase both high-density lipoprotein (HDL) cholesterol and its subfraction, HDL-2, which contributes most to lowering cardiovascular risk.[14,15] Virtually all of the epidemiological data on the cardioprotective effects of oestrogen relate to orally administered conjugated equine oestrogens. The effects of oestrogen on lipoprotein metabolism are however, dependent on the structure of the molecule, the dose administered and on the route of delivery. While some believe that non-oral administration will avoid most of the metabolic side-effects of oestrogen,[16] others argue that for most oestrogens, transdermal delivery will induce favourable lipid changes, albeit to a lesser extent than obtained with oral administration.[5] Clinical evidence suggests that on the whole, non-oral delivery lowers total and LDL cholesterol, while inducing only small increments in HDL cholesterol.[17]

One interesting difference between oral and non-oral modes of delivery is seen in triglycerides. While triglyceride levels are invariably increased by oral oestrogens at doses used for the treatment of vasomotor symptoms or osteoporosis, this negative impact is avoided with other routes of administration.[17] However, it has been reported elsewhere that ethinyl oestradiol and conjugated equine oestrogens appear to increase triglycerides whether the route of delivery is oral or parenteral.[16]

It has been suggested that changes in the HDL/LDL ratio may account for only 30–50 per cent of the protective effect of oestrogen.[4] Other effects may include beneficial changes in arterial blood flow, coagulation and fibrinolysis, and insulin and glucose metabolism.[18,19] Improvements in blood flow may be mediated through the binding of oestrogen to specific receptors in arterial walls, giving rise to increased production of prostacyclin and subsequent vasodilatation. A similar hormone–receptor interaction between oestrogen and platelets circulating in blood may reduce platelet aggregation by decreasing their production of thromboxane A_2.

Results from a large prospective cohort study carried out in the United States showed the beneficial effect of oestrogen on CHD to be primarily among current users.[20] Another recent study found that oestrogen treatment of post-menopausal women can reduce or prevent symptoms of myocardial ischaemia.[21] The authors suggest that a combination of peripheral effects and direct effects on heart and coronary artery function is the most likely mechanism. This is supported by evidence of a reduced risk in oestrogen users of short duration, along with the lower risk seen in current users compared with past users.

Adding a progestogen

Epidemiological data on the effects of combined therapy on cardiovascular disease risk are scarce. Clinical studies indicate that synthetic progestogens currently used in combined preparations tend to oppose the beneficial effects of oestrogen on serum lipid profiles,[14] suggesting that adding a progestogen either sequentially or continuously might reduce the cardioprotection afforded by oestrogen alone. A recent review of this topic however, suggested that with the cyclic use of progestogen in the lowest possible doses, the oestrogenic actions on lipids and lipoproteins can be largely preserved.[22] Also to be considered is the possibility that progestogens may oppose the adverse effect of oral oestrogen on triglyceride levels.[18] Indeed, results from one cross-sectional study measuring triglyceride levels in HRT users and controls suggest that combined therapy could have a more favourable effect overall on lipid profile than unopposed therapy.[23]

The net effect of combined oestrogen and progestogen preparations on plasma lipids and lipoproteins will depend ultimately on the dose and relative potency of the drugs. Progestogens derived from 19-nortestosterone tend to reduce HDL cholesterol, and in higher doses increase LDL cholesterol levels. In contrast, progestogens derived from 17-hydroxyprogesterone, including medroxyprogesterone acetate, exert only minor effects on plasma lipoproteins. However, recently published results from the *Postmenopausal Estrogen-Progestin Interventions (PEPI) Trial*, carried out in the United States, show that the beneficial effect of conjugated oestrogen on HDL cholesterol in post-menopausal women is substantially decreased when medroxyprogesterone acetate is added either cyclically or continuously, while a much smaller reduction in benefit is seen with the cyclic action of micronized progesterone.[24]

Evidence supporting a biologically plausible mechanism by which oestrogen might reduce the risk of stroke is scarce. It has been suggested that oestrogen may reduce risk through a lowering of blood pressure; however, the biological effect of oestrogen on blood pressure is unclear and the results of studies in post-menopausal women are contradictory.[25]

WHAT IS THE EVIDENCE FOR HRT AND REDUCED ISCHAEMIC HEART DISEASE AND STROKE?

Since 1970, over 30 epidemiological studies have looked at cardiovascular disease in relation to HRT use. A reduction in risk has been reported for a variety of end-points including non-fatal and fatal myocardial infarction (MI), fatal CHD, coronary stenosis, and sudden death. In the discussion which follows, studies are considered according to their main end-points (CHD or stroke) and design (case-control, cohort, or cross-sectional). The results from these studies are expressed in terms of relative risks (RR) and in general relate to ever use of oestrogen.

Case-control studies of HRT and coronary heart disease

Case-control studies assessing the effects of oestrogen therapy have inherent problems with both recall bias (cases might be expected to recall use of oestrogens better than controls, which would tend to underestimate a protective effect) and selection bias (would tend to overestimate a protective effect). The use of hospital controls might also tend to underestimate a protective effect of oestrogen, given that physicians are less likely to prescribe HRT to women who are ill. Bearing this in mind, the better designed case-control studies conducted to date provide fairly good evidence of a protective effect of oestrogen.

The most recently published meta-analysis on this topic lists thirteen case-control studies which included CHD as an end-point.[26] Of the seven studies which used community or population control groups, all but one suggested a protective effect of oestrogen use on the risk of CHD (mainly MI) with relative risks ranging between 0.3 and 0.9. The other case-control study not using diseased controls, reported a slight but non-significant increase in risk (RR = 1.09; 95 per cent confidence interval (CI) 0.65–1.82) associated with oestrogen use for a combined end-point of MI and stroke.[8] Of the five case-control studies which used diseased controls, one showed a non-significant reduction of 40 per cent in risk, two showed no protective effect, and the remaining two reported non-significant increases in risk.

Cross-sectional studies of HRT and coronary heart disease

Three cross-sectional studies which assessed the degree of coronary pathology and recent oestrogen use among women undergoing angiography, found relative risks ranging between 0.4 and 0.6. Combining results from the three studies yields a RR of 0.41 (95 per cent CI 0.34–0.50).[3] The large study by Sullivan *et al.*[27] which compared post-menopausal oestrogen use among 1444 cases with 70 per cent arterial stenosis with that in 744 controls (0 per cent stenosis), estimated the odds ratio for coronary artery disease (CAD) for oestrogen users relative to non-users, to be 0.44 (95 per cent CI 0.29–0.67) after adjustment for various risk factors. These findings are corroborated by evidence from a more recent angiographic study which suggests a substantial (87 per cent) reduction in the prevalence of CAD associated with oestrogen use.[28] While these angiographic studies essentially have a case-control design, they avoid the problems of recall bias, response bias, and control selection. However, it may be that oestrogen users are more likely to be sent for angiography than non-users with similar symptoms, which would over-estimate any protective effect associated with oestrogen use.

Cohort studies of HRT and coronary heart disease

The longitudinal cohort studies designed to investigate the relationship between HRT use and risk of cardiovascular disease have yielded results of striking consistency. Fifteen prospective cohort studies are quoted in the most recently published meta-analysis carried out by Grady and colleagues.[26] All but one of these studies showed a protective effect of oestrogen use on various disease end-points (mainly CHD), with relative risks ranging between 0.2 and 0.8. The *Framingham study* which has been criticised for having major methodological weaknesses, one of which was including angina as an end-point, reported a relative risk of 1.8 for all cardiovascular disease.[29] When only MI was considered, the apparent increase in risk was not statistically significant.

Four cohort studies included no internal control group, using instead external population rates for comparison purposes.[9,10,30,31] Three of these yielded relative risks between 0.30 and 0.48 for fatal CHD, all of which were statistically significant, while the study by Falkeborn *et al.*[10] reported a 20–30 per cent reduction in risk of acute myocardial infarction associated with oestrogen use, again, statistically significant. The remaining 11 cohort studies include eight community-based studies,[20,29,32–37] and three studies which were conducted in clinical settings.[38–40] The clinically-based studies yielded the lowest relative risks, which ranged between

0.16 and 0.33.[38,40] The corresponding range for the community-based studies is 0.37 to 0.7,[32,37] with two outliers being the *Rancho Bernardo Study* where after adjustment for risk factors, no protective effect was suggested,[34] and the *Framingham Study*.[29]

One of the largest prospective studies carried out to date, the *Nurses' Health Study*, with a total of 32 317 participants, reported a 40 per cent reduction in the risk of major coronary disease for current oestrogen users (RR = 0.56; 95 per cent CI 0.40–0.80), with a 20 per cent reduction for former oestrogen users (RR = 0.83).[20] This finding, coupled with the absence of a substantial effect of duration of use, suggests that at least part of the mechanism of cardioprotection may be relatively short-lived.

A study carried out by Sullivan *et al.* looked at the effect of oestrogen use on survival in women with angiographically documented coronary artery disease of defined severity.[40] All-cause mortality over a 10-year period was found to be significantly lower in women with coronary artery disease who used oestrogen replacement therapy than in those who never used oestrogen; current oestrogen use was associated with an 84 per cent reduction in the risk for recurrent disease (RR = 0.16; 95 per cent CI 0.04–0.66). The authors conclude that ORT after the menopause prolongs survival when coronary artery disease is present.

Studies of combined HRT and coronary heart disease

Only a handful of studies have looked at the risk of CHD associated with the use of combined oestrogen and progestogen therapy,[7–10] one of which was a randomized controlled trial.[7] In the latter, which included 84 pairs of subjects followed up for 10 years, combined therapy users were found to have a substantial but non-significant reduction in CHD risk (RR = 0.3); however, the small size of this study limits the usefulness of its results. A case-control study by Thompson and colleagues found a slight but non-significant increase in risk among women who had received more than one prescription for combined therapy in the past (RR = 1.16); the end-point however, included stroke as well as myocardial infarction.[8] The most recent evidence to emerge comes from the large Swedish follow-up study in which women prescribed a particular brand of opposed HRT were found to have a significantly lowered RR of acute MI (RR = 0.53; 95 per cent CI 0.30–0.87), a reduction comparable to that seen in women taking oestrogen alone.[10] Despite the lack of an internal comparison group, these results are nevertheless encouraging and lend support to the argument that the use of cyclical progestogen in low doses may largely preserve any cardioprotective effect of oestrogen.

Meta-analyses of HRT and coronary heart disease

The above studies have been reviewed extensively in recent publications, with at least four reviews using meta-analytic techniques to estimate the overall magnitude of effect on CHD risk.[3,26,41,42] While the earliest meta-analysis (based on 18 published studies and 3345 cases) found an overall relative risk of 0.81 (95 per cent CI 0.76–0.85),[41] the other three yielded summary estimates between 0.55 and 0.65, with narrow confidence intervals.

Case-control studies of HRT and stroke

The three case-control studies of post-menopausal oestrogen use and stroke carried out to date, yielded relative risk estimates of between 0.6 and 1.2, all of which were non-significant.[26] Another case-control study which had a combined end-point of myocardial infarction and stroke, found a slight non-significant increase in risk (RR = 1.16).[8]

Cohort studies of HRT and stroke

At least thirteen cohort studies have investigated the possible association between post-menopausal oestrogen use and stroke.[26,11] Apart from the *Framingham Study*[29] which found a significant increase in risk (RR = 2.3), and the study by Petitti and colleagues[43] which reported a small non-significant increase in risk associated with current use (RR = 1.2), all studies showed either a reduction in risk or no change. Five cohort studies reported significant risk reductions with relative risk estimates ranging between 0.24 and 0.9; the former risk estimate however, relates to oestrogen use in relatively young women with hypoestrogenism.[38]

One of the largest of the cohort studies, the *Nurses' Health Study*, yielded results which suggested that neither current nor former use of oestrogen is associated with any change in the risk of stroke.[20] However, women in this cohort were relatively young, and the period of post-menopausal oestrogen use was fairly short. One recently published study showed a decrease in stroke risk which was just significant (RR = 0.69; 95 per cent CI 0.47–1.00).[44] A similar reduction in risk was found among women who had used oestradiol or conjugated oestrogens in a study carried out by Falkeborn and colleagues (RR = 0.72; 95 per cent CI 0.58–0.88).[11] By the end of the six year follow-up period however, the risk of stroke among ever users (20 per cent of whom were current users) had returned to baseline, suggesting that any beneficial effect may be relatively short-lived.

Although some of these cohort studies included women who had used combined oestrogen and progestogen,[9,11,38] only the most recent of these provided a separate risk estimate for combined therapy users.[11] Women prescribed a combined oestradiol-levonorgestrel brand had a 40 per cent decrease in stroke risk (RR = 0.61; 95 per cent CI 0.40–0.88).

Meta-analysis of HRT and stroke

Grady and colleagues combined the results from three case-control studies, and those from seven cohort studies with internal controls, to yield a summary risk estimate of 0.96 (95 per cent CI 0.82–1.13).[26] It is worth noting however, that five cohort studies, all of which had shown reductions in the risk of stroke, were excluded from the meta-analysis because of the lack of an internal control group, or because of inappropriate subject or control groups.[9,30,31,38,39] In addition, results from another cohort study (also with no internal control group), showing beneficial effects on the risk of stroke, have since been published.[11]

OTHER EFFECTS OF HRT, INCLUDING THOSE ON BREAST CANCER AND OSTEOPOROSIS

The effectiveness of HRT in relieving oestrogen deficiency-related symptoms of the menopause has been well established. Decisions about long-term use must involve a careful weighing-up of the reductions in risk of both cardiovascular disease and osteoporosis against the possible adverse effect on breast cancer risk.[26,45,46] A recent cost-effectiveness study of HRT concluded that in terms of net health benefits, the reduction in cardiovascular disease would have greatest impact on the risk-benefit equation and would overshadow any small increase in breast cancer which may be associated with long-term use.[46] Assuming a 50 per cent reduction in CHD risk and a 25 per cent decrease in stroke risk over a 10 year treatment period (starting at age 50), and persisting for five years post-treatment, the estimated average increase in life expectancy is 11 weeks. With the more modest assumption of decreases of 25 per cent and 12½ per cent in the risks of CHD and stroke respectively, the estimated net health benefit is five weeks.

HRT and breast cancer

Studies of the effect of post-menopausal oestrogen on breast cancer have suggested a modest increase in risk associated with long-term use. This side-effect may however, heavily influence women's perceptions of the overall balance of benefits and risks, and may reduce the level of acceptability of treatment. To date no less than six meta-analyses have been published on the relationship between oestrogen use and breast cancer. Those which looked specifically at long-term use suggest an increase of about 30 per cent in risk following 15 years of use.[26,47–49] While all meta-analyses consistently rule out any effect of ever use of oestrogen on breast cancer risk, the most recent suggests a significant increase in risk associated with current use (RR 1.40; 95 per cent CI 1.20–1.63).[49] The authors suggest that a component of the increased risk associated with long-term use may be caused by a higher proportion of current users in the long-duration categories.

One meta-analysis also considered the association between combined therapy use and breast cancer risk, specifically addressing the hypothesis that the addition of a progestogen to oestrogen therapy reduces the risk of breast cancer.[49] While a previous meta-analysis[48] had suggested that combined therapy was not associated with an increase in breast cancer risk, the analysis by Colditz *et al.*[49] yielded comparable relative risk estimates for users of combined preparations and users of unopposed oestrogen. These two analyses however, were based on only a handful of studies.

HRT and osteoporosis

The other important long-term benefit of HRT use, for which there is both good observational and clinical evidence, is its effect in reducing the risk of osteoporosis. Epidemiological studies have consistently demonstrated an association between the use of oestrogen replacement and a reduction in the risk of fracture of the hip, spine, and radius. A study carried out by Weiss and colleagues suggested a 50 per cent reduction in the risk of hip fracture following five years use of oestrogen.[50] More recently, a similar reduction in fracture risk was reported by Swedish researchers, although this benefit of treatment was found to be concentrated in women who received potent oestrogens before the age of 60.[51] Furthermore, among this group of women, 40 per cent of oestrogen use was opposed by a progestogen, a finding which corroborates clinical evidence that combined regimens are effective in preserving bone mineral density.[52] Until very recently, the issue of duration of effect after treatment is stopped had not been directly addressed. New evidence from the *Framingham Study* suggests that in women aged 75 years and over who used oestrogen for at least seven years in the past, the residual protective effect of treatment on fracture risk is negligible.[53] This has worrying implications for oestrogen's role in preventing the burden of osteoporotic hip fractures, given that the majority of these occur in women over the age of 75.

CONCLUSIONS

- Almost all of the evidence concerning the long-term effect of HRT on cardiovascular disease comes from observational studies in women using unopposed oestrogen therapy.
- On the basis of available evidence it is probable that HRT provides some protection against coronary heart disease but the reduction in risk is likely to be much more modest than the 50 per cent frequently quoted. The evidence to support a beneficial effect on stroke is less conclusive.
- The level of protection is likely to depend on the type, dose, and route of delivery of both the oestrogen and progestogen components of therapy.
- The potential of HRT as a lipid lowering medication in the treatment of hyperlipidaemic post-menopausal women needs to be clarified.
- Further research is needed to establish the place of HRT in the secondary prevention of coronary heart disease.
- The balance of evidence justifies the use of unopposed oestrogen replacement to reduce the burden of cardiovascular disease in hysterectomized women; however, available data relating to the effects of combined oestrogen-progestogen preparations are insufficient to recommend treatment of non-hysterectomized women for this purpose.

REFERENCES

1. Gordon T, Kannel WB, Hjortland MC, McNamara PM. Menopause and coronary heart disease: the Framingham study. Ann Intern Med 1978; **89**: 157–61.
2. Witteman J, Groben D, Kok F, Hofman A, Valkenberg A. Increased risk of atherosclerosis in women after the menopause. BMJ 1989; **298**: 642–4.
3. Stampfer MJ, Colditz GA. Estrogen replacement therapy and coronary heart disease: a quantitative assessment of the epidemiolgic evidence. Preventive Medicine 1991; **20**: 47–63.
4. Lobo RA. Cardiovascular implications of oestrogen replacement therapy. Obstet Gynecol 1990; **75** (suppl): 18s-25s.
5. Sitruk-Ware R. Do estrogens protect against cardiovascular disease? In Sitruk-Ware R, Utian WH, ed. The menopause and hormonal replacement therapy: facts and controversies. New York: Marcel Dekker, 1991: pp. 161–79.
6. Wren BG. The effect of oestrogen on the female cardiovascular system. Med J Aust 1992; **157**: 204–8.
7. Nachtigall LE, Nachtigall RH, Nachtigall RD, Beckman EM. Estrogen replacement therapy II: a prospective study in the relationship to carcinoma and cardiovascular and metabolic problems. Obstet Gynecol 1979; **54**: 74–9.
8. Thompson SG, Meade TW, Greenberg G. The use of hormonal replacement therapy and the risk of stroke and myocardial infarction in women. J Epidemiol Community Health 1989; **43**: 173–8.
9. Hunt K, Vessey M, McPherson K. Mortality in a cohort of long-term users of hormone replacement therapy: an updated analysis. Br J Obstet Gynaecol 1990; **97**: 1080–6.
10. Falkeborn M, Persson I, Adami H-O, Reinhold B, Eaker E, Lithell H, *et al*. The risk of acute myocardial infarction after oestrogen and oestrogen-progestogen replacement. Br J Obstet Gynaecol 1992; **99**: 812–18.
11. Falkeborn M, Persson I, Terent A, Adami H-O, Lithell H, Bergstrom R. Hormone replacement therapy and the risk of stroke: Follow-up of a population-based cohort in Sweden. Arch Intern Med 1993; **153**: 1201–9.
12. American College of Physicians. Guidelines for counseling postmenopausal women about preventive hormone therapy. Ann Intern Med 1992; **117**: 1038–41.
13. Meade TW, Berra A. Hormone replacement therapy and cardiovascular disease. Br Med Bull 1992; 48 (2): 276–308.
14. Bush TL, Miller VG. Effects of pharmacologic agents used during menopause: impact on lipids and lipoproteins. In Mishell DR Jr, ed. Menopause: physiology and pharmacology. Chicago: Year Book Medical Publishers, 1987: pp. 187–208.
15. LaRosa JC. Women, lipoproteins and cardiovascular disease risk. Int J Fertil 1992; **37** (suppl 2): 63–71.
16. Basdevant A. Steroids and lipid metabolism: Mechanism of action. Int J Fertil 1992; **37** (suppl 2): 93–7.
17. Samsioe G. Lipid profiles in estrogen users: is there a key marker for the risk of cardiovascular disease? In Sitruk-Ware R, Utian WH, ed. The menopause and hormonal replacement therapy: facts and controversies. New York: Marcel Dekker, 1991: pp. 181–200.
18. Crook D, Stevenson JC. Commentary: progestogens, lipid metabolism and hormone replacement therapy. Br J Obstet Gynaecol 1991; **98**: 749–50.
19. Bourne T, Hillard TC, Whitehead MI, Crook D, Campbell S. Oestrogens, arterial status and postmenopausal women. Lancet 1990; **335**: 1470–1 (letter).

20. Stampfer MJ, Colditz GA, Willett WC, Manson JE, Rosner B, Speizer FE, Hennekens CH. Postmenopausal estrogen therapy and cardiovascular disease: ten-year follow-up from the Nurses' Health Study. New Engl J Med 1991; **325**: 756–62.

21. Rosano GMC, Sarrel PM, Poole-Wilson PA, Collins P. Beneficial effect of oestrogen on exercise-induced myocardial ischaemia in women with coronary artery disease. Lancet 1993; **342**: 133–6.

22. Jensen J. Effects of sex steroids on serum lipids and lipoproteins. Bailliere's Clinical Obstetrics and Gynaecology 1991; **5**: 867–87.

23. Nabulsi AA, Folsom AR, White A, Patsch W, Heiss G, Wu K, Szklo M. Association of hormone-replacement therapy with various cardiovascular risks factors in postmenopausal women. N Engl J Med 1993; **328**: 1069–75.

24. The Writing Group for the PEPI Trial. Effects of estrogen or estrogen/progestin regimens on heart disease risk factors in postmenopausal women. The Postmenopausal Estrogen/Progestin Interventions (PEPI) Trial. JAMA 1995; **273**; 199–208.

25. Hazzard WR. Estrogen replacement and cardiovascular disease: serum lipids and blood pressure effects. Am J Obstet Gynecol 1989; **161**: 1847–53.

26. Grady D, Rubin SM, Petitti DB, Fox CS, Black D, Ettinger B, Ernster VL, Cummings SR. Hormone therapy to prevent disease and prolong life in postmenopausal women. Ann Intern Med 1992; **117**: 1016–37.

27. Sullivan JM, Vander Zwaag R, Lemp GF, Hughes JP, Maddock V, Kroetz FW, et al. Postmenopausal estrogen use and coronary atherosclerosis. Ann Intern Med 1988; **108**: 358–63.

28. Hong MK, Romm PA, Reagan K, et al. Effects of estrogen replacement therapy on serum lipid values and angiographically defined coronary artery disease in postmenopausal women. Am J Cardiol 1992; **69**: 176–8.

29. Wilson PWF, Garrison RJ, Castelli WP. Postmenopausal estrogen use, cigarette smoking, and cardoivascular morbidity in women over 50: the Framingham Study. N Engl J Med 1985; **313**: 1038–43.

30. Byrd BF Jr, Burch JC, Vaughn WK. The impact of long term estrogen support after hysterectomy. A report of 1016 cases. Ann Surg 1977; **185**: 574–80.

31. MacMahon B. Cardiovascular disease and non-contraceptive oestrogen therapy. In Oliver MF, ed. Coronary heart disease in young women. New York: Churchill Livingstone, 1978: pp. 197–207.

32. Bush TL, Barrett-Connor E, Cowan LD, Criqui MH, Wallace RB, Suchindran CM, et al. Cardiovascular mortality and noncontraceptive use of estrogen in women: results from the Lipid Research Clinics Program Follow-up Study. Circulation 1987; **75**: 1102–9.

33. Petitti DB, Perlman JA, Sidney S. Noncontraceptive estrogens and mortality: long-term follow-up of women in the Walnut Creek Study. Obstet Gynecol 1987; **70**: 289–93.

34. Criqui MH, Suarez L, Barrett-Connor E, McPhillips J, Wingard DL, Garland C. Postmenopausal estrogen use and mortality. Results from a prospective study in a defined homogenous community. Am J Epidemiol 1988; **128**: 606–14.

35. Avila MH, Walker AM, Jick H. Use of replacement estrogens and the risk of myocardial infarction. Epidemiol 1990; **1**: 128–33.

36. Henderson BE, Paganini-Hill A, Ross RK. Decreased mortality in users of estrogen replacement therapy. Arch Intern Med 1991; **151**: 75–8.

37. Wolf PH, Madans JH, Finucane FF, Higgins M, Kleinman JC. Reduction of cardiovascular disease-related mortality among postmenopausal women who use hormones: evidence from a national cohort. Am J Obstet Gynecol 1991; **164**: 489–94.

38. Hammond CB, Jelovsek FR, Lee KL, Creasman WT, Parker RT. Effects of long-term estrogen replacement therapy. I. Metabolic effects. Am J Obstet Gynecol 1979; **133**: 525–36.

39. Lafferty FW, Helmuth DO. Post-menopausal estrogen replacement: the prevention of osteoporosis and systemic effects. Maturitas 1985; **7**: 147–59.
40. Sullivan JM, Vander Zwaag R, Hughes JP, Maddock V, Kroetz FW, Ramanathan KB, *et al.* Estrogen replacement and coronary artery disease. Effect on survival in post-menopausal women. Arch Intern Med 1990; **150**: 2557–62.
41. La Vecchia C, Volpi A. 1988. Patologia cardiovasculare e climaterio femminile: conoscenze disponibili e problemi metodologici. In Bottiglioni F, de Aloysio D, ed. II Climaterio Femminile: Esperienze Italiane di un Decennio. Bologna: Monduzzi Editore, 1988: pp. 219–22.
42. Bush TL. Extraskeletal effects of estrogen and the prevention of artherosclerosis. Osteoporosis International 1991; **2**: 5–11.
43. Petitti DB, Wingerd J, Pellegrin F, Ramcharan S. Risk of vascular disease in women. Smoking, oral contraceptives, noncontraceptive estrogens and other factors. JAMA 1979; **242**: 1150–4.
44. Finucane FF, Madans JH, Bush TL, Wolf PH, Kleinman JC. Decreased risk of stroke among postmenopausal hormone users: results from a national cohort. Arch Intern Med 1993; **153**: 73–9.
45. Adami H-O. Long-term consequences of estrogen and estrogen-progestin replacement. Cancer Causes and Control 1992; **3**: 83–90.
46. Daly E, Roche M, Barlow D, Gray A, McPherson K, Vessey M. Hormone replacement therapy: an analysis of benefits, risks and costs. Brit Med Bull 1992; **48**: 368–400.
47. Steinberg KK, Thacker SB, Smith SJ, *et al.* A meta-analysis of the effect of estrogen replacement therapy on the risk of breast cancer. JAMA 1991; **265**: 1985–90.
48. Sillero-Arenas M, Delgado-Rodriguez M, Rodigues-Canteras R, Bueno-Cavanillas A, Galvez-Vargas R. Menopausal hormone replacement therapy and breast cancer: A meta-analysis. Obstet Gynecol 1992; **79**: 286–94.
49. Colditz GA, Egan KM, Stampfer MJ. Hormone replacement therapy and risk of breast cancer: results from epidemiolgic studies. Am J Obstet Gynecol 1993; **168**: 1473–80.
50. Weiss NS, Ure CL, Ballard JH, Williams AR, Daling JR. Decreased risk of fractures of the hip and lower forearm with postmenopausal use of oestrogen. N Engl J Med 1980; **303**: 1195–8.
51. Naessen T, Persson I, Adami H-O, Bergstrom R, Bergkvist L. Hormone replacement therapy and the risk for first hip fracture—a prospective, population-based cohort study. Ann Intern Med 1990; **113**: 95–103.
52. Munk-Jensen N, Pors Nielsen S, Obel Eb, Eriksen PB. Reversal of postmenopausal vertebral bone loss by oestrogen and progestogen: a double blind placebo-controlled study. BMJ 1988; **296**: 1150–2.
53. Felson DT, Zhang Y, Hannan MT, Kiel DP, Wilson PWF, Anderson JJ. The effect of postmenopausal estrogen therapy on bone density in elderly women. N Engl J Med 1993; **329**: 1141–6.

11 Haemostasis

Chris Silagy

Cigarette smoking, hypertension, and lipid abnormalities are traditionally regarded as the major risk factors associated with the development of cardiovascular disease. However, in recent years the list of other potential risk factors has grown substantially; a review in 1981 identified 246 risk factors.[1] Two reasons may help explain this increase. Firstly, the traditional risk factors alone do not entirely account for the wide variation observed in the rate of cardiovascular disease within and between communities. Secondly, there has been a marked improvement in the understanding of the pathogenesis of cardiovascular disease.

A number of haemostatic parameters have emerged as possible important cardiovascular risk factors in their own right:

Haemostatic factors implicated as possible cardiovascular risk factors

Fibrinogen	Factor VIII:C
Fibrinolytic activity	Plasminogen
Factor II-VII-X activity	Plasma viscosity
Factor VII	

Of these, fibrinogen, factors VII, VIII, and plasminogen-activator have received the most attention.[2] This is not surprising given that clotting factors, blood flow, and the pliability of red blood cells are all known to be important in the evolution of ischaemic vascular diseases.[3] Furthermore, there is now an accumulating body of epidemiological evidence to support these claims, largely based on prospective studies.[4-10]

This chapter examines the role and importance of haemostatic factors in cardiovascular disease by addressing four questions:

1. **Is there a biologically plausible basis for haemostatic parameters being involved in the pathogenesis of cardiovascular disease?**
2. **Is there good epidemiological evidence to support various haemostatic parameters as being independent risk factors for cardiovascular disease ?**
3. **Is there evidence for reduction in risk following appropriate intervention(s) targeted at these parameters ?**
4. **Assuming that some of the haemostatic parameters are shown to be independent risk factors, what is their relevance and applicability to routine clinical practice ?**

BIOLOGICAL PLAUSIBILITY

Atherogenesis is a complex process mediated by a number of different mechanisms.[11,12] Haemostatic factors have been implicated as playing a role at various key stages.[12] For example, fibrinogen is thought to be involved in the early stages of plaque formation.[13,14] Fibrinogen, fibrin and other fibrinogen degradation products have all been found deposited in the initial intimal lesion.[13] It is postulated that some or all of these products may cause damage to the endothelial cells lining vessel walls, stimulate the proliferation of vascular smooth muscle cells, and release substances which cause inflammatory cells to appear and provoke further cell proliferation.[12] In addition, fibrinogen may itself contribute to the thickening of the intimal layer.[13]

,As the atheromatous lesion develops, fibrinogen continues to play an important role by influencing platelet adhesion and aggregation. The platelet aggregates which are formed become incorporated into the developing lesion. To produce clinically manifest disease requires additional platelet deposition and thrombus formation. Haemostatic factors which are involved in the coagulation sequence play an important role in this latter process.[12]

An increase in the blood viscosity will favour local thrombosis, particularly in arteries which are already narrowed.[12] The blood viscosity is principally determined by the haematocrit, aggregability of the blood, viscosity of the plasma component, and the fibrinogen concentration.[10] Hence, any increase in the fibrinogen concentration will tend to produce a hypercoagulable state resulting in a favourable environment for thrombus formation.[12]

EPIDEMIOLOGICAL EVIDENCE

Association with other risk factors

As early as the mid 1960s it was demonstrated that the concentration of fibrinogen rises after a stroke or myocardial infarction.[15,16] This occurs because fibrinogen is an acute phase protein, the concentration of which increases in response to any inflammation or tissue necrosis.[14] However, by the early 1970s, clinical observations emerged which suggested that the presence of a high level of plasma fibrinogen long before the onset of a cardiovascular event may itself be involved in determining the subsequent course of various ischaemic diseases (including ischaemic heart disease, ischaemic cerebrovascular disease, and peripheral vascular disease).[17,18] The initial evidence to support this hypothesis was the strength of the association seen in cross-sectional analyses between conventional risk factors (such as age, smoking, hyperlipidemia, hypertension, and obesity) and various haemostatic factors.

The *Northwick Park Heart Study*,[2] studied a total of 1601 white men and 707 white women aged 18–64 years who were recruited between 1972 and 1978 from three defined occupational groups in north-west London. From analysis of the baseline data it became clear that fibrinolytic activity (FA), which is a measure of the ability to breakdown clots (expressed as 100/dilute clot lysis time in hours) was significantly reduced among smokers, those in higher social classes, and the obese. In both sexes fibrinolytic activity increased with exercise and alcohol consumption. Furthermore, fibrinolytic activity appeared to be greater in women using oral contraceptives than those who were not. As expected, fibrinogen concentrations were found to behave in the reverse way; concentrations rose with age, obesity, oral contraceptive use, and smoking.

Some of these findings have been confirmed in subsequent analyses based on different populations. The correlation between five haemostatic factors and the three traditional risk factors (hypertension, smoking and cholesterol) was examined in a group of 792 Swedish men (all aged 54 years) from Gothenburg.[15] The level of fibrinogen was positively related to all three of the traditional risk factors. However, unlike the *Northwick Park Heart Study*, fibrinolytic activity was unrelated to any of the conventional risk factors, as was factor VIII coagulant activity. The *Swedish Study* also found plasminogen and factor II-VII-X activity (which measures the interaction between these factors) to be positively and significantly correlated with the level of serum cholesterol. Factor II-VII-X activity was also found to be positively correlated with the systolic blood pressure and negatively associated with smoking, although the latter of these failed to reach statistical significance.

The *Framingham Study* provides even more persuasive evidence linking cigarette smoking and fibrinogen levels.[7] Kannel and his co-workers observed that the level of fibrinogen in ex-smokers was similar to that in non-smokers, suggesting a reversible effect. The fibrinogen concentration among women in the *Framingham Study* was also significantly related to most of the other cardiovascular risk factors (haematocrit, cholesterol, glucose, relative weight and blood pressure). In men, other than the relationship observed between smoking, fibrinogen was only related to blood pressure.

In the *Scottish Heart Health Study*[19] of 8824 middle aged men and women fibrinogen was positively associated with age, smoking, total cholesterol, and body mass index, and negatively associated with alcohol consumption. Early menopause and the level of systolic blood pressure were positively associated with the concentration of fibrinogen in women; a history of contraceptive pill use was negatively associated with the level of fibrinogen.

More recently, several other cardiovascular risk factors such as exercise[20] and stress,[21] have been shown to be associated with the level of fibrinogen. This raises the possibility that fibrinogen is either causally involved in the mechanism by which these risk factors exert their effect or is acting as a confounder. The difficulty is to distinguish between these two alternatives. For example, the apparent relationship seen in some studies between exercise and fibrinogen concentration may simply reflect differences in smoking rates.[19]

Relationship between haemostatic factors and cardiovascular disease outcome

Several case-control studies have shown that people either with proven coronary heart disease or extensive angiographic evidence suggestive of atheromatous disease[22,23] are more likely to have a raised fibrinogen concentration than age-sex matched controls. In the *Oxfordshire Community Stroke Project*,[24] the odds ratio for developing a transient ischaemic attack or minor ischaemic stroke was 1.8

among people with elevated levels of fibrinogen after adjustment for all other risk factors. Other case-control studies, however, have failed to confirm these findings.[25,26] Part of the reason for this discrepancy may reflect the observation that fibrinogen concentration rises following a stroke or infarct which may affect interpretation of results, depending on the time of measurement. Although this may be less of a problem among patients who experience a transient ischaemic episode or minor stroke, it is conceivable that some distortion of haemostatic parameters may still occur.

More powerful evidence mainly linking fibrinogen but also several of the other haemostatic parameters to the development of cardiovascular disease comes from long-term cohort studies, of which at least five have been published to date (Table 11.1). Of these, the *Northwick Park Heart Study*[2,6] has probably been the most publicized. The final data from this study, published in 1986,[6] were based on a sub-group of 1511 white men aged between 40 and 64 years at the time of recruitment who had been followed for a mean duration of 6.7 years. A total of 109 first major events of ischaemic heart disease had been recorded, of which 68 were fatal. Among those people with a fibrinogen level in the upper third of the population there was a three fold increase in the risk of ischaemic heart disease compared with those in the lowest third of the population. A similar increase in the risk of ischaemic heart disease was seen when factor VII activity was grouped in the same way.

Even after the influence of other risk factors had been taken into account, using multiple logistic regression techniques, a strong independent association was found between the levels of fibrinogen, factor VII and the occurrence of ischaemic heart disease. This association was particularly marked during the first five years of the study when these two factors appeared to play a more important role than even the serum cholesterol. However, after five years the picture changed slightly. The importance of factor VII (but not fibrinogen) as an independent risk factor declined and the contribution of serum cholesterol rose.

One of the interesting questions raised by the *Northwick Park Study* was the possible role of factor VII in the causal pathway leading to ischaemic heart disease since it has been shown that high dose oestrogen-based contraceptives increase the levels of factor VII.[6] This may help account for the association seen between usage of these contraceptives and the increased rate of ischaemic heart disease.

Many other large prospective studies have provided further evidence to support and even extend the claims made by the *Northwick Park Study* about the importance of haemostatic factors as independent risk factors for cardiovascular disease. In the *Gothenburg Study* from Sweden, the fibrinogen concentration was found not only to be strongly related to the occurrence of myocardial infarction, but also to stroke.[4] However, unlike the *Northwick Park Study* the association between fibrinogen and myocardial infarction was weakened when the contribution of other risk factors were also taken into account using multivariate techniques. None of the other haemostatic parameters examined (factor II-VII-X, factor VIII: C, plasminogen, and fibrinolytic activity) were found to be significantly associated with the incidence of either end-point.[4]

Table 11.1 Prospective cohort studies linking haemostatic parameters to the development of cardiovascular disease

Study	Population	Follow-up duration	Haemostatic factors studied	Principal results
Gothenburg Study[4] (1984)	792 men 54 years at entry	13.5 years	Fibrinogen Fibrinolytic Activity Plasminogen Factor II-VII-X Factor VIII:C	Fibrinogen only was an independent risk factor for both MI and stroke (although only the latter persisted when other risk factors were taken into account). Results were partly explained by differences in smoking habits.
Leigh[5] (1985)	297 men 40–69 years	7.3 years	Fibrinogen	Positively related to risk of MI. Confirmed by multivariate analyses.
Northwick park study[6] (1986)	1511 white men 40–64 years at entry	10 years	Fibrinogen Factor VII	Both clotting factors were independent predictors of CVD risk within 5 years (at least as strong as cholesterol). After this time only fibrinogen retained its predictive power.
Framingham study[7] (1987)	1315 men and women 47–49 years	12 years	Fibrinogen	Fibrinogen was a risk factor for CVD but diminishes with age. Strongly linked to smoking. May provide another mechanism for the CVD effect of smoking.
Caerphilly & Spedwell[8] Collaborative Heart Disease Study (1991)	4860 men and women 45–59 years at entry	3–5 years	Fibrinogen Plasma viscosity White blood cell count	All 3 parameters are important. WBC count is definitely an independent risk factor as is either fibrinogen or viscosity, or possibly both.
Gottingen risk, incidence and prevalence study[9] (1992)	5239 men 40–60 years	5 years	Fibrinogen	Fibrinogen was a strong predictor for CV risk in univariate analysis; weaker in a multivariate model after accounting for LDL, but still statistically significant.
Prospective cardiovascular Munster study[10] (1987)	1674 men 40–65 years	2 years	Fibrinogen	Higher CVD event rate in higher compared with lower fibrinogen tertile. Non-significant due to small numbers of events. Final study results not yet available.

Abbreviations used:
MI – myocardial infarction; CVD – cardiovascular disease; LDL - low density lipoprotein; WBC – white blood cell; NA – not applicable
Year in brackets represents the year in which the final results of the study were published.

A small study in general practice by Stone and Thorp[5] followed 297 men for an average duration of 7.3 years. The fibrinogen concentration correlated significantly with the subsequent incidence of myocardial infarction; multivariate models confirming fibrinogen to be at least as important as the more conventional risk factors.

In a collaborative study involving the towns of Caerphilly and Speedwell in the UK,[8] fibrinogen was again found to be independently predictive of ischaemic heart disease after adjusting for other risk factors. Viscosity and white blood cell count were also found to be important predictors of risk. Their contribution to correctly predicting future risk was strengthened even further when all three were included together.

More recently, the large *Gottingen Risk, Incidence and Prevalence Study* (GRIPS) involving a cohort of 5239 middle aged men followed for an average of five years, found fibrinogen to be a strong predictor for subsequent risk of cardiovascular events in both univariate and multivariate models. In the multivariate model, fibrinogen ranked fifth in order of importance after low denisity lipoprotein (LDL), familial disposition, lipoprotein (a), and high density lipoprotein (HDL), but ahead of age, smoking, glucose, and blood pressure.[9]

Additional evidence is available from the Framingham cohort in the United States.[7] One thousand three hundred and fifteen participants who had not previously experienced a cardiovascular event and agreed to have their fibrinogen levels measured at the time of the tenth biennial examination were followed for the ensuing 14 years. The risk of developing cardiovascular disease increased progressively in relation to the initial fibrinogen levels. However this association became weaker in men with advancing age. Once again, a complex interplay emerged between the impact of cigarette smoking and fibrinogen. Whilst both these factors appear to contribute to the development of cardiovascular disease in cross-sectional analyses, in multivariate models the effect of smoking appeared to be largely accounted for by the fibrinogen concentration.

This difficulty in teasing out the relative contribution of smoking versus fibrinogen raises the issue of confounding and is one of the main reasons that the haemostatic story remains somewhat contentious. It is not possible to confirm a causal role for fibrinogen (or any other haemostatic parameters) in the pathogenesis of cardiovascular disease from these type of prospective studies alone. This is further amplified by the attention drawn recently in several studies to the apparent relationship between certain social influences, including social class and job stress, and fibrinogen levels.[21,27]

In the *Whitehall Study*[27] of 1274 male and female Civil Servants aged 35–54 years, fibrinogen concentration was significantly higher among men in lower grades of employment. This was also borne out in multiple regression analyses. Job stress, but not behaviour type or physical activity was also found to be significantly related to the level of fibrinogen concentration. Data from the *Gothenburg Study*[21] produced slightly different results, suggesting that a relationship between fibrinogen concentration and social factors was only evident in non-smokers and disappeared when multiple regression techniques were used. However, looking at the results from these two studies together, it appears likely that psychosocial factors have an influence on the coagulation system.

To resolve these issues it would be necessary to undertake intervention trials specifically designed to treat specific haemostatic risk factors whilst controlling the potential confounding conventional risk factors. The logistics of this are formidable, and to date no such study has been undertaken.

Preliminary results from the *Prospective Cardiovascular Munster Study* (PROCAM), which is following a cohort of middle aged men using a design similar to the *Framingham Study*, have found reductions of similar magnitude in the incidence of coronary events amongst people in the lowest tertile of fibrinogen compared with those in the upper tertile.[10] These reductions have not reached statistical significance in view of the small number of events which have occurred so far.

When the results from six of the seven prospective studies were combined in a recent meta-analysis, the summary odds ratio for the incidence of cardiovascular events between the upper versus lower tertile of fibrinogen as 2.3 (95 per cent confidence interval 1.9 to 2.8).[28] The remarkable degree of uniformity across the studies is shown graphically in Figure 11.1. The *Stone and Thorp Study*[5] was excluded from the analysis because of the small number of events observed.

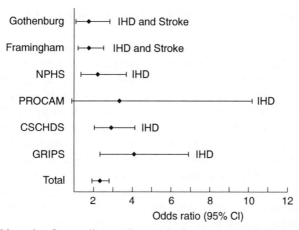

Fig. 11.1 Odds ratios for cardiovascular events in persons with fibrinogen levels in the upper tertile compared to the lower tertile. Odds ratios and 95 per cent confidence intervals in prospective epidemiological studies. IHD = ischaemic heart disease. CSCHDS = the Caerphilly and Speedwell collaborative heart disease study; GRIPS = the G'ttingen risk, incidence, and prevalence study; NPHS = Northwick Park heart study; PROCAM = prospective cardiovascular Munster study. (From Ernst E, Resch KL. Ann Intern Med 1993; **118**: 956–63.)

EVIDENCE OF REVERSIBILITY

Is it possible to reduce the level of fibrinogen ?

A number of different agents have been shown to modify the level of plasma fibrinogen in humans. These include: several of the fibrates (eg. clofibrate, bezafibrate, fenofibrate, ciprofibrate), propranolol, celiprolol, stanazol, ticlodipine, defibrotide, and calcium dobesilate.[13] Although most of these agents have only been evaluated in small numbers of patients many of whom had coexisting diseases, and for short periods of time, the percentage reduction in fibrinogen levels (from baseline) has ranged from 11 per cent to as high as 43 per cent among people with hyperfibrinogenamia.[13]

Non-drug interventions, particularly dietary modification, have been much less successful in reducing plasma fibrinogen levels.[13]

Does reducing fibrinogen lead to a reduction in cardiovascular disease?

The answer is we don't know. As yet there have been no long-term, randomized, controlled trials designed to address this question. Until more specific and safe fibrinogen lowering drugs become available it would be difficult to distinguish between fibrinogen lowering effects and other actions (eg. lipid-lowering, antihypertensive, antiplatelet) of the currently available agents.

RELEVANCE TO CLINICAL PRACTICE

At present we do not have adequate justification to recommend treatment of hyperfibrinogenemia (or other haemostatic parameters). Since these factors appear to be important in determining cardiovascular risk their role in routine clinical practice needs to be addressed. One of the major stumbling blocks at present is the need for readily available and reliable measurement methods. For example, fibrinogen fluctuates in response to physiological changes and is technically difficult to measure. Currently, its measurement is restricted mainly to research laboratories. One strategy suggested to overcome this is to use the erythrocyte sedimentation rate (ESR) as a surrogate measure of fibrinogen since it has been shown in at least one study to be an independent predictor of myocardial infarction.[29] The difficulty with this approach is that whilst the ESR correlates to some extent with the level of fibrinogen, it does not account for all the variation seen. A further stumbling block is the lack of consensus about the 'cut-off' point that determines implications for subsequent risk in a given individual. Finally, appropriate effective and safe methods of intervention need to be established. Until each of these issues is addressed, the role of fibrinogen as a risk factor will remain largely theoretical.

SUMMARY

- Haemostatic factors (particularly fibrinogen, factor VII, and fibrinolytic activity) appear to play an important role in the development of cardiovascular disease and its various clinical manifestations.
- Haemostatic factors appear to be involved in the underlying aetiology of

atherosclerosis at a number of different stages from the early intimal lesion through to promoting thrombus formation.

- Some of the conventional risk factors appear to be associated with haemostatic parameters. This may be the mechanism by which their contribution to the development of cardiovascular disease is mediated. This is likely to be the case for cigarette smoking, and possibly social class, physical activity, and stress.
- An elevation in the concentration of fibrinogen appears to consistently predict the probability of developing coronary heart disease, stroke, and peripheral vascular disease in the future. The predictive strength of other haemostatic variables is less consistent.
- The increase in risk conferred by an elevation in fibrinogen appears to persist after accounting for other risk factors.
- Although various therapies have been shown to reduce fibrinogen levels by between 11 per cent and 43 per cent in the short-term these usually have other favourable cardiovascular effects (such as lowering lipids or blood pressure) which would make it difficult to distinguish the relative effects on cardiovascular disease.
- Currently there is no evidence from randomized, controlled trials to demonstrate that lowering fibrinogen reduces cardiovascular risk.
- Fibrinogen levels are difficult to measure and vary considerably in response to physiological influences.
- Even though fibrinogen concentration may be an accurate risk factor for the development of future cardiovascular disease, its utility in clinical practice is hampered by these practical constraints and lack of any trial evidence for a benefit as a result of reducing it.
- Until these limitations are overcome, fibrinogen is not a practical or useful risk marker in the primary care setting.

REFERENCES

1. Hopkins PN, Williams RR. A survey of 246 suggested coronary risk factors. Atherosclerosis 1981; **40**: 1–52.
2. Meade TW, Chakrabarti R, Haines AP, North WRS, Stirling Y. Characteristics affecting fibrinolytic activity and plasma fibrinogen concentrations. BMJ 1979; **1**: 153–6.
3. Ernst E. Plasma fibrinogen—an independent cardiovascular risk factor. J Intern Med 1990; **227**: 365–72.
4. Wilhelmsen L, Svardsudd K, Korsan-Bengtsen K, Larrson B, Welin L, Tibblin G. Fibrinogen as a risk factor for stroke and myocardial infarction. N Engl J Med 1984; **311**: 501–5.
5. Stone MC, Thorp JM. Plasma fibrinogen—a major coronary risk factor. J Roy Coll Gen Pract 1985; **35**: 565–69.
6. Meade TW, Brozovic M, Chakrabarti, Haines AP, Imeson JD, Mellows S, *et al* Haemostatic function and ischaemic heart disease: principal results of the Northwick Park Heart Study. Lancet 1986; **ii**: 533–37.

7. Kannel WB, D'Agostino RB, Belanger AJ. Fibrinogen, cigarette smoking and risk of cardiovascular disease: insights from the Framingham study. Am Heart J 1987; **113**: 1006–10.
8. Yarnell JWG, Baker IA, Sweetnam PM, Bainton D, O'Brien JR, Whitehead PJ, *et al.* Fibrinogen, viscosity, and white blood cell count are major risk factors for ischaemic heart disease. Circulation 1991; **83**: 836–44.
9. Cremer P, Nagel D, Bottcher B, Seidel D. Fibrinogen: Ein koronarer Risikofactor. Diagnose Labor. 1992; **65**: 815.
10. Balleisen L, Schulte H. Assmann G, Epping PH, Van De Loo J. Coagulation factors and the progress of coronary heart disease. Lancet 1987; **1**: 461.
11. Fuster V, Badimon L, Badimon JJ, Chesebro JH. The pathogenesis of coronary artery disease and the acute coronary syndromes (Part 1). N Engl J Med 1992; **4**: 242–50.
12. Fuster V, Badimon L, Badimon JJ, Chesebro JH. The pathogenesis of coronary artery disease and the acute coronary syndromes (Part 2). N Engl J Med 1992; **4**: 310–18.
13. Cook NS, Ubben D. Fibrinogen as a major risk factor in cardiovascular disease. TiPS 1990; **11**: 444–51.
14. Ernst E. Fibrinogen—an idependent risk factor for cardiovascular disease. BMJ 1991; **303**: 596–97.
15. Eisenberg S. Blood viscosity and fibrinogen concentration following cerebral infarction. Circulation 1966; **33/34** (S2): 10–14.
16. Dormandy J, Ernst E, Matrai A, Flute PT. Haemorheological changes following acute myocardial infarction. Am Heart J 1982; **104**: 1364–7.
17. Korsan-Bengtsen K, Wilhelmsen L, Tibblin G. Blood coagulation and fibrinolysis in a random sample of 788 men 54 years old. Thrombos Diathes Haemorrh (Stuttg) 1972; **28**: 99–108.
18. Meade TW, North WRS, Chakrabarti R, Stirling Y, Haines AP, Thompson SG, *et al.* Haemostatic function and cardiovascular death: early results of a prospective study. Lancet 1980; **i**: 1050–4.
19. Lee AJ, Smith WC, Lowe GDO, Tunstall-Pedoe H. Plasma fibrinogen and coronary risk factors: The Scottish Heart Health Study. J Clin Epidemiol 1990; **43**: 913–19
20. Connelly JB, Coopr JA, Meade TW. Strenuous exercise, plasma fibrinogen, and factor VII activity. Br Heart J 1992; **67**: 351–54.
21. Rosengren A, Wilhlemsen L, Welin L, Tsipogianni A, Teger-Nilsson A, Wedel H, *et al.* Social influences and cardiovascular risk factors as determinants of plasma fibrinogen concentration in a general population sample of middle-aged men. BMJ 1990; **300**: 634–8.
22. Lowe GDO, Drummond MM, Lorimer AR, Hutton I, Forbes CD, Prentice CRM, *et al.* Relationship between extent of coronary artery disease and blood viscosity. BMJ 1980; **i**: 673–74.
23. Nicolaides AN, Bowers R, Horbourne T, Kidner PH, Besterman EM. Blood viscosity, red-cell flexibility, haematocrit and plasma-fibrinogen in patients with angina. Lancet 1977; **ii**: 943–5.
24. Qizilbash N, Jones L, Warlow C, Mann J. Fibrinogen and lipid concentrations as risk factors for transient ischaemic attacks and minor ischaemic strokes. BMJ 1991; **303**: 605–9.
25. Naimi S, Goldstein R, Proger S. Studies of coagulation and fibrinolysis of the arterial and venous blood in normal subjects and patients with atherosclerosis. Circulation 1963; **27**: 904–18.
26. Lofmark R. Fibrinogen derivatives and recurrent myocardial infarction. Acta Med Scand 1982; **212**: 293–94.

27. Markowe HLJ, Marmot MG, Shipley MJ, Bulpitt CJ, Meade TW, Stirling Y, *et al.* Fibrinogen: a possible link between social class and coronary heart disease. BMJ 1985; **291**: 1312–14.
28. Ernst E, Resch KL. Fibrinogen as a cardiovascular risk factor: a meta-analysis and review of the literature. Ann Intern Med. 1993; **118**: 956–63.
29. Bottinger LE, Carlson LA. Risk factors for ischaemic vascular death in the Stockholm prospective study. Atherosclerosis 1980; **36**: 389–408.

12 Antioxidants

Chris Silagy and David Mant

There is now considerable biochemical and experimental animal evidence in support of oxidative modification of lowdensity lipoprotein (LDL) playing an important causative role in atherosclerosis.[1] More recently, this has been strengthened by some impressive epidemiological evidence.[2-5] The oxidative process depends on the presence of free radicals. The main contribution of antioxidants appears to be in scavenging these free radicals and converting them to inactive substances.[6] As a result, antioxidants have been postulated as potential protective agents which help to guard against atherosclerosis and its clinical manifestations.

Antioxidants can be classified into two main groups: (i) naturally occurring and (ii) synthetic. A number of intracellular enzymes, such as catalase and glutathione, have antioxidant properties. Outside the cell, vitamins E and C, beta carotene, selenium, lycopene, retinol, and cryptoxanthine, all exist as naturally occurring antioxidants. Of these, probably vitamin E, vitamin C, and betacarotene appear to be the most important in humans. The plasma levels of these compounds appear to correlate closely with the level of dietary intake. Vitamin E is found in liver, egg yolks, cereal grains, nuts, and vegetable oils. It is fat soluble and closely linked to circulating lipids. Beta carotene is also fat soluble and is present in carrots and green vegetables. Vitamin C, on the other hand, is water soluble and found in various fruits and vegetables.

In this chapter the role of antioxidants in cardiovascular disease prevention is examined by addressing the following six questions:

1. How does oxidative modification of LDL occur and how may antioxidants interfere with this process ?
2. How is oxidized LDL related to the development of atheroma ?
3. What experimental evidence exists from animal studies to suggest that antioxidants may play a preventive role in cardiovascular disease ?
4. What epidemiological evidence is there to link antioxidant status with the risk of coronary heart disease (CHD)?
5. Is there any evidence that antioxidant supplementation reduces the risk of coronary heart disease ?
6. What are the implications of antioxidants for cardiovascular disease prevention in clinical practice ?

HOW DOES OXIDATIVE MODIFICATION OF LDL OCCUR, AND HOW MAY ANTIOXIDANTS INTERFERE WITH THIS PROCESS?

Free radical formation is a by-product of normal cellular metabolism. It results from a complex chain reaction in which oxy radicals interact with polyunsaturated fatty acids to produce a lipid radical.[7] This lipid radical can further interact with oxygen to form a peroxyl radical which is highly reactive and capable of attacking other lipid molecules. This can potentially become a runaway process which consumes valuable polyunsaturated fatty acids. It only stops when two peroxyl radicals combine to form an inactive product.

LDL is particularly susceptible to oxidative modification.[8] However, LDL carries within it a number of natural antioxidants (vitamins E, C, and betacarotene) which can prevent the formation of free radicals by competing for the peroxyl radicals much faster than polyunsaturated fatty acids.[7] As a result they can minimize or prevent the extent to which LDL is oxidized. The importance of this naturally occurring 'protective system' is that oxidized LDL appears to be potentially much more atherogenic than native (unoxidized) LDL.[1]

HOW IS OXIDIZED LDL RELATED TO THE DEVELOPMENT OF ATHEROMA?

The peroxide modified components of LDL appear to affect the development of atherosclerosis by multiple mechanisms.[1] Firstly, they can be taken up by macrophages and transformed into foam cells which are loaded with lipids. This transformation is believed to be the initiating step in the development of atherosclerosis.[1] Secondly, they appear to be cytotoxic for cells of the artery wall. Thirdly, they release substances which attract and promote the adherence of other cells on endothelial surfaces.

WHAT EXPERIMENTAL EVIDENCE EXISTS FROM ANIMAL STUDIES TO SUGGEST THAT ANTIOXIDANTS MAY PLAY A PREVENTIVE ROLE IN CHD?

There is extensive experimental evidence in animal models to confirm the importance of oxidative modification in the pathogenesis of atherosclerosis. Vitamin E appears to be the most important determinant of resistance to LDL modification. For example, atherosclerotic-like lesions appear to occur with increased frequency in rodents, piglets, and primates who have chronic marginal deficiencies of vitamin E.[9] Furthermore, it is possible to prevent experimentally induced atheroma in hyperlipidemic rabbits and hens by administration of vitamin E.[10] Synthetic antioxidants have been shown to have similar effects. Of these, probucol, which is also a hypolipidemic drug, has been studied the most.[11,12] It was capable of inhibiting the extent of atherosclerosis far beyond the levels expected from its cholesterol lowering effect.

Antioxidants probably have several other favourable properties that contribute to the prevention of cardiovascular disease. These include their ability to stabilize cell membranes and thereby salvage ischaemic myocardial tissue. In addition several of the antioxidants have been shown to interfere with platelet aggregation both *in vitro* and *in vivo*, although the clinical significance of this remains unclear.[13]

WHAT EPIDEMIOLOGICAL EVIDENCE IS THERE TO LINK ANTIOXIDANT STATUS WITH THE RISK OF CHD?

The epidemiological evidence in support of a relationship between antioxidant status and the development of (CHD) comes from two main sources. Firstly, within population data (both retrospective and prospective) and secondly, cross cultural comparisons of populations with different CHD mortality rates.

Within population studies—retrospective data

Data comparing the difference in levels of antioxidant vitamins between people with and without (CHD) has produced conflicting results. In the *Kuopio Risk Factor Study* no difference was found between plasma vitamin C levels or the vitamin E/cholesterol ratio among people with and without symptomatic or demonstrable evidence of CHD.[14] The *Eastern Finland Heart Study* also found no difference in concentrations of vitamins A and E between people who died from CHD and matched healthy controls.[15] At least four other studies[16–19] have produced similar results, failing to provide evidence in support of an association between antioxidant vitamins and cardiovascular morbidity and mortality.

More recent studies have produced more promising results. The largest of these was a case control study conducted by Riemersma, *et al*[3] who studied 110 people with angina (identified from a positive response to a chest pain questionnaire) and 394 age-matched controls. Plasma concentrations of vitamins C, E, and carotene were all significantly inversely related to the risk of angina. No significant relationship was found between vitamin A and the risk of developing CHD,. The association between the vitamin E concentration and the risk of developing angina persisted even after adjustment for cigarette smoking with an odds ratio of 2.68 for developing angina among people in the highest quintile of vitamin E concentration compared with those in the lowest quintile.

Adjustment for smoking is important since it appears almost certain that cigarette smoking acts as a confounder in the relationship between antioxidants and development of cardiovascular disease.[20] Reports from cross-sectional studies indicate that plasma antioxidant levels are significantly lower in smokers than non-smokers.[20,21] The levels in ex-smokers are to similar to those of non-smokers within about five years of cessation. The relationship between vitamin E and the risk of developing angina is further strengthened when corrected for the prevailing plasma lipid level.[3]

Within population studies—prospective data

Prospective data from the *United States Nurses' Health Survey* involving 87 000 women supports these findings.[4] In that study vitamin E and beta carotene intakes (as well as plasma levels) were both inversely correlated with the risk of developing CHD. Amongst those with the highest calculated intakes the risk was reduced 30–40 per cent. Other antioxidants, such as selenium, showed little or no association with the risk of developing heart disease, irrespective of whether one examined intake or plasma levels. Therefore, it appears that vitamin E is possibly the most clinically important of the naturally occurring antioxidants.

Cross cultural studies

In 1991 evidence from a large cross cultural comparison of ischaemic heart disease mortality rates in 16 different European countries provided probably the most persuasive epidemiological evidence to date of the role that antioxidants may be playing in prevention of cardiovascular disease.[2] Essential antioxidants were identified from plasma samples obtained from approximately 100 subjects in each of the European communities that were participating in a large *WHO/ MONICA* study. Among these communities there is a six-fold difference in the age-specific mortality rates from ischaemic heart disease which cannot be adequately explained by differences in conventional risk factors (such as hypertension, smoking, elevated lipids). Interestingly, the lipid standardized concentration of vitamin E emerged as the strongest predictor of heart disease across these different communities. When multiple regression techniques were used, the lipid standardized plasma vitamin E concentration accounted for 62 per cent of the difference in mortality rates. These results indicate that the vitamin E concentration may be of greater quantitative importance than the conventional risk factors in predicting the risk of ischaemic heart disease.

Despite these findings there remain a number of unanswered questions. For example, is there any change in antioxidant levels with age. Preliminary evidence suggests that between early adulthood and the sixth decade of life there is little change.[22] Beyond this age the data is scarce. Assuming that this observation is true, it suggests that the latter stages of atherosclerosis may be less dependent on antioxidants than the earlier ones. It is also unclear as to which antioxidants are most important for the prevention of cardiovascular disease in humans, what dose levels to use, when and for how long. The effect of other risk factors (such as hypertension, obesity, stress, physical activity) on antioxidant levels is also not known. All these questions will need to be addressed in the future.

IS THERE ANY EVIDENCE THAT ANTIOXIDANT SUPPLEMENTATION REDUCES THE RISK OF CHD?

Probably the major limiting factor in the antioxidant jigsaw at present is the lack of evidence in humans that intervention with antioxidant supplementation reduces risk. Although there is the animal data demonstrating the efficacy of probucol, there have been no comparable studies in humans.[11,12] Some evidence exists to show that dietary supplementation with antioxidants can increase the plasma levels of these substances, although the magnitude of this effect is relatively small.[23] Among smokers it has been possible to show that vitamin E supplementation at least partially reverse indices of sustained oxidant stress.[24] Whether this translates into reducing the risk of CHD is unclear.

To date, one large randomized placebo-controlled trial of alphatocopherol and betacarotene, given to 29 133 male smokers (aged 50–69 years) in Finland over a five to eight year period found fewer deaths from ischeamic heart disease and stroke amongst participants treated with alphatocopherol, but a significant increase in the rate of death from haemorrhagic stroke.[25] This last observation was ascribed to the antiplatelet effects of alphatocopherol. Amongst the group treated with betacarotene, the rate of death from ischaemic heart disease and stroke were both significantly greater than in the placebo treated group. Furthermore, the rate of death from lung cancer, as well as overall mortality, was significantly higher in the three anti-oxidant groups than those receiving placebo.

In contrast, preliminary results from a small subset of participants in the trial of aspirin and beta carotene being conducted amongst 22 000 males physicians in the United States, suggest that beta carotene significantly reduces the risk of cardiovascular sequelae in men with stable angina or who have had coronary artery bypass grafts.[26] The results of the full trial, expected to finish later in 1995, may shed further light on the potential role of beta carotene in preventing the morbidity and mortality associated with cardiovascular disease. Further large scale clinical trials examining the effect of other antioxidants (including vitamins C and E), both in men and women, are planned or in progress.[23] When the results from these current trials become available, they will need to be systematically reviewed in conjunction with the limited existing data in order to assess more reliably the role of antioxidants in the treatment and prevention of cardiovascular disease in the future.

WHAT ARE THE IMPLICATIONS OF ANTIOXIDANTS FOR CHD PREVENTION IN CLINICAL PRACTICE?

Until this occurs the value of antioxidants as risk markers and modifiers will remain in a similar category to that of the haemostatic parameters. Measurement is difficult and currently limited to research laboratories. Data on reproducibility is scarce. Cut off values for determining 'at risk' sub-groups have not yet been established. Each of these issues will need to be addressed in detail before antioxidants can play a prominent role in routine clinical practice.

One practical concern is the increasing proportion of the population who are already taking vitamin supplements for their purported beneficial health effects. Even though these agents are readily available throughout the community and appear to be relatively harmless, the benefits of using them are still not sufficiently established for this form of self-medication to be justified on medical grounds.

SUMMARY

- Low density lipoproteins are particularly susceptible to oxidative modification by free radicals. This occurs as part of normal cellular metabolism but can be prevented by antioxidants which convert free radicals to inactive compounds.
- Oxidized low density lipoprotein plays an important role in atherogenesis, especially in the early stages of formation of lesions.
- There is evidence indicating that animals deficient in certain antioxidants are more prone to developing atherosclerosis. Conversely, administration of anti-oxidants to animals with experimentally induced atherosclerosis can prevent further progression.
- In humans, epidemiological studies have shown an increased odds ratio for the risk of developing ischaemic heart disease among people with low plasma concentrations of vitamin E. This persists after adjustment for cigarette smoking, which has been shown to be a confounding factor.
- Differences in antioxidant levels (particularly vitamin E) appear to explain much of the variation in mortality rates from ischaemic heart disease between different communities.
- The currently available evidence from randomized controlled trials provides conflicting evidence about the effects of using antioxidant supplementation to reduce cardiovascular risk.
- A considerable proportion of the population already take antioxidant vitamins. This practice needs to be closely monitored in light of the lack of information about dosages, levels requiring treatment, duration, and timing of treatment.
- Before the role of antioxidants in cardiovascular disease prevention is finalized, further clinical trials are required to determine the risk to benefit ratio amongst different patient groups.

REFERENCES

1. Steinberg D. Antioxidants in the prevention of human atherosclerosis. Circulation 1992; **85**: 2338–44.
2. Gey KF, Puska P, Jordan P, Moser UK. Inverse correlation between plasma vitamin E and mortality from ischaemic heart disease in cross-cultural epidemiology. Am J Clin Nutr 1991; **53**: 326–34.

3. Riemersma RA, Wood DA, Macintyre CCA, Elton RA, Gey KF, Oliver MF. Risk of angina pectoris and plasma concentrations of vitamins A, C, and E and carotene. Lancet 1991; **337**: 1–5.

4. Stampfer MJ, Hennekens CH, Manson JE, Colditz GA, Rosner B, Willett WC. Vitamin E consumption and the risk of coronary disease in women N Engl J Med 1993; **328**: 1444–9.

5. Salonen JT. Selenium in ischaemic heart disease. Int J Epidemiol 1987; **570**: 269–82.

6. Sinclair AJ, Barnett AH, Lunec J. Free radicals and antioxidant systems in health and disease. Br J Hosp Med 1990; 43(5): 334–44.

7. Parthasarathy S, Rankin SM. Role of oxidized low density lipoprotein in atherogenesis. Prog Lipid Res 1992; **31**: 127–43.

8. Steinberg D, Parthasarathy S, Carew TE, Khoo JC, Witztum JL. Beyond cholesterol: modifications of low-density lipoportein that increase its atherogenicity. N Engl J Med 1989; **320**: 915–24.

9. Nelson JS. Pathology of vitamin E deficiency. In (Machlin LJ. ed.) Vitamin E, a comprehensive treatise. New York: Dekker, 1980, pp. 397–428.

10. Wilson RB, Middleton CC, Sun GY. Vitamin E antioxidants and lipid peroxidation in experimental atherosclerosis of rabbits. J Nutr 1978; **108**: 1858–67.

11. Carew TE, Schwenke DC, Steinberg D. Antiatherogenic effect of probucol unrelated to its hypocholesterolaemic effect: evidence that antioxidants in vivo can selectively inhibit low-density lipoprotein degradation in macrophage-rich fatty streaks and slow the progression of atherosclerosis in the Watanabe heiritable hyperlipidemic rabbit. Proc Natl Acad Sci USA 1987; **84**: 7725–9.

12. Quinn MT, Parasarathy S, Fong LG, Steinberg D. Oxidatively modified low-density lipoproteins: a potential role in recruitment and retention of monocyte/macrophages during atherogenesis. Proc Natl Acad Sci USA 1987; **84**: 2995–8.

13. Salonen JT. Antioxidants and platelets. Ann Med 1989; **21**: 59–62.

14. Salonen JT, Salonen R, Seppanen K, Kantola M, Parviainen M, Alfthan G, et al. Relationship of serum selenium and antioxidants to plasma lipoproteins, platelet aggregability and prevalent ischaemic heart disease in Eastern Finnish men. Atherosclerosis 1988; **70**: 155–60.

15. Salonen JT, Salonen R, Pentilla I, Herranen J, Jauhiainen M, Kantola M, et al. Serum fatty acids, apolipoproteins, selenium and vitamin antioxidants and the risk of death from coronary artery disease. Am J Cardiol 1985; **56**: 226–31.

16. Roussouw JE, Labadarios D, Jooste PL, Shephard GS. Lack of a relationship between plasma pyridoxal phosphate levels and ischaemic heart disease. Sth African Med J 1985; **67**: 539–41.

17. Lapidus L, Andersson H, Bengtsson C, Bosaeus I. Dietary habits in relation to incidence of cardiovascular disease and death in women: 12-year follow-up of participants in the population study of women in Gothenburg, Sweden. Am J Clin Nutr 1986; **44**: 444–48.

18. Gey KF, Stahelin HB, Puska P, Evans A. Relationship of plasma level of vitamin C to mortality from ischaemic heart disease. Ann N Y Acad Sci 1987; **498**: 110–13.

19. Kok FJ, de Bruijn AM, Vermeeeren R, Hoffman A, van Laar A, de Bruin M, et al. Serum selenium, vitamin antioxidants, and cardiovascular mortality: a 9 year follow-up study in the Netherlands. Am J Clin Nutr 1987; **45**: 462–8.

20. Stryker WS, Kaplan LA, Stein EA, Stampfer MJ, Sober A, Willett WC. The relation of diet, cigarette smoking, and alcohol consumption to plasma beta-carotene and alpha-tocopherol levels. Am J Epidemiol 1988; **127**: 283–96.

21. Duthie GG, Short CT, Robertson JD, Walker KA, Arthur JR. Plasma antioxidants, indices of lipid peroxidation and coronary heart disease risk factors in a Scottish population. Nutr Res 1992; **12**(S1): 61–7.

22. Comstock GW, Menkes MS, Schober SE, Vuilleumier JP, Helsing KJ. Serum levels of retinol, beta-carotene, and alpha-tocopherol in older adults. Am J Epidemiol 1987; **127**: 114–13.
23. Steinberg D (and workshop participants). Antioxidants in the prevention of human atherosclerosis. Summary of the proceedings of a national heart, lung and blood institute workshop: September 5–6, 1991, Bethesda, Maryland. Circulation 1992; **85**: 2338–44.
24. Hoshino E, Shariff R, Gossum AV. Vitamin E suppresses increased lipid peroxidation in cigarette smokers. J Parent Nutr 1990; **14**: 300–5.
25. The alpha-tocopherol, beta carotene cancer prevention study group. The effect of vitamin E and beta carotene on the incidence of lung cancer and other cancers in male smokers. N Engl J Med 1994; **330**: 1029–35.
26. Gaziano JM, Hennekens CH. Vitamin antioxidants and cardiovascular disease. Current Opinion in Lipidology 1992; **3**: 291–4.

13   Prevention of stroke

Jonathan Mant

INTRODUCTION

There is considerable overlap between the risk factors for coronary heart disease and stroke. The major modifiable risk factors for stroke are smoking[1] and hypertension[2] (see Chapters 1 and 2). Other modifiable risk factors include alcohol consumption[3] and lack of exercise.[4] Diabetes[5] and coronary heart disease[6] are also risk factors. Lowering serum cholesterol does not appear to protect against stroke.[7]

Risk factors which relate largely to cerebrovascular disease rather than coronary heart disease include atrial fibrillation,[8] a past history of a transient ischaemic attack (TIA)[9] or stroke, and presence of carotid artery stenosis. Three interventions which can modify the risk of stroke in these circumstances include the use of antiplatelet agents such as aspirin, the use of anticoagulants for people in atrial fibrillation, and the use of carotid endarterectomy for patients with carotid artery stenosis. The aim of this review is to explore the role of these three interventions in the prevention of stroke by considering three questions:

1. **What is the role of antiplatelet agents in the prevention of stroke?**
2. **Should patients with non-rheumatic atrial fibrillation be given aspirin or warfarin?**
3. **Which patients benefit from carotid endarterectomy, and how should they be identified in general practice?**

WHAT IS THE ROLE OF ANTIPLATELET AGENTS IN THE PREVENTION OF STROKE?

Primary prevention of stroke in low risk patients

The contribution that the use of antiplatelet agents such as aspirin can make to the prevention of stroke has been clarified by an overview of randomized controlled trials performed by the Antiplatelet Trialists' Collaboration.[10] Three studies were identified which had investigated the effect of antiplatelet agents on incidence of stroke and myocardial infarction in people without pre-existing risk factors for cardiovascular disease, including the US physicians' health study with over 22 000 participants,[11] and a study on British male doctors with over 6000 participants.[12] These studies show that while prophylactic aspirin does offer some protection against myocardial infarction, the benefit appears to be offset by an increased risk of haemorrhagic stroke, with the result that overall, there was no significant reduction in the number of vascular deaths. Thus, there is insufficient evidence at present to recommend the use of aspirin in the primary prevention of cardiovascular disease in low risk patients.

Secondary prevention in patients who have had a transient ischaemic attack or stroke

The Antiplatelet Trialists' Collaboration identified 18 trials with over 1ᴦ 000 patients in total which have explored the role of antiplatelet agents in patients who have had a TIA or stroke. Their results are shown in Table 13.1. Treatment with an antiplatelet agent reduces the relative risk of a subsequent non-fatal myocardial infarction by 34 per cent and of a non-fatal stroke by 20 per cent . However, given that people who have already had a stroke or TIA are at much greater risk of a further non-fatal stroke than a non-fatal heart attack, the absolute benefits of treatment are greater in terms of prevention of stroke rather than myocardial infarction: treatment of 1000 patients will prevent 20 non-fatal strokes over a three year period and nine heart attacks. In terms of lives saved, treating 59 patients with an antiplatelet agent for three years will prevent one death.

Table 13.1 Effect of anti-platelet therapy on patients with previous stroke or TIA—results from Antiplatelet Trialists' Collaboration

	Non-fatal MI	Non-fatal stroke	Vascular death	Any death
Event rate in treatment group	109/5654 (1.9%)	479/5837 (8.2%)	497/5837 (8.5%)	675/5837 (11.6%)
Event rate in control group	163/5681 (2.9%)	600/5870 (10.2%)	562/5870 (9.6%)	780/5870 (13.3%)
Relative risk reduction	34%	20%	11%	13%
Benefit per 1000 patients treated for 3 years (in events prevented)	9	20	11	17
Number needed to treat for 3 years to prevent one event	111	50	91	59

The overview by the Antiplatelet Trialists' Collaboration includes antiplatelet agents other than aspirin, such as sulphinpyrazone and ticlopidine and the addition of dipyridamole. The Collaboration did not find any major differences of effect between these different agents. A separate meta-analysis which compared the results achieved by aspirin against placebo as compared to aspirin with dipyridamole against placebo, in the secondary prevention of stroke suggested that the addition of dipyridamole conferred extra benefit.[13] However, this conclusion needs to be interpreted with caution, since it was not based on studies which directly compared the two approaches. Trials which provide direct comparisons of aspirin alone against aspirin and dipyridamole in the secondary prevention of stroke have not been of sufficient size to allow firm conclusions to be drawn.

While it has been established that aspirin is effective in the secondary prevention of stroke, it is not clear what is the optimal dose to be used. The dosage used in the trials included in the Antiplatelet Trialists' Collaboration varied between 50 mg and 1500 mg daily. Matchar *et al* in an overview of trials comparing aspirin to placebo following stroke or TIA found no relationship between dose and protective effect.[14] The *Swedish Aspirin Low-dose Trial* (SALT)[15] found that a 75 mg dose of aspirin led to a 18 per cent reduction in risk of stroke or death in patients who had previously suffered a TIA or minor stroke—an order of magnitude that is similar to the pooled results of the Antiplatelet Trialists' Collaboration. There have been two trials which have compared different doses of aspirin in the context of secondary prevention of stroke: the *United Kingdom TIA* (UK-TIA) *aspirin trial* (1200 mg/day vs 300 mg/day),[16] and the *Dutch TIA trial* (283 mg/day vs 30 mg/day).[17] Neither trial found any significant differences in terms of vascular outcomes, but in both trials side effects were lower in the group that had received the lower dose of aspirin.

One area of current controversy is the extent to which the pathology of a past stroke (that is infarct or haemorrhage) should be elucidated before starting a patient on aspirin. Aspirin does appear to confer a slightly increased risk of intracerebral haemorrhage,[10] and it is not unreasonable to assume that someone who has suffered one intracerebral haemorrhage is at greater risk of a further one. Therefore, it may be appropriate to perform a CT scan on a patient with a stroke to exclude a haemorrhage before starting aspirin therapy. However, the ability of a CT scan to discriminate between infarction and haemorrhage declines with time. Two weeks after a stroke, a CT scan may be unable to distinguish between these pathologies. Indeed, intracerebral haemorrhage may be incorrectly classified as an infarction.[18] Thus, to make a pathological diagnosis, a CT scan needs to be performed early. However, given that over 80 per cent of strokes are caused by an infarct rather than a haemorrhage,[19] it can be argued that from a population perspective it is more cost-effective to treat all patients with stroke with aspirin, without performing a CT scan.[20]

Patients who have suffered a TIA or ischaemic stroke should be offered aspirin therapy. There is no current evidence to recommend alternative antiplatelet regimes over and above aspirin alone, but alternatives have a role where there are clear contra-indications to aspirin therapy, such as definite allergy or significant gastric symptoms. Medium dose aspirin (75–325 mg) has been most widely tested; the lower dosages appear to be as effective as the higher while causing less side-effects, and are therefore probably the best to use.[10] While it is not ideal to prescribe aspirin to someone who has had a previous intracerebral haemorrhage, absence of CT confirmation of the underlying pathology is not generally held to preclude the use of aspirin in someone who has suffered a stroke.

Use of aspirin in patients with non-rheumatic atrial fibrillation

There have been two trials of aspirin against placebo for the prevention of stroke in patients with atrial fibrillation—the *Stroke Prevention in Atrial Fibrillation Study* (SPAF),[21] and the *Copenhagen AFASAK Study*,[22] and one study, the *European Atrial Fibrillation Trial* (EAFT), which has looked specifically at the secondary prevention of stroke in patients with atrial fibrillation.[23] Pooling of the results from SPAF and AFASAK suggest that aspirin reduces the relative risk of an adverse outcome (stroke, systemic embolism, or death) in patients with atrial fibrillation by 28 per cent.[24] The estimated relative risk reduction in EAFT was lower (17 per cent), but because of the higher risk of stroke in patients who have already suffered a stroke or TIA, the absolute benefits are likely to be greater. Aspirin appears to be an effective treatment to prevent stroke in patients with atrial fibrillation, but its role needs to be considered in the light of what is known about the effectiveness of anticoagulants in such patients (see below).

SHOULD PATIENTS WITH NON-RHEUMATIC ATRIAL FIBRILLATION BE GIVEN ASPIRIN OR WARFARIN?

Evidence of effect of warfarin

There is strong evidence that warfarin is an effective means of preventing stroke in patients with non-rheumatic atrial fibrillation. An analysis of pooled individual patient data from five randomized controlled trials[24] found that treatment with warfarin leads to a 68 per cent reduction in the risk of stroke, a 33 per cent reduction in the risk of death, and a 48 per cent reduction in the risk of stroke, systemic embolism, or death. These relative risk reductions are greater than those achieved by aspirin (see above), but it must be borne in mind that indirect comparisons of this nature can be misleading, since there will have been different selection criteria for trials involving warfarin as compared to trials involving aspirin.

Direct comparison of warfarin to aspirin

There have been three published trials which randomized patients with non-rheumatic atrial fibrillation to receive either aspirin or warfarin.[22,23,25] These trials are summarised in Table 13.2. All three suggest that warfarin is superior to aspirin. EAFT and SPAF-2 give similar estimates of the relative risk of a stroke on warfarin as compared to aspirin—60 per cent and 70 per cent respectively. AFASAK found the stroke rate to be similar in patients on aspirin to those on placebo, and therefore compared the stroke rate of patients on warfarin (2 per cent per annum) to patients on aspirin or placebo (5.5 per cent per annum). This gives a lower estimate of relative risk than the other studies (i.e. suggests a greater benefit of warfarin relative to aspirin).

Table 13.2   Summary of trials which provide direct comparison of aspirin to warfarin in patients with atrial fibrillation

	SPAF-2	AFASAK	EAFT
No. of subjects randomized to receive aspirin or warfarin	1100 patients with AF	671 patients with AF	455 patients with AF and history of TIA or minor stroke in previous 3 mths
Length of follow-up	mean 2–3 yrs	2 yrs	mean 2.3 yrs
Primary outcome	ischaemic stroke or systemic embolism	TIA, stroke (fatal or non-fatal), or systemic embolism	death from vascular disease, non-fatal stroke, MI, or systemic embolism
RR of primary outcome on warfarin as compared to aspirin (95% confidence interval)	70% (43%–114%)	Not given directly. RR on warfarin as compared to aspirin or placebo is 36%	60% (41%–87%)

SPAF-2, stroke prevention in atrial fibrillation study; AFASAK, Copenhagen study; EAFT, European atrial fibrillation trial; RR, relative risk

Warfarin is more effective than aspirin in preventing stroke in patients with non-rheumatic atrial fibrillation, but leads to a greater risk of haemorrhage. The decision whether to prescribe aspirin or warfarin is critically dependent upon two factors: the risk that a patient will suffer a stroke off treatment (the 'baseline' risk), and the risk that a patient will suffer a major haemorrhage on treatment. The magnitude of both risks will depend upon individual patient factors, but can be estimated by using data from the trials and other epidemiological studies.

What is the risk of stroke off treatment?

Follow-up of the Framingham cohort has shown atrial fibrillation is an important risk factor for stroke—a stroke is four to five times as likely in someone with atrial fibrillation as opposed to someone without the condition.[8] Given that both the incidence of stroke[26] and the incidence of atrial fibrillation[8] rise with age, atrial fibrillation is a particularly important risk factor in the elderly. It has been estimated that it accounts for 16 per cent of strokes in people aged 70–79, and 31 per cent of strokes in people aged over 80.[8]

From analysis of the pooled data of the five trials that looked at the role of warfarin in atrial fibrillation, the individual risk of a patient with atrial fibrillation having a stroke is dependent upon age, previous history of stroke or TIA, hypertension, and diabetes.[24] A history of recent cardiac failure may also be an independent risk factor for stroke in patients with atrial fibrillation.[27] With regard to investigations, echocardiography has emerged as a useful investigation for predicting risk of stroke: presence of left atrial dilatation or left ventricular dysfunction increases risk, and absence of these features reduces risk.[28]

Presence or absence of these different risk factors will lead to wide differences in an individual's risk of a stroke. A person under the age of 65 with atrial fibrillation but no other risk factors for stroke has an annual risk of stroke of around 1 per cent.[24] In contrast, the risk for a patient with three or more risk factors may be as high as 19 per cent.[28]

It is important to have some idea of the individual patient's risk of stroke since this will affect the absolute benefit of treatment. If 1000 patients with a 1 per cent risk of stroke are treated, this will prevent about seven strokes per annum. On the other hand, treating 1000 patients with an 19 per cent risk of stroke will prevent around 120 strokes per annum. However, this ignores the risk of haemorrhage on warfarin, which also needs to be taken into account.

What is the risk of a major haemorrhage on warfarin?

In the trials that looked at the effect of warfarin in atrial fibrillation, the annual frequency of major bleeding events (intracranial bleeding, or a bleed requiring hospitalisation or two units of blood) in the patients receiving warfarin was low: 1.3 per cent, as compared to 1 per cent in the control group. This is likely to reflect the tight anticoagulation control and careful selection of patients included in the trials.[29] Indeed, the follow-up of out-patients treated with warfarin outside trial conditions suggests that the rate of major bleeding per year of therapy may be much higher, with estimates ranging as high as 18 per cent.[29] Patient factors that appear to increase the risk of haemorrhage include serious comorbidity and age.[30] Not surprisingly, the lower the mean prothrombin time ratio (PTR) at which the blood is maintained and the more stable the PTR is over time, the lower the risk of serious bleeding.[31]

Given that the clinical issue is usually whether to prescribe warfarin or aspirin, rather than warfarin or nothing, the most relevant data on risk of haemorrhage are provided by direct comparison of warfarin to aspirin. The largest study to do this (see Table 13.2) to date has been SPAF-2,[25] which found that the annual rate of haemorrhage on warfarin was 1.7 per cent in patients under the age of 75, and 4.2 per cent in patients over the age of 75. This compares with an annual rate of haemorrhage on aspirin of 0.9 per cent in the under 75s, and 1.6 per cent in the over 75s. The risk of a haemorrhage will also depend upon the target international normalized ratio (INR). In SPAF-2, the target INR was 2–4.5, and the mean INR was 2.7. This is higher than the other sudies, which reported lower haemorrhage rates.

Should we use aspirin or warfarin?

Aspirin or warfarin therapy needs to be considered for all patients with non-rheumatic atrial fibrillation. Which is chosen will depend upon weighing up the potential benefit (greater protection against stroke) and potential harm (greater risk of haemorrhage) of warfarin for each patient. The greater the risk of stroke for an individual, the more that person is likely to benefit from treatment with warfarin. One way in which the harm and benefit can be compared is to consider how many strokes would be prevented per major haemorrhage caused by switching from aspirin to warfarin. If more strokes were prevented than haemorrhages caused, then the risk-benefit ratio would tend to favour warfarin, especially since major haemorrhages, unless they are intracranial, will have a better prognosis than stroke. An illustration of such calculations is shown in Table 13.3. Table 13.3 shows, for different levels of baseline risk of stroke, what the effect of switching from aspirin to warfarin might be based upon the results of SPAF-2.[25] Thus, for a young person in atrial fibrillation without risk factors for stroke, the risk-benefit analysis appears to favour aspirin in that 500 patients would need to be switched to warfarin from aspirin to prevent one stroke, and four of those 500 patients would suffer a major haemorrhage. Likewise, for an older patient, if one assumes (as was found in SPAF-2) that he is at a higher risk of haemorrhage on warfarin, then, despite his higher risk of stroke, the risk-benefit analysis may favour aspirin, unless he has several risk factors for stroke. On the other hand, younger patients with risk factors for stroke would appear to be better off on warfarin than aspirin.

Risk stratification as in Table 13.3 can only offer an indication of what might be the most appropriate therapy. Other factors will come into account too, such as how easy it is to monitor anticoagulation control, and patient factors, such as risk of falling, mental state, alcohol consumption, and ability to comply with medication and with blood tests. Given the impact that minor bleeds can have on the quality of life on patients with warfarin,[32] and the potential inconvenience of the monitoring, patient preference will play a key role in the final decision.

While there is strong evidence that warfarin is more effective than aspirin at reducing risk of stroke in patients with non-rheumatic atrial fibrillation, because of its increased risk of haemorrhage and requirement for long term monitoring, aspirin will be more appropriate in certain circumstances.

WHICH PATIENTS BENEFIT FROM CAROTID ENDARTERECTOMY, AND HOW SHOULD THEY BE IDENTIFIED IN GENERAL PRACTICE?

Studies that have explored the role of carotid endarterectomy in the prevention of stroke have looked at two main circumstances: patients who have had symptoms attributable to a carotid artery stenosis and patients who have been symptom free, but nevertheless have carotid artery disease.

Table 13.3 Warfarin or aspirin for non-rheumatic atrial fibrillation? A summary of the likely impact of treatment at different levels of patient risk

Baseline risk of stroke	Patient characteristics	Risk of stroke if treated with aspirin	Risk of stroke if switched from aspirin to warfarin	Risk of haemorrhage on aspirin	Risk of haemorrhage on warfarin	NNT to prevent one stroke by switching from aspirin to warfarin	NNT to cause one haemorrhage by switching from aspirin to warfarin	Number of strokes prevented per haemorrhage caused by switching from aspirin to warfarin
1%	age <65; no risk factors for stroke	0.7%	0.5%	0.9%	1.7%	500	125	0.25
4%	age 65–75; no risk factors	2.8%	2.0%	0.9%	1.7%	125	125	1.0
5%	age <65; one or more risk factors	3.5%	2.5%	0.9%	1.7%	100	125	1.25
6%	age 65–75; one or more risk factors	4.2%	2.9%	0.9%	1.7%	77	125	1.6
8%	age >75; one or more risk factors	5.6%	3.9%	1.6%	4.2%	59	38	0.6
19%	at least 3 risk factors	13.3%	9.3%	1.6%	4.2%	25	38	1.5

Risks are per annum. NNT = Number needed to treat. Risk factors for stroke include hypertension, prior stroke or TIA, diabetes.
Estimates of baseline risk are drawn from the Atrial Fibrillation Investigators' overview of 5 trials[24], except the 19% estimate which is drawn from the SPAF data[28]
Aspirin is assumed to cause a 30% reduction in relative risk, regardless of baseline risk; relative risk of stroke on warfarin as compared to aspirin is assumed to be 0.7, regardless of baseline risk.

Carotid endarterectomy in symptomatic patients

There have been three recent randomized controlled trials which have looked at the role of carotid endarterectomy in preventing stroke in people who have suffered a transient ischaemic attack or non-disabling stroke in the territory supplied by the carotid artery. These are the *MRC European Carotid Surgery Trial* (ECST),[33] the *North American Symptomatic Carotid Endarterectomy Trial* (NASCET),[34] and the *Veterans Affairs Study*.[35] The third of these studies was terminated early because of the beneficial results obtained in the other two studies. Both ECST and NASCET found that carotid endarterectomy leads to significant reductions in the risk of stroke for symptomatic patients with severe (70–99 per cent) carotid artery stenosis. The ECST found that after three years of follow-up, 11 per cent of patients in the control group had suffered a fatal or disabling stroke as compared to 6 per cent in the treatment group. This is the equivalent of preventing five fatalities or disabling strokes per 100 operations. The NASCET found that after two years of follow up, 18.1 per cent of control patients had suffered a major stroke or died, compared to 8 per cent in the treatment group—the equivalent of preventing 10 such events per 100 operations. The higher risks of stroke in the control group in the *NASCET Study*, and the consequently greater absolute benefits of surgery probably reflects the different radiological definitions of severe carotid artery stenosis that were used in the two trials.

The ECST also looked at the impact of carotid endarterectomy in symptomatic patients with mild stenosis (0–29 per cent), and found that surgery did not appear to confer any benefit in such patients. Both NASCET and ECST are continuing to enrol symptomatic patients with moderate stenosis (30–69 per cent) to determine whether carotid endarterectomy is indicated in this intermediate group of patients.

The benefits of carotid endarterectomy are crucially dependent upon the skill of the operator. In NASCET, only surgeons that had a 30-day post-operative complication rate for stroke or death of less than 6 per cent were allowed to participate. If the 30-day complication rate is higher, then clearly the benefits of surgery will be diminished—a complication rate approaching 10 per cent would mitigate the possible benefit altogether.[36]

Carotid endarterectomy in asymptomatic patients

The effectiveness of carotid endarterectomy in preventing strokes in people with severe carotid artery stenosis that have had a TIA or minor stroke raises the question: would the operation be of benefit to people with the same underlying pathology who have not had any symptoms? Four randomized trials have reported results addressing this question,[37,38,39,40] and a fifth trial, the ACST (*Asymptomatic Carotid Surgery Trial*) is currently underway.[36] The findings of these studies have been mixed. The *Mayo Clinic Trial* was terminated after 71 patients had been entered into the trial because of a significantly higher rate of adverse outcome (myocardial infarction and TIAs) in patients who underwent surgery that was attributed to the non-use of aspirin in the surgical arm of the trial. The

CASANOVA Study found no difference in outcome between medical and surgical treatment. However, the study was not of sufficient size (410 patients) to exclude the possibility of a clinically important effect of surgery and the study protocol excluded patients with greater than 90 per cent stenosis, who arguably might have been the most likely to benefit from surgery. The *Veterans Affairs Co-operative Study*, which followed up its 444 patients for an average of four years, found a significant reduction in the incidence of TIAs and stroke in the surgical arm of the trial (12.8 per cent vs 24.5 per cent). However, it can be argued that the aim of the operation is primarily to prevent strokes rather than TIAs.[41] The impact on stroke rate alone was less impressive (8.1 per cent vs 12 per cent), especially if one also takes the 1.9 per cent 30-day operative mortality (four deaths from myocardial infarction in 211 patients) into account. The interim results of the *Asymptomatic Carotid Atherosclerosis Study* (ACAS), which is the largest trial with 1662 patients, show that the five year risk of stroke or death in the surgical arm of the trial was 4.8 per cent as compared to 10.6 per cent in the medical arm. This implies that operating on 100 people will prevent 5.8 strokes or deaths in five years.

While the most recent and largest study has demonstrated a beneficial effect of surgery on people with carotid stenosis (greater than 60 per cent), but without symptoms attributable to it, the results of other studies on carotid surgery in asymptomatic patients have been equivocal. Surgery may be justified in asymptomatic patients with proven severe carotid artery stenosis based on carotid arteriography. However, the evidence is not yet available to justify the investigations that would be required to identify such patients, given the risks attached to carotid arteriography (1.2 per cent risk of stroke from the procedure in the ACAS study), and the costs of screening to identify patients (such as by ultrasound) for whom carotid arteriography might be indicated.

How to identify patients with severe stenosis

While it is not yet justified to identify asymptomatic patients with carotid artery stenosis, there is potential benefit in identifying such patients once they have had a TIA or minor stroke. How can this be done in primary care? Unfortunately, the principal clinical sign of carotid stenosis, the presence of a carotid bruit, is a poor predictor of the severity of the stenosis in that neither does its presence rule in a severe stenosis, nor does its absence rule one out.[42] Therefore, referral for carotid endarterectomy needs to be considered in patients who have had a recent TIA or minor stroke in the territory of the carotid arteries, regardless of whether or not a carotid bruit is present. The assessment of the carotid arteries prior to surgery in the clinical trials was done by arteriography. As yet, there is insufficient evidence to suggest that less invasive techniques such as ultrasound are sufficiently accurate to replace arteriography in the surgical work up,[36] though it may be that magnetic resonance angiography may fill this role in the future. The decision as to who should be referred on for assessment for surgery will depend upon patient factors such as concurrent medical conditions and willingness to undergo surgery. Duplex ultrasonography is a useful investigation with which to identify which patients with a history of minor stroke or TIA are likely to have severe ipsilateral carotid artery stenosis, and therefore warrant arteriography.[43]

SUMMARY

- There is strong evidence that medium dose aspirin (75–325 mg) is effective in reducing the risk of stroke in patients who have suffered a transient ischaemic attack or stroke.
- There is strong evidence that warfarin is effective in reducing the risk of stroke in patients with non-rheumatic atrial fibrillation.
- Aspirin is also probably effective in reducing the risk of stroke in patients with non-rheumatic atrial fibrillation, but less so than warfarin.
- Whether individuals with atrial fibrillation are better off on aspirin or warfarin depends upon how likely they are to suffer a stroke, and how great is their risk of haemorrhage on warfarin.
- There is good evidence that carotid endarterectomy is an effective operation to reduce the risk of stroke in people who have had a recent TIA or minor stroke, and who have severe (70–99 per cent occlusion) carotid artery stenosis on the appropriate side.
- The role of carotid endarterectomy is still being evaluated for:
    i. people who have had a recent TIA or minor stroke and have a moderate stenosis (30–69 per cent)
    ii. people who have carotid artery stenosis in the absence of symptoms.

REFERENCES

1. Shinton R, Beevers G. Meta-analysis of relation between cigarette smoking and stroke. BMJ 1989; **298**: 789–94.
2. MacMahon S, Peto R, Cutler J, Collins R, Sorlie P, Neaton J, *et al.* Blood pressure, stroke and coronary heart disease **1**: prolonged differences in blood pressure: prospective observational studies corrected for the regression dilution bias. Lancet 1990; **335**: 765–74.
3. Camargo CA. Moderate alcohol consumption and stroke: the epidemiologic evidence. Stroke 1989; **20**: 1611–26.
4. Shinton R, Sagar G. Lifelong exercise and stroke. BMJ 1993; **307**: 231–4.
5. Fuller J, Shipley M, Rose G, Jarrett RJ, Keen H. Mortality from coronary heart disease and stroke in relation to degree of glycaemia: the Whitehall Study. BMJ 1983; **287**: 867–70.
6. Kannel WB, Gordon T, Wolf PA, McNamara P. Manifestations of coronary disease predisposing to stroke. The Framingham Study. JAMA 1983; **250**: 2942–6.
7. Atkins D, Psaty BM, Koepsell TD, Longstreth Jr WT, Larson EB. Cholesterol reduction and the risk for stroke in men: a meta-analysis of randomized controlled trials. Ann Intern Med 1993; **119**: 136–45.
8. Wolf PA, Abbott RD, Kannel WB. Atrial fibrillation: a major contributor to stroke in the elderly. The Framingham study. Arch Intern Med 1987; **147**: 1561–4.

9. Dennis M, Bamford J, Sandercock P, Warlow C. Prognosis of transient ischemic attacks in the Oxfordshire community stroke project. Stroke 1990; **21**: 848–53.

10. Antiplatelet Trialists' Collaboration. Collaborative overview of randomized trials of antiplatelet therapy—**1**: prevention of death, myocardial infarction, and stroke by prolonged antiplatelet therapy in various categories of patients. BMJ 1994; **308**: 81–106.

11. Steering committee of the physicians' health study research group. Final report on the aspirin component of the ongoing physicians' health study. New Engl J Med 1989; **321**: 129–35.

12. Peto R, Gray R, Collins R, Wheatley K, Hennekens CH, Jamrozik K, *et al.* Randomised trial of prophylactic daily aspirin in British male doctors. BMJ 1988; **296**: 313–16.

13. Lowenthal A, Buyse M. Secondary prevention of stroke: does dipyridamole add to aspirin? Acta Neurol. Belg 1994; **94**: 24–34.

14. Matchar DB, McCrory DC, Barnett HJM, Feussner JR. Medical treatment for stroke prevention. Ann Intern Med. 1994; **121**: 41–53.

15. The SALT Collaborative Group. Swedish aspirin low-dose trial (SALT) of 75mg aspirin as secondary prophylaxis after cerebrovascular ischaemic events. Lancet 1991; **338**: 1345–9.

16. UK-TIA Study Group. The United Kingdom transient ischaemic attack (UK-TIA) aspirin trial: final results. Journal of Neurology, Neurosurgery and Psychiatry 1991; **54**: 1044–54.

17. The Dutch TIA trial study group. A comparison of two doses of aspirin (30 mg vs 283 mg a day) in patients after a transient ischemic attack or minor ischemic stroke. N Engl J Med 1991; **325**: 1261–6.

18. Dennis MS, Bamford, JM, Molyneaux AJ, Warlow CP. Rapid resolution of signs of primary intracerebral haemorrhage in computed tomograms of the brain. BMJ 1987; **295**: 379–81.

19. Bamford J, Sandercock P, Dennis M, Burn J, Warlow C. A prospective study of acute cerebrovascular disease in the community: the Oxfordshire community stroke project 1981–86 **2**: incidence, case fatality rates and overall outcome at one year of cerebral infarction, primary intracerebral and subarachnoid haemorrhage. Journal of Neurology, Neurosurgery & Psychiatry 1990; **53**: 16–22.

20. Ebrahim S. Clinical epidemiology of stroke. Oxford University Press 1990.

21. Stroke prevention in atrial fibrillation investigators. Stroke prevention in atrial fibrillation study: final results. Circulation 1991; **84**: 527–39.

22. Petersen P, Godtfredsen J, Boysen G, Andersen ED, Andersen B. Placebo-controlled, randomized trial of warfarin and aspirin for prevention of thromboembolic complications in chronic atrial fibrillation—the Copenhagen AFASAK Study. Lancet 1989; **i**: 175–9.

23. EAFT (European atrial fibrillation trial) study group. Secondary prevention in non-rheumatic atrial fibrillation after transient ischaemic attack or minor stroke. Lancet 1993; **342**: 1255–62.

24. Atrial fibrillation investigators. Risk factors for stroke and efficacy of antithrombotic therapy in atrial fibrillation—analysis of pooled data from five randomized controlled trials. Arch Intern Med 1994; **154**: 1449–57.

25. Stroke prevention in atrial fibrillation investigators. Warfarin versus aspirin for prevention of thromboembolism in atrial fibrillation: Stroke Prevention in Atrial Fibrillation II study. Lancet 1994; **343**: 687–91.

26. Bamford J, Sandercock P, Dennis M, Warlow C, Jones L, McPherson P, *et al.* A prospective study of acute cerebrovascular disease in the community: the Oxfordshire community stroke project 1981–86. 1. Methodology, demography and incident cases of first ever stroke. Journal of Neurology, Neurosurgery and Psychiatry 1988; **51**: 1373–80.

27. The stroke prevention in atrial fibrillation investigators. Predictors of thromboembolism in atrial fibrillation: 1 clinical features of patients at risk. Annals of Internal Medicine 1992; **116**: 1–5.
28. The stroke prevention in atrial fibrillation investigators. Predictors of thromboembolism in atrial fibrillation: 2 echocardiographic features of patients at risk. Annals of Internal Medicine 1992; **116**: 6–12.
29. Sweeney KG, Gray DP, Steele R, Evans P. Use of warfarin in non-rheumatic atrial fibrillation: a commentary from general practice. British Journal of General Practice 1995; **45**: 153–8.
30. Landefeld CS, Goldman L. Major bleeding in outpatients treated with warfarin: incidence and prediction by factors known at the start of outpatient therapy. American Journal of Medicine 1989; **87**: 144–152.
31. Fihn SD, McDonell M, Martin D, *et al* for the warfarin optimized outpatient follow-up study group. Risk factors for complications of chronic anticoagulation: a multicenter study. Annals of Internal Medicine 1993; **118**: 511–20.
32. Lancaster TR, Singer DE, Sheehan MA, *et al.* The impact of long-term warfarin therapy on quality of life. Evidence from a randomized trial. Archives of Internal Medicine 1991; **151**: 1944–9.
33. European carotid surgery trialists' collaborative group. MRC European carotid surgery trial: interim results for symptomatic patients with severe (70–99 per cent) or with mild (0–29 per cent) carotid stenosis. Lancet 1991; **337**: 1235–43.
34. North American symptomatic carotid endarterectomy trial collaborators. Beneficial effect of carotid endarterectomy in symptomatic patients with high-grade carotid stenosis. N Engl J Med 1991; **325**: 445–54.
35. Mayberg MR, Wilson E, Yatsu F, *et al.* Carotid endarterectomy and prevention of cerebral ischemia in symptomatic carotid stenosis. JAMA 1991; **266**: 3289–94.
36. Barnett H, Meldrum H. Status of carotid endarterectomy. Current Opinion in Neurology 1994; **7**: 54–9.
37. Hobson RW, Weiss DG, Fields WS, *et al.* Efficacy of carotid endarterectomy for asymptomatic carotid stenosis. N Engl J Med 1993; **328**: 221–7.
38. The CASANOVA Study Group. Carotid versus medical therapy in asymptomatic carotid stenosis. Stroke 1991; **22**: 1229–35.
39. Mayo asymptomatic carotid endarterectomy study group. Results of a randomized controlled trial of carotid endarterectomy for asymptomatic carotid stenosis. Mayo Clinic Proceedings 1992; **67**: 513–18.
40. ACAS investigators. Clinical advisory: carotid endarterectomy for patients with asymptomatic internal carotid artery stenosis. Stroke 1994; **12**: 2523–4.
41. Barnett HJM, Haines SJ. Carotid endarterectomy for asymptomatic carotid stenosis. New Engl J Med 1993; **328**: 276–9.
42. Sauve J-S, Laupacis A, Ostbye T, Feagan B, Sackett DL. Does this patient have a clinically important carotid bruit? JAMA 1993; **270**: 2843–5.
43. Hankey GJ, Warlow CP. Symptomatic carotid ischaemic events: safest and most cost-effective way of selecting patients for angiography, before carotid endarterectomy. BMJ 1990; **300**: 1485–91.

14 Secondary prevention of coronary heart disease

Tim Lancaster and Peter Sleight

INTRODUCTION

Survivors of myocardial infarction have a four to eight times increased risk of recurrence and death.[1,2] Coronary artery disease is common, so this represents a high absolute risk. In the *British Regional Heart Study* 14 per cent of 242 men with electrocardiographic signs of definite infarction had reinfarctions over a 4.2 year follow-up, compared with only 2 per cent of those with a normal electrocardiogram at entry to the study.[1] Focusing clinical resources on such patients is attractive because of the health gain that can be achieved from small reductions in their high absolute risk, and because they may be more highly motivated to change damaging behaviours and comply with medical treatment.[3] Unfortunately, effective treatments are not offered as often they could be,[4] perhaps because physicians mistakenly believe that it is too late to improve coronary disease once infarction has occurred.

Medical, surgical, and behavioural interventions all have the potential to help (and harm) patients with coronary disease, and in most cases their efficacy can only be judged by performing randomized clinical trials. Although a number of secondary prevention trials have been performed, there has been confusion about how to interpret them because individual trials have produced inconclusive or conflicting results.[5] This is largely because they have been of inadequate size to detect or reliably exclude moderate, but clinically important, effects. The situation has been clarified in recent years with the development of statistical techniques (meta-analysis) which allow data from individual trials to be combined to provide pooled estimates of treatment effects,[6] and a number of such analyses have been performed in the field of secondary prevention.[5,7,8,9] In addition, information is increasingly available from large 'mega-trials', which provide more reliable answers by enrolling tens of thousands of participants.

In this chapter, experimental studies are considered the strongest evidence for efficacy, but it is important to appreciate their limitations. For some interventions, such as smoking cessation, formal randomized trials are difficult, and to insist on such evidence before making clinical recommendations is not appropriate. On the other hand, when valid trials have been performed, caution is required in generalizing their results to categories of patient who have not been eligible to participate. This criticism has been levelled particularly at trials in myocardial infarction which have frequently excluded women, the elderly and ethnic minorities.[10] In general, however, differences in effect of interventions between these groups are likely to be quantitative rather than qualitative, and it is probably better to assume that the results of trials conducted in one group are applicable to others as well. Finally, how different treatments interact is not fully understood. While there is increasing evidence for the additive effects of pharmacological interventions, studies comparing, for example lifestyle change and drug therapy, are few. With these *caveats*, this chapter considers secondary prevention of ischaemic heart disease in primary care by addressing three questions:

1. **What is the evidence that modifying risk factors improves outcome in survivors of myocardial infarction?**
2. **What is the evidence that pharmacological agents given prophylactically reduce mortality and morbidity in such patients?**
3. **Which patients benefit from revasularization by surgery or angioplasty and how should they be identified and appropriately triaged in general practice?**

WHAT IS THE EVIDENCE THAT MODIFYING RISK FACTORS IMPROVES OUTCOME IN SURVIVORS OF MYOCARDIAL INFARCTION?

Cardiac rehabilitation

Cardiac rehabilitation programmes use various combinations of exercise training and life-style modification with the aim of improving functional capacity and reducing morbidity and mortality. Their best feature may be as a forum for education, confidence building, and group support.

Evaluation is difficult because of differences in the nature of the interventions and the often multiple endpoints used. Compliance with the programmes, when it has been reported, has generally been low.[3] Nevertheless, a meta-analysis of ten trials in which subjects underwent at least six weeks of exercise or exercise plus risk factor management found that they achieved statistically significant reductions of about 25 per cent in both cardiovascular and all-cause mortality, with no significant difference in the rate of non-fatal recurrent infarction.[8] There is, therefore, good evidence for enrolling patients in such programmes where they are available. It is also reasonable to recommend graduated exercise to all patients, though the evidence for benefit of this approach is less clear (see Chapter 5). Trials which have included interventions other than exercise, such as relaxation training and stress management, have reported reductions in cardiac morbidity and/or mortality,[11,12] but it is difficult to separate their effects from other aspects of the treatment programmes. In the *Lifestyle Heart Trial*, for example, reductions in angina and angiographic regression were achieved with an intervention which included smoking cessation, stress management training, and exercise in addition to a rigorous vegetarian diet.[12]

Smoking

Survivors of myocardial infarction who continue to smoke approximately double their risk of dying compared to those who quit.[13] In a number of case control studies and some cohort studies smoking cessation led to an immediate risk reduction,[14,15] suggesting that the effect of smoking may be mediated through thrombotic factors. In other cohort studies, ex-smokers remained at increased risk for many years afterwards;[13,16] misclassification of quitters who relapse is a possible explanation for this discrepancy.[15] Evidence suggests that advice on smoking cessation can reduce cardiac mortality,[17,18,19] although no trial has examined its effect on outcome after MI. Studies of the safety and efficacy of nicotine substitution in patients with known vascular disease are badly needed, since adding this form of therapy to counselling and other strategies increases the quit rate in primary prevention trials.[20]

Cholesterol and other dietary factors

Cholesterol is a risk factor for reinfarction (see Chapter 3). In the placebo group in the *Coronary Drug Project*, the relative risk associated with the highest as compared with the lowest quintile of serum cholesterol was 1.5.[21] Although there has been recent concern about possible increases in noncardiovascular mortality by cholesterol lowering in relatively low risk subjects,[22,23] this is less relevant in secondary prevention, where most deaths will be from cardiovascular causes. Recent overviews of randomized trials concluded that high risk patients benefit from cholesterol-lowering.[5,22,24] Meta-analysis of eight secondary prevention trials, using diet, and or drugs, indicated statistically significant reductions in the risk of non-fatal (25 per cent), fatal (16 per cent), and total (22 per cent) myocardial infarction.[24] Total mortality was also reduced.[5] In addition, angiographic studies showed regression with cholesterol lowering.[12,25,26] Most recently, the first trial (*Scandinavian Simvastatin Survival Study*) to study the effects of a drug from the HMG-CoA reductase inhibitor class, reported striking effects on both cardiovascular and total mortality in patients with angina or previous myocardial infarction with cholesterol of 5.5–8.0 mmol/l after dietary treatment.[27] In the long-term such treatment would save about 30–40 lives per 1000 patients treated. These effects were associated with a mean reduction of 25 per cent in total cholesterol.

There is, therefore, strong evidence for intervention by diet and/or drugs in patients who have manifest vascular disease, either on the basis of threshold cholesterol levels, or perhaps more logically on the basis of overall risk. There is no clear evidence about the most appropriate threshold values and target levels, but the results of the *Scandinavian Simvastatin Survival Trial* provide strong evidence for the recommendation that treatment be given for levels greater than 5.2 mmol/l in patients with established vascular disease.[27] A large British trial (the *MRC/BHF Heart Protection Study*) is now underway to determine the benefits of cholesterol reduction in various categories of high risk patients, randomizing patients with vascular disease or diabetes to receive simvastatin, antioxidant vitamins or placebo for cholesterol levels > 3.5 mmol/l. Physicians who remain unconvinced about the value of lowering cholesterol might consider entering their patients into this study.

Although the efficacy of conventional dietary advice for lowering cholesterol is limited,[28] highly motivated individuals may achieve impressive reductions with diet alone; in the *Lifestyle Heart Trial*,[12] large reductions were attained with a vegetarian diet which included less than 10 per cent of calories as fat. Many patients will be unable to comply with such rigorous programmes, and drug therapy may be required when diet is ineffective. There is increasing evidence that antioxidants contained in fruit and vegetables (vitamins A, E and C) may protect against atheroma formation (Chapter 12), and randomized trials are underway to assess their role in therapy.

Weight reduction

Although there are no randomized trials of the effect of weight reduction on prognosis in survivors of myocardial infarction, overweight patients should benefit from a weight reduction programme because of associated improvements in blood pressure and cholesterol levels.[3]

Blood pressure

Patients who remain hypertensive after myocardial infarction are at increased risk of further events. In primary prevention trials, treatment of hypertension reduced cardiac risk,[29] and indirect evidence suggests that treating persistently elevated blood pressure after myocardial infarction is worthwhile. In the *Hypertension Detection and Follow-up Program* patients with a history of myocardial infarction allocated to the special care group had a 20 per cent reduction in mortality.[3] There is little direct evidence about the most appropriate target levels for treatment in this group. On the basis of results from primary prevention trials, the *British Hypertension Society* recommends initiating treatment for diastolic blood pressure of 90–99 mm Hg or systolic greater than 160 mm Hg in patients with target organ damage.[30] The recommended goals of treatment are reduction of the diastolic to less than 90 mm Hg, and the systolic to less than 160 mm Hg. Others have recommended lower target pressures such as less than 85 mm Hg diastolic and less than 125 mm Hg systolic but there has been concern that over aggressive reductions of blood pressure in patients with known ischaemic heart disease may increase coronary events.[31]

WHAT IS THE EVIDENCE THAT PHARMACOLOGICAL AGENTS GIVEN PROPHYLACTICALLY REDUCE MORTALITY AND MORBIDITY IN SUCH PATIENTS?

Anti-platelet therapy

In the *ISIS-2 Study*, aspirin (160 mg) started at the onset of infarction and continued for four weeks reduced mortality whether or not thrombolytic therapy was used.[32] The most recent overview of clinical trials of antiplatelet therapy by *The AntiPlatelet Trialists' Collaboration* has shown that it is effective in the prevention of recurrent myocardial infarction, stroke, and other vascular events.[33] Vascular events are reduced by 20–25 per cent in the first few years after the index event, and all-cause mortality by 12 per cent. About 25 lives are saved per 1000 patients treated. There is particular benefit in unstable angina. Other antiplatelet agents offer no advantage over aspirin alone. Trials of aspirin which used lower doses (160–325 mg/day) show comparable efficacy and about one third of the toxicity of those that used higher doses (900–1500 mg/day). Reductions in vascular morbidity and mortality have been achieved with doses as low as 75 mg/day.[34,35,36] On the basis of evidence from clinical trials, antiplatelet agents should be prescribed for at least one to two years, but in the absence of side-effects, it is reasonable to continue them indefinitely.

Warfarin

The use of warfarin after myocardial infarction has been debated for many years, but there is now conclusive evidence that it can reduce mortality. In the *Warfarin Re-Infarction Study*[37] total mortality was reduced by 24 per cent and non-fatal reinfarctions by 50 per cent in subjects randomized to take warfarin (target INR 2.8 to 4.8) for two years. This is consistent with the pooled results of earlier studies.[5] More recently, the *ASPECT Study*[38] found significant reductions in recurrent vascular events in patients treated with oral anticoagulants after myocardial infarction. There is little evidence of the relative efficacy of anticoagulation and aspirin from direct comparisons, though trials are underway to address this question. Meanwhile, low dose aspirin is preferred because it is cheaper and simpler to take, with a lower risk of haemorrhage, than warfarin. Anticoagulation may be particularly appropriate in patients with left ventricular thrombus, large anterior infarction or atrial fibrillation. Trials of combined therapy are also in progress and low dose warfarin plus aspirin has been shown to reduce mortality in patients with artificial heart valves.[39]

Betablockade

Since 1972, at least 18 randomized, controlled trials of long-term beta-adrenergic blockade have been conducted in more than 18 000 survivors of acute myocardial infarction.[9] Overviews of the data from these studies suggest that the reduction in mortality is about 20 per cent (about 10 lives saved per 1000 subjects treated).[5,9] Although the relative risk reduction in patients at low risk of recurrence (for example, an inferior infarction without complications) will be less than for a high risk patient, the benefits of this treatment have been seen across all classes of risk. There is little direct evidence on the optimum duration of treatment, as no trial has examined the effect of withdrawing treatment after a period of time. A recent analysis suggests that the drugs may safely be withdrawn after one year in patients who are not defined as clinically high-risk on the basis of recurrent ischaemia, congestive heart failure, or arrythmias.[40] This may be a reasonable clinical strategy given the side-effects of these agents which are contra-indicated or not tolerated in about 50 per cent of patients.

ACE inhibitors

A substantial subgroup of patients develop clinical or subclinical evidence of heart failure after myocardial infarction despite the use of beta-adrenoreceptor antagonists and antiplatelet agents, and their risk of recurrence and death is high. Angiotensin converting enzyme (ACE) inhibitors have previously been shown to improve mortality in patients with established severe heart failure,[41] leading to interest in their prophylactic use after myocardial infarction. The *CONSENSUS 11 Trial* studied the routine administration to patients with suspected infarction of enalaprilat started intravenously on admission to hospital followed by oral enalapril for six months. There was no reduction in mortality, and a non-signficant excess of deaths in the intervention group.[42] In the *SAVE Study*,[43] captopril was administered at a mean of eleven days after infarction to patients who had asymptomatic left ventricular dysfunction (left ventricular ejection fraction less than 40 per cent). Total mortality was reduced by 19 per cent and recurrent myocardial infarction by 25 per cent in the active treatment group. Similar benefits for asymptomatic left ventricular dysfunction were seen in the *SOLVD Study*.[44] In the *AIRE Study*,[45] oral ramipril, started two to nine days after myocardial infarction in patients who showed clinical evidence of heart failure reduced total mortality by 27 per cent.

Most recently, the large (58 050 subjects) *ISIS-4 Trial* studied the effects of oral captopril started on admission for myocardial infarction, and continued for one month afterwards. The treatment was safe and reduced the risk of death by 7 per cent (about five fewer deaths per 1000 patients treated, or 10/1000 in higher risk patients).[46] There is therefore now a good case for one month's routine treatment with an oral ACE inhibitor following myocardial infarction, continuing treatment in those with evidence of ventricular dysfunction or clinical heart failure. Facilities for detecting asymptomatic left ventricular dysfunction are not at present readily available in general practice, but echocardiography may become increasingly used for this purpose in the light of these results.

Hormone replacement therapy

The weight of evidence from observational studies[47] suggests that post-menopausal oestrogen replacement therapy reduces the risk of ischaemic heart disease by about 40 to 50 percent (see Chapter 10). This effect persists with statistical adjustment for other known cardiac risk factors, but as the allocation of treatment was not randomized in these studies, a bias towards offering treatment to healthier women cannot be ruled out. In addition, the evidence for benefit relates to unopposed oestrogen, whereas current practice is usually to treat women who have not undergone hysterectomy with combined oestrogen and progestin therapy to protect against endometrial cancer. This raises the concern that the progestin component may blunt the beneficial effects of the oestrogen by adverse effects on serum lipoproteins. Given this uncertainty, routine use of this treatment for secondary prevention should await results from randomized trials, which are currently planned.[48]

Other drug treatments

Verapamil post-infarction reduced the risk of reinfarction and sudden death in patients without heart failure in one study,[49] but other calcium channel blockers have not been shown to improve prognosis.[5] Prophylactic use of Type one anti-arrythmic drugs increases the death rate after myocardial infarction,[5,50] and they have no place in secondary prevention.

WHICH PATIENTS BENEFIT FROM REVASCULARIZATION BY SURGERY OR ANGIOPLASTY AND HOW SHOULD THEY BE IDENTIFIED AND APPROPRIATELY TRIAGED IN GENERAL PRACTICE?

There are many uncertainties about the most appropriate use of surgery and interventional cardiology after myocardial infarction. Randomized trials in patients with stable angina suggest that coronary artery bypass grafting improves symptoms and also prolongs survival in certain sub-groups at high risk because of extensive coronary disease or poor ventricular function.[51,52,53] Initial results from clinical trials[54] suggest that angioplasty, although less effective at relieving angina and more frequently followed by repeat interventions, yields similar mortality results to surgery. Patients with disabling angina or clinical evidence of impaired cardiac function after myocardial infarction may therefore be candidates for one of these forms of revascularization.

More controversial is the role of revascularization in patients who survive their infarction without marked symptoms. The main problem lies in accurately identifying those at high risk of recurrence and death. Routine cardiac catheterization[55] is expensive and of unknown benefit; although under evaluation in a randomized trial in Denmark. An alternative strategy is to screen with non-invasive tests such as exercise electocardiography or Holter monitoring, reserving angiography for those patients with tests judged to be strongly positive for ischaemia. Recent studies have questioned the accuracy of such tests in predicting risk of recurrent infarction.[56,57] The limitations of risk stratification based on detection of coronary artery narrowing are perhaps not surprising, since angiographic studies show that occlusive thrombus can form on relatively mild stenoses.

Given this uncertainty, strategies are likely to vary from area to area, and clinical management will reflect the availability of cardiac services and individual patient preferences. From the general practitioner perspective, patients not already under hospital care should be referred if they demonstrate adverse clinical variables such as low-level angina, impaired cardiac function, or arrythmias.

SUMMARY

There is clear evidence that mortality can be reduced by secondary prevention measures. In many cases, the benefits are additive: for example, captopril in ISIS-4, and simvastatin in the *Scandinavian Study* reduced mortality despite the fact that other proven treatments such as thrombolysis, aspirin, and beta blockers were also prescribed. How the different treatments will interact in individual patients is less clear, however, and it is therefore important to individualize treatment recommendations. So, for example, while some highly motivated individuals may reduce their risk by behaviour change alone,[12] drug treatment may be more effective for patients who are less successful at modifying their habits. General practice management is likely to be more effective if protocols and a recall system for systematic review are in place. Future research is important to define the comparative benefits of life-style change, drug therapy and revascularization procedures, and to determine the best ways of delivering this care in general practice.

RECOMMENDATIONS FOR MANAGEMENT AFTER MYOCARDIAL INFARCTION:

- offer systematic follow-up according to agreed protocols
- offer routine advice on smoking cessation, healthy eating, and weight control
- encourage exercise and refer to cardiac rehabilitation programmes if available
- monitor blood pressure and aim to reduce systolic to less than 160 mm Hg and diastolic to less than 90 mm Hg in patients with recordings consistently greater than these levels
- measure serum cholesterol and consider diet and or drug treatment for levels greater than 5.2 mmol/l, or consider entering patients into randomized trials
- prescribe aspirin (75–325 mg daily) routinely and continue indefinitely if tolerated
- consider warfarin for large anterior myocardial infarction or ventricular thrombus
- prescribe betablockers for at least one year if no contraindication
- prescribe ACE inhibitors for patients with clinical or echocardiographic evidence of ventricular dysfunction
- refer patients with low-level angina, arrthymias, or heart failure for cardiological evaluation.

REFERENCES

1. Shaper AG, Pocock SJ, Walker M., *et al*. Risk factors for ischaemic heart disease: the prospective phase of the British regional heart study. J Epidemiol Community Health 1985; **39**: 197–209.
2. Weinblatt E, Shapiro S, Frank CW, Sager RV. Prognosis of men after myocardial infarction: mortality and first recurrence in relation to selected parameters. Am J Public Health. 1968; **58**: 1329–47.
3. Siegel D, Grady D, Browner WS, Hulley SB. Risk factor modification after myocardial infarction. Ann Intern Med 1988; **109**: 213–18.

4. Eccles M, Bradhshaw C. Use of secondary prophylaxis against myocardial infarction in the north of England. BMJ 1991; **302**: 91–2.

5. Lau J, Antman EM, Jimenez-Silva J, *et al.* Cumulative meta-analysis of therapeutic trials for myocardial infarction. N Engl J Med 1992; **327**: 248–54.

6. Peto R. Why do we need systematic overviews of randomized trials? Stat Med 1987; **6**: 233–40.

7. Law MR, Wald NJ, Thompson SG. By how much and how quickly does reduction in serum cholesterol concentration lower risk of ischaemic heart disease? BMJ 1994; **308**: 367–72.

8. Oldridge NB, Guyatt GH, Fischer ME, Rimm AA. Cardiac rehabilitation after myocardial infarction: combined experience of randomized clinical trials. JAMA 1988; **260**: 945–50.

9. Yusuf S, Peto R, Lewis J, Collins R, Sleight P. Beta blockade during and after myocardial infarction: an overview of the randomized trials. Prog Cardiovas Dis 1985; **27**: 335–71.

10. Gurwitz JH, Col NF, Avorn J. The exclusion of the elderly and women from clinical trials in acute myocardial infarction. JAMA 1992; **268**: 1417–22.

11. Kallio V, Hamalainen H, Hakkila J, Luurila OJ. Reduction in sudden deaths by a multi-factorial intervention programme after acute myocardial infarction. Lancet 1979; **2**: 1091–4.

12. Ornish D, Brown SE, Scherwitz LW *et al.* Can lifestyle changes reverse coronary heart disease? Lancet 1990; **336**: 129–33.

13. Cook DG, Shaper AG, Pocock SJ, Kussick SJ. Giving up smoking and the risk of heart attacks. A report from the British regional heart study. Lancet 1986; 1376–80.

14. Reid DD, Hamilton PJS, McCartney P, Rose G. Smoking and other risk factors for coronary heart-disease in British Civil Servants. Lancet 1976; **2**: 979–84.

15. Rosenberg L, Palmer J, Shapiro S. Decline in the risk of myocardial infarction among women who stop smoking. N Engl J Med 1990; **322**: 213–17.

16. Doll R, Peto R. Mortality in relation to smoking: 20 years' observations on male British doctors. BMJ 1976; **2**: 1525–36.

17. Rose GA, Hamilton PJS, Colwell L, Shipley MJ. A randomized controlled trial of anti-smoking advice: 10-year results. J Epidemiol Community Health. 1982; **36**: 102–108.

18. Holme I, Hjermann I, Hegleland A, Leren P. The Oslo Study: diet and antismoking advice: additional results from a 5-year primary preventive trial in middle-aged men. Prev Med 1985; **14**: 279–92.

19. The Multiple Risk Factor Intervention Trial Research Group. Mortality rates after 10.5 years for participants in the multiple risk factor intervention trial. JAMA 1990; **263**: 1795–801.

20. Silagy C, Mant D, Fowler G. Meta-analysis on efficacy of nicotine replacement therapies in smoking cessation. Lancet 1994; **343**: 139–42.

21. Coronary drug project research group. Natural history of myocardial infarction in the Coronary Drug Project: long-term prognostic importance of serum lipid levels. Am J Cardiol 1978; **42**: 489–98.

22. Davey Smith G, Song F, Sheldon TA. Cholesterol lowering and mortality: the importance of considering initial level of risk. BMJ 1993; **306**: 1367–73.

23. Muldoon MF, Manuck SB, Matthews KA. Lowering cholesterol concentrations and mortality: a quantitative review of primary prevention trials. BMJ 1990; **301**: 309–14.

24. Roussow JE, Lewis B, Rifkind BM. The value of lowering cholesterol after myocardial infarction. N Engl J Med 1990; **323**: 1112–9.

25. Watts GF, Lewis B, Brunt JNH, *et al.* Effects on coronary artery disease of lipid-lowering diet, or diet plus cholestyramine, in the St Thomas' atherosclerosis regression study (STARS). Lancet 1992; **339**: 563–9.

26. Blankenhorn DH, Nessim SA, Johnson RL *et al*. Beneficial effects of combined colestipol-niacin therapy on coronary atherosclerosis and coronary venous bypass grafts. JAMA 1987; **257**: 3233–40.
27. Scandinavian Simvastatin Survival Study Group. Randomised trial of cholesterol lowering in 4444 patients with coronary heart disease. Lancet 1994; **344**: 1383–9.
28. Ramsay LE, Yeo WW, Jackson PR. Dietary reduction of serum cholesterol concentration: time to think again. BMJ 1991; **303**: 953–7.
29. Collins R, Peto R, Macmahon S, *et al*. Blood pressure, stroke, and coronary heart disease, part 2, short-term reductions in blood pressure: overview of randomized drug trials in their epidemiological context. Lancet 1990; **335**: 827–38.
30. Sever P, Beevers G, Bulpitt C *et al*. Management guidelines in essential hypertension: report of the second working party of the British Hypertension Society. BMJ 1993; **306**: 983–7.
31. Fletcher AE, Bulpitt CJ. How far should blood pressure be lowered? N Engl J Med 1992; **326**: 251–4.
32. ISIS-2 Collaborative Group.Randomised trial of intravenous streptokinase, oral aspirin, both, or neither among 17 187 cases of suspected myocardial infarction. Lancet 1988; **2**: 349–60.
33. Antiplatelet Trialists' Collaboration. Collaborative overview of randomized trials of antiplatelet therapy–1: prevention of death, myocardial infarction, and stroke by prolonged antiplatelet therapy in various categories of patients. BMJ 1994; **308**: 81–106.
34. Juul-Moller S, Evardsson N, Jahnmatz B *et al*. Double-blind trial of aspirin in primary prevention of myocardial infarction in patients with stable chronic angina pectoris. Lancet 1992; **340**: 1421– 4.
35. The RISC group. Risk of myocardial infarction and death during treatment with low dose aspirin and intravenous heparin in men with unstable coronary artery disease. Lancet 1990; **336**: 827–30.
36. The SALT Collaborative Group. Swedish aspirin low-dose trial (SALT) of 75mg aspirin as secondary prophylaxis after cerebrovascular ischaemic events. Lancet 1991; **338**: 1345–9.
37. Smith P, Arnesen H, Holme I. The effect of warfarin on mortality and reinfarction after myocardial infarction. N Engl J Med 1990; **323**: 147–52.
38. Aspect Research Group. Effect of long-term oral anticoagulant treatment on mortality and cardiovascular morbidity after myocardial infarction. Lancet 1994; **343**: 499–503.
39. Turpie AG, Gent M, Laupacis A, *et al*. A comparison of aspirin with placebo in patients treated with warfarin after heart-valve replacement. N Engl J Med 1993; **329**: 524–9.
40. Viscoli CM, Horwitz RI, Singer BH. Beta-blockers after myocardial infarction: influence of first-year clinical course on long-term effectiveness. Ann Intern Med 1993; **118**: 99–105.
41. The CONSENSUS Trial Study Group. Effects of enalapril on mortality in severe congestive heart failure: results of the Cooperative North Scandinavian Enalapril Survival Study. (CONSENSUS). N Engl J Med 19987; **316**: 1429–35.
42. Swedberg K, Held P, Kjeckshus J, Rasmussen K, RydenL, Wedel H. Effects of the early administration of enalapril on mortality in patients with acute myocardial infarction—results of the cooperative New Scandinavian enalapril survival study 11 (CONSENSUS 11). N Engl J Med 1992; **327**: 678–84.
43. Pfeffer MA, Braunwald E, Moye LA *et al*. Effect of captopril on mortality and morbidity in patients with left ventricular dysfunction after myocardial infarction—results of the survival and ventricular enlargement trial. N Engl J Med 1992; **327**: 669–77.

44. The SOLVD Investigators. Effect of enalapril on mortality and the development of heart failure in asymptomatic patients with reduced left ventricular ejection fractions. N Engl J Med 1992; **327**: 685–91.

45. The Acute Infarction Ramipril Efficacy (AIRE) Investigators. Effect of ramipril on mortality and morbidity of survivors of acute myocardial infarction with clinical evidence of heart failure. Lancet 1993; **342**: 821–8.

46. ISIS-4 Collaborative Group. ISIS-4: A randomized factorial trial assessing early oral captopril, oral mononitrate, and intravenous magnesium sulphate in 58 050 patients with suspected acute myocardial infarction. Lancet 1995; **345**: 669–85,

47. Stampfer MJ, Colditz GA. Estrogen replacement therapy and coronary heart disease: a quantitative assessment of the epidemiologic evidence. Prev Med 1991; **20**: 47–63.

48. Goldman L, Tosteson ANA. Uncertainty about postmenopausal oestrogen. Time for action, not debate. N Engl J Med 1991; **325**: 800–2.

49. The Danish Study Group on verapamil in myocardial infarction. Effect of verapamil on mortality and major events after acute myocardial infarction (The Danish verapamil infarction trial 11-DAVIT 11). Am J Cardiol 1990; **66**: 779–85.

50. The Cardiac Arrhythmia Suppression Trial (CAST) Investigators. Preliminary report: effect of encainide and flecainide on mortality in a randomized trial of arrrhythmia suppression after myocardial infarction. N Engl J Med 1989; **321**: 406–12.

51. The Veterans Administration Coronary Artery Bypass Surgery Cooperative Study Group. Eleven-year survival in the veterans administration randomized trial of Coronry bypass surgery for stable angina. N Engl J Med 1984; **311**: 1333–9.

52. Passamani E, Davis KB, Gillesie MJ, Killip T, CASS Principal Investigators and Their Associates. A randomized trial of coronary artery bypass surgery: survival of patients with a low ejection fraction. N Engl J Med 1985; **312**: 1665–71.

53. Varnauskas E, European coronary surgery study group. Twelve-year follow-up of survival in the randomized European Coronary Artery Surgery Study. N Engl J Med 1988; **319**: 332–7.

54. RITA Trial Participants. Coronary angioplasty versus coronary srtery bypass grafting: the randomised intervention treatment of angina (RITA)Trial. Lancet 1993; **341**: 573–80.

55. Kulick DL, Rahimtoola SH. Risk stratification in survivors of myocardial infarction: routine cardiac catheterization and angiography is a reasonable approach in most patients. Am Heart J. 1991; **121**: 641–55.

56. Mickley H, Pless P, Nielsen JR, Beming J, Moller M. Transient myocardial ischaemia after a first acute myocardial infarction and its relation to clinical characteristics, predischarge exercise testing and cardiac events at one-year follow-up. Am J Cardiol. 1993; **71**: 139–44.

57. Moss AJ, Goldstein RE, Hall WJ et al. Detection and significance of myocardial ischaemia in stable patients after recovery from an acute coronary event. JAMA. 1993; **269**: 2379–85.

15 Multiple risk

John Muir and David Mant

INTRODUCTION

'The combined effect of all risk factors on risk is striking. The difference in incidence between the highest and lowest deciles (of multivariant risk) is thirty-fold for men and seventy-fold for women.' This quotation, taken from an early report of the *Framingham Study* in 1967,[1] indicates why it is important not to consider individual risk factors in isolation. Many commonly recognized risk factors for ischaemic heart disease, such as smoking, blood pressure, and diet, exert a largely independent effect on risk and their overall effect is cumulative. The Framingham investigators recognized not only the epidemiological importance of their observation but also its implication for clinical practice: 'Programmes require a rational method for identifying persons at high risk so as to focus attention on them and to avoid needlessly alarming persons at lower risk, because of a single stigma. By the same token, it is important not to provide false reassurance to persons with multiple marginal risk factors who may be at a much greater than average risk'.[2]

This chapter discusses the interactive nature of coronary heart disease (CHD) risk factors and explores five areas of uncertainty:

1. **How do risk factors interact?**
2. **What CHD risks should we assess?**
3. **How can we calculate multiple CHD risk in general practice?**
4. **How valuable is multiple CHD risk assessment?**
5. **Is multiple risk intervention sensible?**

HOW DO RISK FACTORS INTERACT?

Risk of vascular events attributable to different independent risk factors and disease states are cumulative. Figure 15.1 was developed from the *Multiple Risk Factor Intervention Trial* (MRFIT) and illustrates the risk of cardiovascular death over a six year period for males aged 46–57 years according to blood pressure, blood cholesterol and smoking status.[3] Each individual risk factor exerts no more than a four-fold increase in risk, but a smoker with a diastolic blood pressure and a total cholesterol in the highest quintile is at 11 times the risk of cardiovascular death of a non-smoker with a diastolic blood pressure and a total cholesterol in the lowest quintile, suggesting that the increase in risk associated with these three risk factors is at least additive. This observation has been confirmed in a formal analysis of the MRFIT data by Silbeberg which indicates that, for most risk factors, the cumulative risk is more than additive but less than multiplicative.[4]

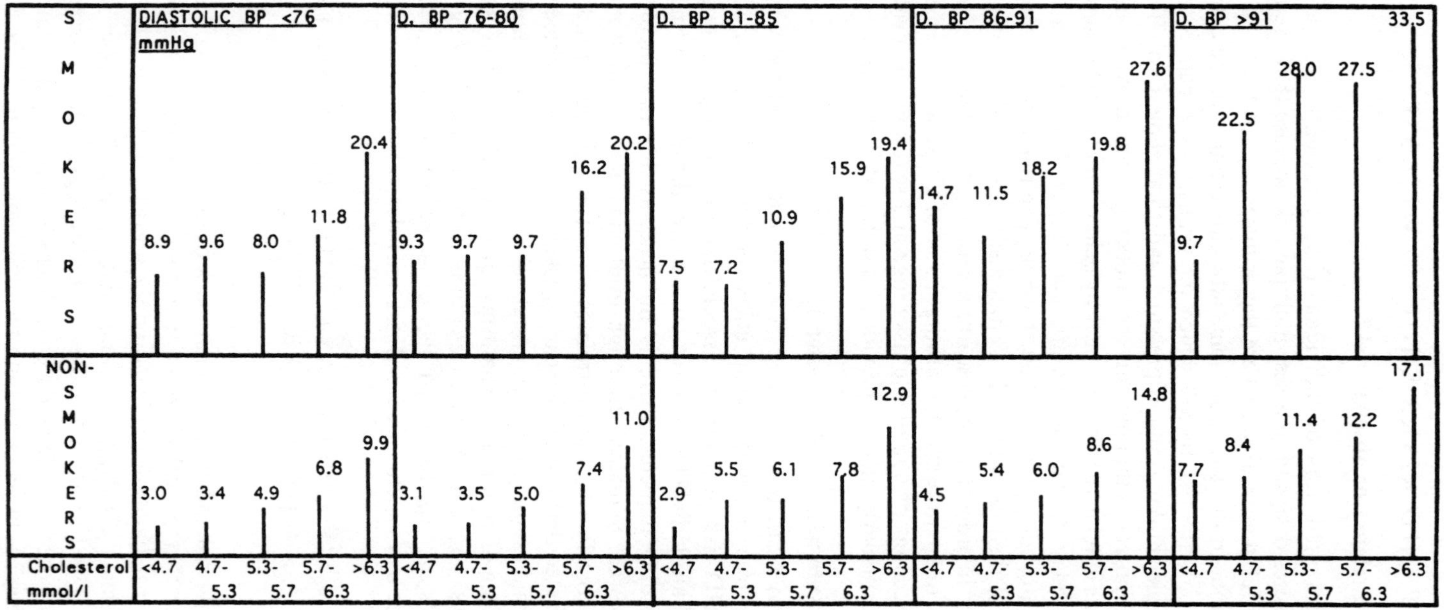

Fig. 15.1 Six year cardiovascular disease mortality rates per 1000 men aged 46–57 years in relation to diastolic blood pressure, smoking, and blood cholesterol. (From Kannel WB, Neaton JD, Wentworth MPH, Thomas HE, *et al.* Overall coronary heart disease mortality rate in relation to major risk factors in 325 348 men screened for the multiple risk factor intervention trial (MRFIT). Am Heart J 1986; **112**: 825–36.)

WHAT CHD RISKS SHOULD WE ASSESS?

Are we interested in relative or absolute risk?

The most important predictors of individual risk, particularly age, are often omitted from measures designed to assess multiple risk because they are thought to be less than helpful in clinical use where the primary objective is to encourage life-style modification. In this situation, some advocate estimating the cumulative relative risk using only the risk factors which the primary care team is trying to modify—for example smoking, blood pressure, and total cholesterol. The main advantage of this approach is that patients are not being asked to swim against the tide—improvements in relative risk from healthy behaviour cannot be annulled by an intervening birthday. Critics of this approach argue that this is a form of subterfuge—that informing patients about their relative risk is misleading unless they are informed of their absolute risk. Critics also point out that if cumulative risk is being assessed in order to allocate scarce resources, measurement of absolute risk is essential. In order to assess the absolute risk of CHD with precision it is necessary to take account of immutable risks (age and sex) and any evidence of existing disease (particularly angina, previous infarct, and diabetes).

Do we have to measure weight and cholesterol?

Predictive risk factors can be omitted if they are closely correlated with other factors and do not exert an independent effect on risk. For example, although weight predicts CHD risk, it is closely associated with blood pressure and the development of clinical diabetes mellitus. If we are already measuring blood pressure and recording diabetes, there is no necessity for risk prediction to measure weight as well. Similarly, although total cholesterol is often measured as an 'independent' risk factor, it too correlates with other risk factors and Shaper, *et al* have demonstrated that overall risk can be assessed with reasonable precision by clinical history and examination without taking blood to measure cholesterol.[5] As our understanding of common mechanisms for the development of ischaemic heart disease grows, and our ability to measure such mechanisms (e.g. insulin resistance) increases, the number of risk factors we have to measure to obtain a reasonably accurate assessment of overall risk may decrease.

HOW CAN WE CALCULATE MULTIPLE RISK IN GENERAL PRACTICE?

Visual charts

The simplest multiple risk indicator is a chart such as that shown in Fig. 15.1. This has the advantages that no calculations or gadgets are required, the potential benefit of risk factor reduction is evident, and the absolute as well as relative risks are apparent. The main disadvantage is inflexibility—Fig. 15.1 applies to males aged 46–57 years. The European Societies of Cardiology, Atherosclerosis, and Hypertension Task Force have devised a chart, based on Framingham data, which shows risk from ages 30–70 years for both men and women (Fig. 15.2). The risks shown are for exact ages, blood pressures and cholesterol—risk increases as a person approaches the next category. Both the effect of changing risk status and the effect of lifetime exposure to a risk factor can be read directly from the chart, although it is slightly less easy to interpret than Fig. 15.1.

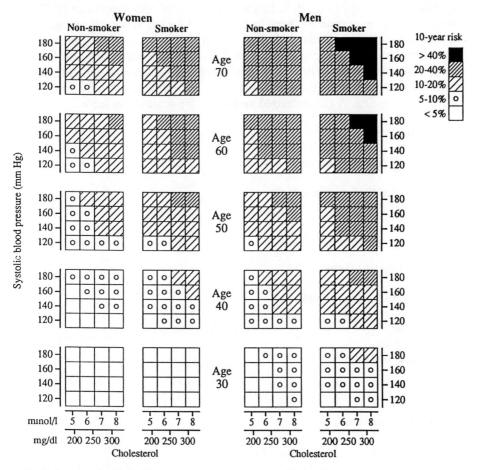

* To find a person's absolute 10-year risk of a CHD event, find the table for their sex, age and smoking status. Inside the table, find the cell nearest to their systolic blood pressure (mm Hg) and cholesterol (mmol/l or mg/dl).

* To find a person's relative risk, compare their risk category with other people of the same age. The absolute risk shown here may not apply to all populations, especially those with a low CHD incidence. Relative risk is likely to apply to most populations.

* Risk is at least one category higher in people with overt cardiovascular disease. People with diabetes, familial hyperlipidaemia or a family history of premature cardiovascular disease are also at increased risk.

Fig. 15.2 European task force CHD chart showing 10 years risk of CHD event, expressed as an approximate percentage, in relation to age, sex, total cholesterol, systolic blood pressure, and smoking habit. (From Recommendations of European Task Force of the European Society of Cardiology, European Atherosclerosis Society, and European Society of Hypertension. European Heart J 1994; **15**: 1300–31.)

British Regional Heart Study risk score

This assessment method, based on follow-up of the 7735 males aged 40–59 years in the *British Regional Heart Study*, is available in two versions. The full score involves measurement of ten factors, including total cholesterol, and requires an ECG. The simpler, six factor version has been recommended for use in general practice.[5] The application of the score is shown in Fig. 15.3. It is the assessment method of choice for making strategic decisions about allocation of health resources. Its drawback for use as a motivational tool in primary care is that it calculates absolute rather than relative risk with the result that benefits from life-style change tend to be obscured by the effect of ageing. A computerized version of the score is available.

Calculation:

Years of cigarette smoking   _____   x 7   _____

Mean blood pressure (mmHg):   _____   x 6.5   _____
(systolic + 2 x diastolic) / 3

Previous diagnosis of IHD: + 270

Chest pain on exertion: + 150

Parent died of heart trouble: + 85

Diabetic: + 150   _____

TOTAL SCORE: ========

Interpretation:

Score	Event risk/1000/year	Decile
647	1.8	10
713	2.4	20
766	3.1	30
812	3.9	40
865	4.8	50
898	5.8	60
944	7.1	70
1000	9.2	80
1091	13.5	90

Fig. 15.3 The British regional heart study (Shaper) modified score. (From Shaper AG, Pocock SJ, Phillips , Walker M. Identifying men at high risk of heart attacks: strategy for use in general practice. BMJ 1986; **293**: 474–79.)

Dundee risk-disk

The front and back of the manual version of the Dundee risk calculator[6] are illustrated in Fig. 15.4. Again, a computer version is also available and the

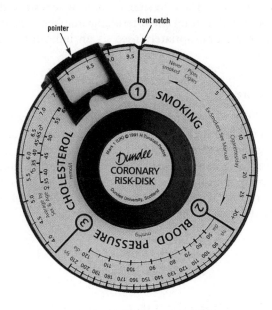

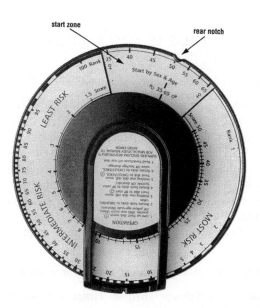

Fig. 15.4 The Dundee risk-disk: front and rear views. (From Tunstall-Pedoe H. The Dundee coronary risk-disk for management of change in risk factors. BMJ 1991; **303**: 744–7.)

mathematical equation on which it is based is explained in Appendix 1. It is based on data relating to the follow-up of 5203 men aged 40–59 years screened in the early 1970s in Scotland. The disk is also recommended for predicting relative risk in women (with an additional step to take account of the age-specific changes in cholesterol levels in women). The assessment is otherwise restricted to 'changeable' risk factors—blood pressure, total cholesterol, the number of cigarettes smoked—and it is therefore more appropriately used as an indicator of relative than of absolute risk.

The Framingham score

The calculation of the Framingham score is shown in Appendix 2. The main advantage over its rivals is that it is based on data for women as well as for men. It is also relatively simple to use and it provides both relative and absolute risk estimates which can be compared with the average risk of a subject of the same age and sex. The main limitations of the Framingham calculation for use in UK general practice are that it requires knowledge of HDL cholesterol and ECG changes and that it is based on an American population with a middle class bias.

SUMMARY

The advantages and disadvantages of the four options described are summarized and compared in Table. 15.5.

HOW VALUABLE IS MULTIPLE CHD RISK ASSESSMENT?

Should we abandon multiple risk assessment in clinical care?

In the OXCHECK cohort,[7] 86 per cent (678/790) of the patients who were in the top decile of relative risk as identified by the Dundee risk-disk, would have been identified anyway because they were smokers, had high blood pressure, or were known to suffer from CHD or diabetes. On this evidence it has been shown that only marginal gain (in terms of mortality reduction) is achieved from adopting a preventive strategy which involves screening for additional risk factors.[8] Regarding cholesterol, in particular, it has been argued in Chapter 3 that primary prevention using individual intervention cannot at present be recommended. The clinical benefit of calculating multiple risk remains unproven.

Should we abandon multiple risk assessment for resource allocation?

The Coronary Prevention Group—British Heart Foundation guidelines on cardiovascular risk assessment encourage general practitioners to assess multiple

Table 15.5 Comparison of multiple risk assessment tools for use in general practice

	Visual Chart	Modified BRHS score	Dundee risk-disk	AHA Framingham score
Application to men and women?	Yes	No	Yes	Yes
Ease of use	+++	+	++	+
Good for assessing absolute risk	Yes	Yes	No	Yes
Motivational potential	+++	+	+++	+
Risk factors included	Smoking Blood pressure Cholesterol	Age Smoking years Blood pressure Personal History Family History	Smoking Blood pressure Total cholesterol*	Age Total cholesterol HDL cholesterol Smoking Blood pressure Personal history ECG

* If cholesterol not measured, risk can be estimated on basis of smoking and blood pressure alone.

risk to decide on the allocation of practice resources.[9] A computer simulation of the application of these guidelines to a general practice population indicated that at an acceptable workload threshold, 41 per cent of heavy smokers and 34 per cent of those with systolic blood pressure greater than or equal to 180 mm Hg were not selected for 'special care'.[10] Although this may be consistent with the objective of cost effective resource use to prevent heart disease, it clearly ignores the effect of smoking on respiratory disease and of blood pressure on stroke. Multiple risk assessment to allocate resources based on cardiovascular disease alone is hard to justify.

IS MULTIPLE RISK INTERVENTION SENSIBLE?

Although there can be no reasonable doubt that in order to get an accurate assessment of individual risk, it is necessary to consider more than one risk factor, this does not necessarily mean that it is sensible to try to organize interventions designed to modify risk on a 'multiple' basis. Every general practitioner is aware of the difficulty of dealing with multiple problems within a consultation and, where possible, will seek to deal with one issue at a time. It is therefore of interest to assess the effectiveness of interventions designed to deal simultaneously with multiple risks.

Trials outside UK general practice

There have been five randomized control trials of multiple risk factor intervention in which the end-point was the cardiovascular disease mortality rate. Three were in Scandinavia (in the towns of Göteborg,[11] Oslo,[12] and Helsinki[13]), the *Multiple Risk Factor Intervention Trial* (MRFIT)[14] was in the United States, and the *WHO Factories Trial* took place in 80 factories in different countries in Europe.[15] In addition, there have been three major community intervention trials—the *North Karelia project*,[16] the *Minnesota project*,[17] and the *Stanford Heart Disease Prevention Project*.[18] The studies all commenced in the 1970s and reported their principal findings in the 1980s. The interpretation of these trials has been the subject of hot debate, not least because of marked reductions in CHD mortality in the control populations in MRFIT, Göteborg, and North Karelia. However, three general conclusions can be drawn:

1. Given a motivated population and sufficient resources it is possible to intervene successfully on more than one risk factor at a time. In the Oslo study, mean serum and cholesterol levels were 15 per cent lower, and tobacco consumption 47 per cent lower in the intervention than in the control group.[13]
2. The success of an intervention depends very much on the setting in which it takes place. In the *WHO European Collaborative Group Study*, which involved 61 000 men aged 40–59 from 80 factories in Belgium, Italy, Poland, and the UK, there were major differences in success rates between countries.[16] In Belgium, a

reduction of 25 per cent in CHD incidence was achieved in the intervention compared with the control group,[19] whereas the intervention achieved almost no success in the UK.[20]

3. Individual health education is synergistic with, but may depend on, multiple risk intervention in the community. The *Stanford Heart Disease Prevention Project* evaluated the effect of media health education (TV, radio, newspaper articles and adverts, billboards, and mail literature).[18] One intervention town also had one-to-one health education for a sub-group of those at highest risk. The media intervention was successful in reducing saturated fat intake, cigarette smoking, blood pressure and total cholesterol. The sub-group receiving intensive face-to-face input did better only in terms of reported tobacco consumption.

Trials in UK general practice

Two randomized control trials have recently reported on the effectiveness of nurse administered health checks in reducing ischaemic heart disease risk factors in primary care—the *OXCHECK trial*[21] and the *British Family Heart Study*.[22] The results of the two studies were very similar if patients not attending follow-up are included in the analysis. The health checks were ineffective in promoting smoking cessation. The average (mean) total cholesterol level was 2–3 per cent lower in the intervention than in the control groups. There was a reduction in blood pressure, but this may have represented a real reduction or an accommodation to measurement in the intervention group. There is ,however, no dispute that blood pressure screening is desirable. The lack of effect of smoking intervention calls into question the wisdom of trying to intervene on more than one risk factor at a time and of dealing simultaneously with issues of addiction and life-style.

Should we abandon multiple risk intervention?

The results of multiple intervention in the UK general practice context have been disappointing. The failure of the smoking cessation programme in the UK health check trials is of particular importance in the light of evidence of effectiveness of smoking cessation advice in other primary care settings. However, there are examples of intervention programmes from Europe and America where advice on smoking cessation has been combined successfully with interventions to modify dietary fat intake and other risk factors such as exercise. Much appears to depend on the available resources. There is also an issue of selectivity: multiple intervention appears to be most successful in those at highest overall risk. In the end, the decision about whether to concentrate on unifactorial or multifactorial intervention must be pragmatic. It is incomplete care to treat hypertension with drugs without trying to help patients to modify their diet and stop smoking. However, it is equally inappropriate to ignore the evidence that both professionals and patients may find it very difficult to deal effectively with more than one issue at one time.

If multiple intervention is considered appropriate, there is certainly a case on pragmatic and scientific grounds for considering serial rather than parallel interventions.

CONCLUSIONS

- A clear distinction must be made between multiple risk assessment and calculation, multiple risk screening, and multiple (compared with sequential) risk intervention. The benefits of each must be assessed independently.
- Accuracy of individual CHD risk assessment can be increased by taking account of more than one risk factor.
- The best method of multiple risk factor assessment depends on whether it is more important to measure absolute or relative risk. Age, sex and clinical history must be included if assessment of absolute risk is important.
- There is no evidence that multiple risk calculation is of clinical benefit for primary or secondary prevention of CHD in general practice.
- Multiple risk calculation for CHD is a limited strategy for making resource allocation decisions in primary care as two key risk factors (smoking and blood pressure) are also important risk factors for other diseases.
- When multiple intervention seems to be appropriate (e.g. a hypertensive patient who is also obese and a heavy smoker) a pragmatic decision must be made on whether it is better to deal with each risk factor sequentially or in parallel.

REFERENCES

1. Truett J, Cornfield J, Kannel W. A multivariate analysis of the risk of coronary heart disease in Framingham. J Chronic Dis 1967; **20**: 511–24.
2. Kannel WB, McGee D, Gordon T. A general cardiovascular risk profile: The Framingham study. Am J Cardiol 1976; **38**: 46–51.
3. Kannel WB, Neaton JD, Wentworth MPH, Thomas HE, Stamler J, Hulley SB, *et al.* Overall and coronary heart disease mortality rates in relation to major risk factors in 325,348 men screened for the MRFIT. Am Heart J 1986; **112**: 825–36.
4. Silberberg J. Estimating the benefits of cholesterol lowering: are risk factors for CHD multiplicative? J Clin Epidemiol 1990; **43**: 875–9.
5. Shaper AG, Pocock SJ, Phillips, Walker M. Identifying men at high risk of heart attacks: strategy for use in general practice. BMJ 1986; **293**: 474–79.
6. Tunstall-Pedoe H. The Dundee coronary risk-disk for management of change in risk factors. BMJ 1991; **303**: 744–7.
7. OXCHECK Study Group. Prevalence of risk factors for heart disease the OXCHECK trial: implications for screening in primary care. BMJ 1991; **302**: 1057–60.
8. Silagy C, Mant D, Carpenter L, Muir J, Neil A. Modelling different strategies to prevent coronary heart disease in primary care. J Clin Epidemiol 1994; **9**: 993–1001.
9. Working group of Coronary Prevention Group and British Heart Foundation. An action plan for preventing coronary heart disease in primary care. BMJ 1991; **303**: 748–50.

10. Randall T, Muir J, Mant D. Choosing the preventive workload in general practice: practical application of the coronary prevention group guidelines and Dundee coronary risk-disk. BMJ 1992; **305**: 227–31.
11. Wilhelmson L, Berglund G, Elmfeldt D, Tibblin H, *et al.* The multifactor primary prevention trial in Göteborg, Sweden. Eur Heart J 1986; **7**: 279–88.
12. Hjermann I, Velve Byre K, Holme I, Leren P. Effect of diet and smoking intervention on the incidence of coronary heart disease. Lancet 1981; **ii**: 1303–10.
13. Strandberg TE, Salomaa VV, Naukkarinen VA, Vanhanen HT, *et al.* Long-term mortality after 5-year multifactorial primary prevention of cardiovascular disease in middle-aged men. JAMA 1991; **266**: 1225–129.
14. Multiple Risk Factor Intervention Trial Research Group. Mortality rates after 10.5 years for participants in the Multiple risk factor intervention trial. JAMA 1990; **263**: 1795–801.
15. WHO European Collaborative Group. European collaborative trial of multifactorial prevention of coronary heart disease: Final report on the 6-year results. Lancet 1986; **i**: 869–72.
16. Tuomilehto J, Geboers J, Salonen J, Nissinen A, Kuulasmaa K, Puska P. Decline in cardiovascular mortality in North Karelia and other parts of Finland. BMJ 1986; **293**: 1068–71.
17. Murray DM, Lueprker RV, Pirie PL, Grimm RH, Bloom E, Davis MA, Blackburn H. Systematic risk factor screening and education: a community-wide approach to prevention of coronary heart disease. Prev Med 1986; **15**: 661–672.
18. Farquhar JW, Maccoby N, Wood PD, Alexander JK, Breitrose H, Brown BW Jr, *et al.* Community education for cardiovascular health. Lancet 1977; **ii**: 192–5.
19. Kornitzer M, De Backer G, Dramaix M, Kittel F, Thilly C, Graffar M, Vuylsteek K. Belgian heart disease prevention project: incidence and mortality results. Lancet 1983; **i**: 1066–70.
20. Rose G, Tunstall-Pedoe HD, Heller RF. UK heart disease prevention project: incidence and mortality results. Lancet 1983; **i**: 1062–66.
21. The ICRF OXCHECK Study Group report by Muir J, Mant D, Jones L, Yudkin P. The effectiveness of health checks conducted by nurses in primary care: one year results from the OXCHECK study. BMJ 1994; **308**: 308–12.
22. Family Heart Study Group. Randomised controlled trial evaluating cardiovascular screening and intervention in general practice: principal results of British family heart study: BMJ 1994; **308**: 313–20.

APPENDIX

Multiple logistic function formula and modifications

Five year risk of coronary heart disease

$$= \frac{1}{1 + e^{-(a + b_1x_1 + b_2x_2 + b_3x_3 + b_4x_4)}}$$

Coefficients (SEs)
a $\ = -10\cdot117\ (0\cdot745) =$ constant*
$b_1 = 0\cdot06510\ (0\cdot0114)$ $x_1 =$ age in years*
$b_2 = 0\cdot010543\ (0\cdot00270)\ x_2 =$ systolic blood pressure (mm Hg)
$b_3 = 0\cdot009378\ (0\cdot00131)\ x_3 =$ cholesterol (mg/100 ml)**
$b_4 = 1\cdot00$ $x_4 =$ smoking code (see below)***

Smoking codes
Never smoked $= 0\cdot0$ (preset)
Ex-smoker or pipe or cigar smoker $= 0\cdot1453\ (0\cdot224)$
Cigarettes per day:

1-9	$= 0\cdot4483\ (0\cdot274)$	20	$= 0\cdot9333\ (0\cdot247)$
10	$= 0\cdot9242\ (0\cdot283)$	21-29	$= 1\cdot263\ (0\cdot303)$
11-19	$= 1\cdot019\ (0\cdot228)$	$\geqslant30$	$= 1\cdot431\ (0\cdot285)$

Modifications for Dundee coronary risk-disk:
*Constant "a" reset for fixed age 50:
   $-10\cdot117 + (50 \times 0\cdot0651) = -6\cdot8624$.
This value is constant for men but is modified in women by age:
   $35 = +0\cdot5719;\ 40 = +0\cdot3875;\ 45 = +0\cdot1922;$
   $50 = +0\cdot0156;\ 55 = -0\cdot1047;\ 60 = -0\cdot2219;$
   $65 = -0\cdot3156$

**Cholesterol:
$b_3 = 0\cdot3627;\ x_3 =$ cholesterol (mmol/l)

***Cigarette dose-response rationalised to:
   1-4/day $= 0\cdot406$
   5-9/day $= 0\cdot406 +$ (No of cigarettes -5) $(0\cdot0813)$
   10-29/day $= 0\cdot8125 +$ (No of cigarettes -10) $(0\cdot0312)$
   $\geqslant30$/day $= 1\cdot437$.

Appendix 1   The Dundee risk-disk: how it calculates the cumulative risk. (From Tunstall-Pedoe H. The Dundee coronary risk-disk for management of change in risk factors. BMJ 1991; **303**: 744–7.)

1. Find points for such risk factor

2. Score each risk factor box

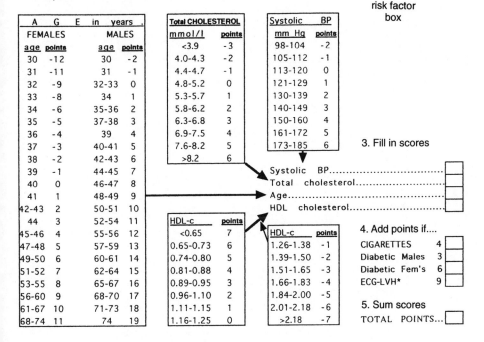

A G E in years				Total CHOLESTEROL		Systolic BP	
FEMALES		MALES		mmol/l	points	mm Hg	points
age	points	age	points	<3.9	-3	98-104	-2
30	-12	30	-2	4.0-4.3	-2	105-112	-1
31	-11	31	-1	4.4-4.7	-1	113-120	0
32	-9	32-33	0	4.8-5.2	0	121-129	1
33	-8	34	1	5.3-5.7	1	130-139	2
34	-6	35-36	2	5.8-6.2	2	140-149	3
35	-5	37-38	3	6.3-6.8	3	150-160	4
36	-4	39	4	6.9-7.5	4	161-172	5
37	-3	40-41	5	7.6-8.2	5	173-185	6
38	-2	42-43	6	>8.2	6		
39	-1	44-45	7				
40	0	46-47	8				
41	1	48-49	9				
42-43	2	50-51	10				
44	3	52-54	11	HDL-c	points		
45-46	4	55-56	12	<0.65	7	HDL-c	points
47-48	5	57-59	13	0.65-0.73	6	1.26-1.38	-1
49-50	6	60-61	14	0.74-0.80	5	1.39-1.50	-2
51-52	7	62-64	15	0.81-0.88	4	1.51-1.65	-3
53-55	8	65-67	16	0.89-0.95	3	1.66-1.83	-4
56-60	9	68-70	17	0.96-1.10	2	1.84-2.00	-5
61-67	10	71-73	18	1.11-1.15	1	2.01-2.18	-6
68-74	11	74	19	1.16-1.25	0	>2.18	-7

3. Fill in scores

Systolic BP.............................□
Total cholesterol.....................□
Age..□
HDL cholesterol......................□

4. Add points if....

CIGARETTES 4 □
Diabetic Males 3 □
Diabetic Fem's 6 □
ECG-LVH* 9 □

5. Sum scores

TOTAL POINTS...□

6. Look up risk (probability percent) corresponding to total points

Pts.	5 yr.	10 yr.	Pts.	5 yr.	10 yr.	Pts.	5 yr.	10 yr.	Pts.	5 yr.	10 yr.
≤1	<1	<2	9	2	5	17	6	13	25	14	27
2	1	2	10	2	6	18	7	14	26	16	29
3	1	2	11	3	6	19	8	16	27	17	31
4	1	2	12	3	7	20	8	18	28	19	33
5	1	3	13	3	8	21	9	19	29	20	36
6	1	3	14	4	9	22	11	21	30	22	38
7	1	4	15	5	10	23	12	23	31	24	40
8	2	4	16	5	12	24	13	25	32	25	42

7. Compare to average (probability percent) risk over ten years

AGE	WOMEN	MEN	AGE	WOMEN	MEN	AGE	WOMEN	MEN
30-34	<1	3	55-59	12	16	55-59	12	16
35-39	<1	5	60-64	13	21	60-64	13	21
40-44	2	6	65-69	9	30	65-69	9	30
45-49	5	10	70-74	12	24	70-74	12	24
50-54	8	14						

Appendix 2 American Heart Association coronary heart disease risk prediction score (Framingham score). (From Anderson KM, Wilson PWF, Odell PA, Kannel WB. An updated coronary risk profile: a statement for health professionals. Circulation 1991; **83**: 356–62. Reformatted by J Muir with the permission of WB Kannel.)

Part 2
Evidence for the effectiveness of implementation

16 Community-based interventions

Michael Rayner

INTRODUCTION

There is some debate about what constitutes community-based coronary heart disease (CHD) prevention, and amongst those who would say they are involved in it there is disagreement about how it should be carried out.[1] However, all agree that it involves activities which take place outside of traditional medical settings such as hospitals or general practitioners' surgeries. Doctors and other health professionals may be involved but not invariably so.

Many commentators have pointed out that there are two main approaches to preventing CHD in communities: the population and the high-risk strategies.[2] The former focuses on reducing risk factor levels in the population as a whole while the latter aims to reduce the risk of individuals identified as being at high risk (see Chapter 21). Community-based prevention programmes generally use a combination of both population and high-risk approaches but normally place greater emphasis on the population approach.[3]

Community-based prevention programmes can involve action within a wide variety of settings: primary health care, schools, and workplaces but also supermarkets, leisure centres, and youth clubs. A number of different professionals can be involved including general practitioners, nurses, dietitians, teachers, and journalists; and these can work for a range of different organisations such as the health service, voluntary bodies, commercial organisations, the media, and both local and national government.

Community-based prevention programmes are normally, but not invariably, designed to reduce levels of more than one risk factor in the target population. Health education is usually the principal intervention method: the aim being to persuade people to change behaviour related to CHD risk. The health educators seek to change smoking and eating habits but also physical activity and stress related behaviour. Various educational methods are used ranging from one-way methods of communicating health advice such as videos, leaflets and posters to more interactive forms of communication such as verbal advice and counselling. In schools the teaching occurs mainly within classes, in other settings the educators generally work with individuals rather than groups.

Whilst health education is normally regarded as fundamental, other intervention methods are increasingly regarded as equally important, if not more so. These methods, often described as 'healthy public policy',[1] include a wide range of activities designed to facilitate behavioural change. They can be divided into three categories.

Firstly, there are measures which provide people with better information with which to make decisions about their health. Such measures are not necessarily educational—for example improvements in the accuracy and understandability of food labelling in general might help people to make more informed choices about the foods they eat, without necessarily influencing them to eat particular foods. Secondly, there are measures that affect the price of goods and services relative to income. It follows from the basic precepts of economics that, other things being equal, increasing the price of cigarettes will reduce their consumption. Thirdly, there are measures which affect the availability of these goods and services. Such measures are often associated with price changes but not invariably so. It may be possible to increase participation in a sport such as swimming by building more swimming pools.

These 'healthy public policy' measures, together with health education, constitute health promotion as espoused by the World Health Organisation and enshrined in the Ottawa Charter for Health Promotion.[4]

What role is there for primary health care personnel in community-based CHD prevention? This chapter seeks to clarify that role. The specific questions which it aims to address are as follows:

1. **What evidence is there that a community-based approach to CHD prevention is effective?**
2. **What is the range of possible action with a community-based approach to CHD prevention?**
3. **What action should the Government take to reduce CHD rates in the UK?**
4. **What role can primary care play in community-based CHD prevention?**

WHAT EVIDENCE IS THERE THAT A COMMUNITY-BASED APPROACH TO CHD PREVENTION IS EFFECTIVE?

Most of the evidence for a community-based approach to CHD prevention comes from large scale projects, some of which have involved whole regions or even whole countries.

Large scale CHD prevention programmes began with the *North Karelia Project* in Finland[5] and the *Stanford Heart Disease Prevention Program's Three Community Study* in the United States during the mid 1970s.[6] These were initiated in the light of cohort studies such as the *Framingham Study* which had revealed three key aspects of the epidemiology of CHD. They had shown, firstly, that the effect of blood cholesterol and blood pressure on risk of CHD is continuous and, secondly, that most cases of the disease come from the middle of the risk factor distribution. Both of these features of the epidemiology of CHD suggest that to reduce rates of the disease in populations where rates are high, an intervention programme aimed at the whole population is needed. Thirdly, the cohort studies had shown that the risk factors for CHD are multiplicative in their action rather than additive suggesting a multifactorial approach to CHD prevention might be more cost-effective than a strategy focusing on a single risk factor.

Seven major community-based CHD prevention programmes were started in the 1970s: the two already mentioned, the *National Research Program* in Switzerland,[7] the *CHAD Program* in Israel,[8] the *Schleiz Project* in the German Democratic Republic,[9] the *Eberbach Weisloch Project* in the Federal Republic of Germany[10] and the *Martignacco Project* in Italy.[11,12]

In the late 1970s and early 1980s, five more major community-based studies were started, three in the US and two in Europe. In the light of their experience with the *Three Community Study* the Stanford group began the larger scale *Five-City Project* in the late 1970s.[13] This was followed by the launch of the *Minnesota Heart Health Program*[14] and of the *Pawtucket Heart Health Program*[15] in the early 1980s. In Europe the *German Cardiovascular Prevention Study*[16] and *Heartbeat Wales*[17] both began in the early 1980s. During the late 1980s, a third generation of community-based prevention programmes were initiated throughout Europe, North America, and Australasia. These were often smaller in scale and focused on particular types of community, such as those with a high proportion of people on a low income.[17,18,19,20] These programmes often had no reference area and were generally much less intensive. An example of this type of programme was the English *Look After Your Heart Programme* launched in 1987.[17]

All these community-based prevention programmes involved a wide range of measures carried out in a variety of different settings designed to reduce a number of risk factors for CHD. Activities undertaken by the *North Karelia Project*, for example, included: media-campaigns using local newspapers and radio to encourage people to eat more fruit and vegetables and to quit smoking; the training of doctors, nurses, social workers, teachers, and representatives of voluntary organisations in providing life-style advice; the reorganization of hypertension control in the area (through the setting up of hypertension clinics and a hypertension register); changes in food labelling and food composition though joint initiatives with the food industry, and control of smoking through increases in the tax on cigarettes.

The results of the community-based prevention programmes have been somewhat equivocal and the conclusions disputed. Normally, changes in mortality, morbidity, and risk factor levels in just one or a few intervention areas have been assessed with reference to a baseline survey carried out prior to implementation of the programme and with changes in one or two reference communities. Compared, therefore, with randomized controlled clinical trials, any inference about the relationship between intervention and outcome is limited.

Nevertheless in most cases, and particularly for the programmes started during the 1970s, there does seem to have been some demonstrable effect of the interventions. Five of the seven programmes begun in the 1970s had a significant effect on smoking, five on cholesterol levels and four on blood pressure (Table 16.1). The results of the first ten years of the *North Karelia Project*, for example, showed that cigarette smoking in men living in North Karelia had fallen by 34 per cent, mean serum cholesterol levels by 11 per cent, and mean diastolic blood pressure levels by 6 per cent: significantly greater than the changes in the control area of Kuopio (8 per cent, 9 per cent and 4 per cent respectively). For women the reductions in blood pressure and serum cholesterol were similar but smoking rose steadily in both North Karelia and Kuopio.[5] Furthermore, between 1974 and 1979 North Karelia experienced a 24 per cent reduction in age-standardized CHD mortality in men and 51 per cent for women, compared with 12 per cent and 24 per cent respectively in the rest of Finland.[21]

Table 16.1 Risk factor changes in the major controlled community prevention programmes for CHD

	Smoking	Blood cholesterol	Blood pressure
Projects started in 1970s			
North Karelia Project (Finland)	+	+	+
Stanford three community study (US)	+	+	+
National research program (Switzerland)	+	–	–
CHAD program (Israel)	+	–	–
Schleiz project (German Democratic Republic)	+	+	+
Eberbach-Weisloch project (Federal Republic of Germany)	NR	+	NR
Martignacco project (Italy)	–	+	+
Projects started in 1980s			
Stanford five-city project (US)	(+)	(+)	(+)
Minnesota heart health program (US)	(+)	–	–
Pawtucket heart health program (US)	–	–	–
German cardiovascular prevention study (Federal Republic of Germany)	+	+	+
Heartbeat Wales (UK)	–	–	–

+ indicates a significant difference between the intervention area(s) and the control area(s); (+) indicates that there were differences between intervention and control areas but these were not consistently significant; NR indicates that differences between intervention areas and control areas were not reported. Adapted from a table produced by E Vartiainen.

The results of the programmes started in the 1980s have generally been less convincing than for those started in the 1970s (Table 16.1). The outcome evaluation of the *Stanford Five-City Project* showed net significant reductions in smoking, blood cholesterol, and blood pressure levels in a cohort sample from the intervention area but not in independent samples.[13] In the *Minnesota Heart Health Program* the only measurable effect was a small net reduction in smoking amongst women and then only in the independent samples not the cohort samples.[22] In the *Pawtucket Heart Health Program* no statistically significant effect was seen on risk factor levels.[23] With *Heartbeat Wales* there was little, if any, net effect of the intervention.[24] The only programme started in the 1980s which has had positive results has been the *German Cardiovascular Prevention Study*. The results of this study are about to be published and will show net changes in blood pressure, blood cholesterol and smoking in the intervention regions.

With the *North Karelia Project* the results were less persuasive in the 1980s than they had been in the 1970s. Between 1979 and 1989 risk factor levels continued to fall in North Karelia but the reductions were similar to those in the control area.[25]

The difference between the results of the community-based prevention programmes in the 1970s and in the 1980s is probably because CHD rates began to fall rapidly in many of the countries where programmes were running during the 1980s, obscuring any particular effect of the programmes. By the mid 1980s CHD rates were falling by more than two per cent per year in the US, UK, and Finland (Fig. 16.1a and b).[26] The reasons for these falls is debated but they were undoubtedly partly due to changes in blood pressure, blood cholesterol, diet, smoking, and/or exercise levels which were, of course, a target of many of the programme activities. Only in Germany, where the decline in mortality from CHD has been less marked and where mortality rates were lower in the first place has the community-based prevention programme demonstrated a net effect.

There is then mixed evidence for the effectiveness of community-based CHD prevention programmes. Moreover, the programmes which appear to have been most effective have been the most intensive and therefore questions have been raised about their cost-effectiveness. There now seems little likelihood that large-scale community-based programmes along the lines of the *North Karelia Project* and *Heartbeat Wales* will be widely replicated. Nevertheless, certain elements of these programmes would be worth introducing elsewhere.

WHAT IS THE RANGE OF POSSIBLE ACTION WITH A COMMUNITY-BASED APPROACH TO CHD PREVENTION?

Adopting a community-based approach to CHD prevention leads to the generation of a wide variety of possibilities for action in a number of settings. To identify the range of possibilities many commentators have used matrices with one axis for the settings or agents and the other for the method of intervention. Table 16.2a, b and c shows three such matrices for interventions in the area of nutrition, smoking, and physical activity. Only non-pharmacological interventions are shown because pharmacological interventions are covered extensively elsewhere in this book.

Some of the cells of the matrices shown in Table 16 are blank because some agents have no direct way of influencing health related behaviour with certain types of measure, for instance primary health care personnel cannot normally influence the price of food and it is probably unreasonable to expect retailers to educate the public in the dangers of smoking while they continue to sell cigarettes. However, agents who can have no direct effect in particular areas can support the action of others who can, for instance the Government currently has little direct control over food labelling, but on the one hand it could use its influence with the European Union to bring in food labelling legislation which takes account of health needs and on the other hand it could encourage food manufacturers and retailers to improve food labelling on a voluntary basis.

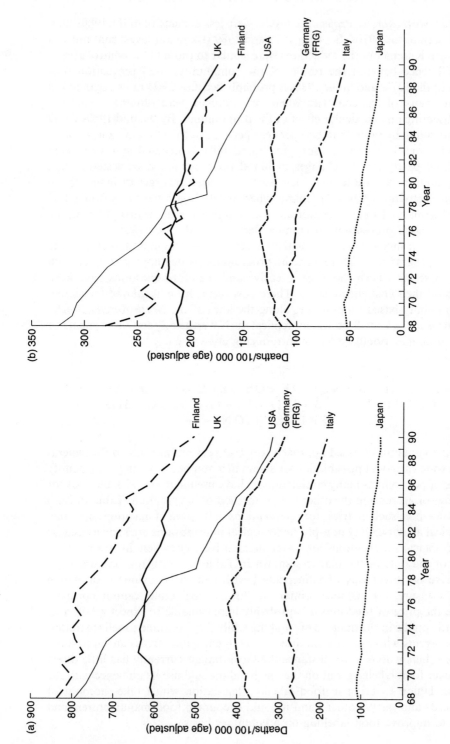

Fig. 16.1 Death rates from CHD for(a) men and (b) women aged 35–74, in 1968–90, in selected countries[26].

For some interventions in some settings there is clear evidence of effectiveness, sometimes drawn from randomized controlled trials (for example school-based health education programmes) and even from meta-analyses of randomized controlled trials. For other interventions the evidence does not, and could never realistically, come from randomized controlled trials but nevertheless is persuasive (for example the beneficial effect of banning cigarette advertising).

WHAT ACTION SHOULD THE GOVERNMENT TAKE TO REDUCE CHD RATES IN THE UK?

For at least three reasons interest in CHD prevention in general, and a community-based approach in particular, increased considerably during the 1970s and 1980s in many developed countries. Firstly, there were the changing patterns of disease— with the continuing decline in infectious diseases and the increase in chronic diseases such as CHD. Rates of CHD peaked in the UK in the late 1970s (see Fig. 16.1). Secondly, there was the growing evidence for a relationship between life-style and risk of CHD together with the early results of intervention studies (including the community-based programmes) which showed that CHD could potentially be prevented. Thirdly, there were the spiralling costs of health care which made governments, in particular, look for more cost-effective ways of reducing the incidence of chronic diseases.

The growing interest in prevention was reflected in various reports issuing from national and international health bodies, which, because of their authority and the publicity given to their findings, in turn fuelled the growing interest. Increasingly these reports argued for a community-based approach to the prevention of CHD. The World Health Organisation played a particularly influential role in this respect.[4,27]

In the UK, government support for community-based CHD prevention lagged behind that in other developed countries. By as late as 1976, the Government report 'Prevention and Health: Everybody's Business' still only briefly acknowledged the potential for CHD prevention and concluded that the role of government was largely limited to health education.[28] Despite its title, this report placed most emphasis on what individuals could do to protect their own health and little on the action others, and in particular the Government itself, could take.

It was not until the early 1980s that the Government began to see a community-based approach to CHD prevention as desirable. A key event was a conference, held in Canterbury, in 1983, organized by a multi-agency advisory group. The report of this conference, published in 1984,[29] took as its starting point the 1982 WHO report on CHD prevention,[27] and made some 20 recommendations for action to be taken by the Government, by the food and agricultural industry, the mass media, the education sector, and the health service. Shortly after the 'Canterbury Conference' the Health Promotion Authority for Wales set up the community-based CHD prevention programme *Heartbeat Wales* as a demonstration project: the aim being to ascertain whether such a programme should be

Table 16.2a Options for improving diet through the action of various agents

Agents	Setting	Health education measures — Education about nutrition	Healthy public policy measures — Information about food	Availability of food	Price of food
General practitioners, practice nurses, health visitors and dietitians	Primary health care	Improve nutrition advice[1,2,3,4]	Provide information about food		
Teachers	Schools	Increase nutrition education[5,6,7]			
School catering staff			Improve menu labelling in canteens	Increase range of 'healthier' foods in canteens[8]	Reduce price of 'healthier' foods in canteens
Occupational health physicians and nurses	Workplaces	Improve nutrition advice[9]			
Workplace catering staff			Improve menu labelling in canteens[10]	Increase range of 'healthier' foods in canteens	Reduce price of 'healthier' foods in canteens
Caterers	Restaurants, cafes, fast food outlets and pubs		Improve menu labelling[11,12]	Increase range of 'healthier' foods. Improve nutritional content of foods	
Food retailers	Supermarkets and other food shops	Improve nutrition education materials	Improve food labelling[13] and advertising	Increase range of 'healthier' foods	Reduce price of 'healthier' foods[14]
Food manufacturers	Primary health care, schools and work places	Improve nutrition education materials			
	Supermarkets and other food shops		Improve food labelling and advertising	Improve nutritional content of foods	

			Improve nutritional content of foods e.g. though changes in production methods	Reduce price of 'healthier' foods e.g. through subsidies[17]
Farmers	Supermarkets and other food shops			
Journalists and reporters	Mass media	Improve reporting of nutritional issues		
Media regulators		Improve food advertising e.g. through changes in codes of practice[15]		
UK Government and European Union	Primary health care, schools and work places	Improve nutrition education materials and training for nutrition educators		
	Supermarkets and other food shops	Improve food labelling[16] and advertising e.g. through changes in legislation	Improve range of 'healthier' foods e.g. through subsidies	

1. Royal College of General Practitioners, Nutrition in General Practice Working Party. Nutrition in general practice 1. Basic principles of nutrition 2. Promoting health and preventing disease. 3. Nutrition in the management of disease. London: RCGP, 1995. (R)
2. Health Education Authority. Nutrition interventions in primary health care. A literature review. London: HEA, 1993. (R)
3. Truswell A S. Review of dietary intervention studies: effect on coronary events and on total mortality. Australian and New Zealand J of Medicine 1994; **24**: 98–106. (SR)
4. Ramsay LE, Yeo W W, Jackson P R. Dietary reduction of serum cholesterol concentration: time to think again. BMJ 1991; **303**: 953–7.(SR)
5. Thomas J. New approaches to achieving dietary change. Current Opinion in Lipidology 1994; **5**: 364–1. (R)
6. Contento I R, Manning A D, Shannon B. Research perspective on school-based nutrition education. J Nut Educ 1992; **24**: 247–60. (R)
7. Young I. Health eating policies in schools: an evaluation of effects on pupils knowledge, attitudes and behaviour. Health Educ J 1993; **52**: 3–9. (R)
8. Caroline Walker Trust Expert Working Group on Nutritional Guidelines for School Meals. Nutritional guidelines for school meals. London: CWT, 1993. (R)
9. Sorenson G, Morris D M, Hunt M K, Herber J R, Harris DR, Stoddard A, Ockene J K. Work-site nutrition intervention and employees' dietary habits: the Treatwell Program. Am J Public Health 1992; **82**: 877–80. (CT)
10. Poulter J, Torrance I. Food and health at work—a review. The costs and benefits of a policy approach. J Human Nutrition Dietetics 1993; **6**: 89–100. (R)
11. Hurren CA, Black AE (ed.). The food network. Achieving a healthy diet by the year 2000. London: Smith Gordon, 1991. (R)
12. Carlson B, Tabacchi M. Meeting consumer nutrition information needs in restaurants. J Nut Ed 1986; **18**: 211–3. (R)
13. Scott V, Worsley A F. Ticks, claims, tables and food groups: a comparison for nutrition labelling. Health Promotion International 1994; **9**: 27–37. (CT)
14. Raven H, Lang T, Dumonteil C. Off our trolley: food retailing the hypermarket economy. London: IPPR, 1994. (R)
15. Dibb S. Children: advertisers' dream, nutrition nightmare? The case for more responsibility in food advertising. London: National Food Alliance, 1993. (R)
16. Ministry of Agriculture, Fisheries and Food. Food Advisory Committee Report on its review of food labelling and advertising 1990. London: HMSO, 1991. (R)
17. Colman D R. Consequences of national and European pricing policy for nutrition and the food industry. In Food and Health. (ed R Cottrell). The Parthenon Publishing Group Ltd.: Carnforth, Lancs: 1987: pp. 119–38. (R)

R indicates reference is a review, SR indicates a systematic review, CT indicates a controlled trial, T indicates a single study without a control group or groups

Table 16.2b Options for smoking control through the action of various agents

Agents	Setting	Health education measures		Healthy public policy measures	
		Education about smoking	Information about smoking	Availability of cigarettes	Price of cigarettes
General practitioners, practice nurses, health visitors	Primary health care and hospitals	Improve anti-smoking/quit-smoking advice.[1,2] Act as exemplars through not smoking[3]		Stop cigarette smoking in health service properties[4,5]	
Teachers	Schools	Improve anti-smoking education.[6,7] Act as exemplars through not smoking		Stop cigarette smoking in schools	
Occupational health physicians and nurses	Workplaces	Improve quit-smoking advice[8]		Stop cigarette smoking in workplaces[9]	
Retailers	Supermarkets and other shops which sell cigarettes			Stop sales of cigarettes to children[10]	

UK Government and European Union

Primary health care, schools, and work places

Improve anti-smoking/quit-smoking education materials and training for health educators

Stop cigarette smoking in public places[14]

Supermarkets and other shops which sell cigarettes

Improve warnings on cigarette packets[11,12]

Increase price of cigarettes e.g. through tax increases[15,16]

Mass media

Stop cigarette advertising[13]

1. Silagy C A, Fowler G H. Systematically reviewing the effectiveness of pharmacological and non-pharmacological smoking cessation methods. J Smoking Related Dis 1994; **5** (Suppl 1): 295–303. (SR)
2. Law M R, Tang J L. An analysis of the effectiveness of interventions to help people stop smoking. Archives of Internal Medicine 1995; in press. (SR)
3. Davis R M. When doctors smoke. Tobacco Control 1993; **2**: 187–8. (R)
4. Amos A. Hospital smoking policies: examples of good practice. Br J Addict 1991; **86**: 704–6. (R)
5. Seymour L, Batten L. I can see clearly now: achieving a smoke-free NHS. Health Education J 1994; **53**: 348–53 (R).
6. Bellew B, Wayne D. Prevention of smoking among schoolchildren: a review of research and recommendations. Health Education J 1991; **50**: 3–7.(R)
7. Bruvold W H. A meta-analysis of adolescent smoking prevention programs. Am J Public Health 1993; 83: 872–80. (SR)
8. Fisher K J, Glasgow R E, Terborg J R. Worksite smoking cessation: a meta-analysis of long-term quit rates from controlled studies. J Occupational Medicine 1990; **32**: 429–39.
9. Bostock Y. A workplace smoking policy. London: Health Education Authority, 1994. (R)
10. Amos A. Selling tobacco to children. BMJ 1990; **301**: 1173–4. (R)
11. Kaiserman M J. The effectiveness of health warning messages. Tobacco Control 1993; **2**: 267–69. (R)
12. Carr-Gregg M R, Gray A J. "Generic" packaging—a possible solution to the marketing of tobacco to young people. Med J Aust 1990: **153**: 685–6. (T)
13. Action on Smoking and Health. Tobacco advertising—the case for a ban. London: ASH, 1993. (R)
14. Bierer M F, Rigotti N A. Public policy for the control of tobacco-related disease. Med Clin North Am 1992; **76**: 515–39. (R)
15. Godfrey C, Maynard A. Economic aspects of tobacco use and taxation policy. BMJ 1988; **297**: 339–43. (T)
16. Townsend J, Roderic P, Cooper J. Cigarette smoking by socioeconomic group, sex and age: effects of price, income and health publicity. BMJ 1994; **309**: 923–7. (R)

Table 16.2c Options for increasing physical activity through the action of various agents

Agents	Setting	Health education measures	Healthy public policy measures	Availability of facilities for physical activity	Price of facilities for physical activity
		Education about physical activity	Information about physical activity		
General practitioners, practice nurses, health visitors	Primary health care	Improve advice on physical activity[1,2,3]	Provide information about physical activity		
Teachers	Schools	Improve education about physical activity[4]		Increase amount of exercise at school	
Occupational health physicians and nurses	Workplaces	Increase advice on physical activity[5]			
Employers				Improve facilities for exercise at work[6]	Subsidise exercise facilities. Give travel allowances for walking and bicycling[7]
Sports and leisure centre staff	Sports and leisure centres	Increase advice on physical activity		Improve facilities for exercise	

UK Government and European Union	
Primary health care, schools and work places	Improve education materials about physical activity and training for educators
Sports and leisure centres	Increase facilities for exercise[8]
Roads and streets	Improve facilities for walking and cycling[9]

1. Campbell M J, Browne D, Waters W E. Can general practitioners influence exercise habits? Controlled trial. BMJ 1985; 290: 1044-6. (CT)
2. Iliffe S, See Tai, S, Gould M, Thorogood M, Hillsdon M. Prescribing exercise in general practice. BMJ 1994; 309: 494-5. (R)
3. Biddle S, Fox K, Edmunds L. Physical activity promotion in primary health care in England. London: Health Education Authority, 1994. (R)
4. Armstrong N. Promoting physical activity in schools. Health Visitor 1993; 66: 362-4. (R)
5. Health of the Nation Workplace Task Force. Health of the Nation Workplace Task Force Report. London: Department of Health, 1993. (R)
6. Association for Public Health. Policy statement on transport: transport and health the next move. London: APH, 1994. (R)
7. Cyclists' Touring Club. What price cycling? A guide to cycling mileage allowances. Information sheet. London: CTC, 1993. (R)
8. Royal College of Physicians. Medical aspects of exercise - benefits and risks. London: RCP, 1990. (R)
9. British Medical Association. Cycling: towards health and safety, Oxford: Oxford University Press, 1992. (R)

implemented throughout the UK. And in 1987, without waiting for the results of *Heartbeat Wales*, the joint Department of Health/Health Education Council's *Look After Your Heart Programme* was launched in England along similar lines but with less resources.[17]

During the 1980s a community-based approach to CHD prevention became almost universally accepted as important and in 1992 Government policy on health promotion reflected this consensus with the publication of the Health of the Nation white paper[30] and the equivalent programmes for Scotland, Wales and Northern Ireland.[31,32,33] The *Health of the Nation Programme* has specific targets for a reduction in rates of CHD and stroke. It also identifies 'areas for action' and those who should be involved, ranging from the Government itself to health professionals, the media, employers, schools, etc. While the main focus of the *Health of the Nation Programme* is on health education it does advocate some other measures in areas such as food labelling, food advertising and smoking in public places.

In parallel with the growing recognition of the value of community-based CHD prevention the relationship between life-style and health has become increasingly accepted as a focus for government action. The adverse health effects of smoking had been recognized by the early 1960s, and through the activities of organizations such as the pressure group Action on Smoking and Health (ASH) and the Royal College of Physicians[34,35] the issue remained on the public agenda. In consequence the Government took some action to limit smoking—not only through health education—but also with other measures such as restricting the advertising of cigarettes (for example banning television advertising in 1965) and through raising the tax on tobacco.

In the area of diet the Government was slower to recognize a relationship with health and more reluctant to advocate or take any action. By the early 1970s the Government had accepted the need for some individuals to reduce their fat, saturated fat, cholesterol, and calorie intake, as evidenced by the 1974 report on diet and coronary heart disease of its Committee on Medical Aspects of Food Policy (COMA),[36] but this report was vague in its recommendations and saw no need for specific government measures.

In 1983, the National Advisory Committee on Nutrition Education (NACNE) set up by the Health Education Council published a report which included quantified targets for fat, saturated fat, added sugar, salt, and fibre levels.[37] Then in 1984 COMA[38] published its report with similar quantified dietary goals. Both the NACNE and COMA reports made detailed recommendations for the action that health professionals, food manufacturers, food retailers and the Government itself could take to improve the national diet, some of which have been implemented. The latest report on diet and CHD from COMA reiterates the need for action on the part of all sectors.[39]

With exercise there has long been some acceptance of its health benefits[28] but hardly any government action to increase participation. Various expert reports have made specific recommendations for government measures, for example that published by the Royal College of Physicians in 1990.[40] The Health of the Nation white paper promised government targets and a plan of action and a consultation paper has just been published.[41]

This brief history of Government involvement in CHD prevention in the UK aims to show an increasing acceptance of the need for a community based approach—but always with an emphasis on health education as opposed to other health promotion measures.

WHAT ROLE CAN PRIMARY CARE PLAY IN COMMUNITY-BASED CHD PREVENTION INITIATIVES?

During the late 1980s and early 1990s there was a proliferation of small-scale community-based CHD prevention projects in the UK, particularly under the umbrella of the Government's *Look After Your Heart Programme*. Some of these projects adopted a multi-factorial, multi-disciplinary approach but many others have been concerned with reducing the level of a single risk factor in a single setting.

There has been little attempt to survey this local activity, or to evaluate its impact. A review of 16 of 279 such projects funded under a scheme set up by the *Look After Your Heart Programme* in 1987[42] provides details of: a pack about the health benefits of walking; healthy eating guidelines for school caterers; a health week involving a 'health fair'; a fun run; and an 'inter-agency co-ordinated programme of heart disease prevention activities' over a whole county (*Look After Your Heart-Avon*[43]). The review thus demonstrates enormous variety in the intervention methods used, personnel involved, target groups, time-scale and costs involved, but it provides virtually no evidence that any of these projects actually helped to reduce CHD rates, or even risk factors for CHD, in the localities in which they were carried out. Similarly, a survey of CHD prevention projects throughout Europe carried out in 1991 found a wide range of different activities being carried out by a variety of different agencies—both governmental and non-governmental.[44] Few of these initiatives were subject to any rigorous evaluation.

Turning again to Table 16, these matrices attempt to map the wide range of possible community-based activity that may have a beneficial effect on CHD rates. Health professionals have an important part to play in this activity because of their acknowledged expertise in health-related issues. Even outside of traditional medical settings they can have an important supporting role. For example, they could help improve the nutritional quality of meals provided in schools and workplaces (by pointing out the health benefits of doing so, by identifying healthier alternatives to the foods currently provided, and by advising on methods of monitoring progress.) They could seek to ensure that the law on sale of cigarettes to children is enforced in their area. They could argue for better facilities for exercise, etc.

In particular primary health care personnel, both individually and collectively through representative bodies, are in a powerful position to request Government action on health issues such as advertising of tobacco, food labelling, and transport policy.

SUMMARY

- There is evidence that a community-based approach to CHD prevention is effective, but the evidence mainly comes from large-scale programmes which may not be cost-effective to replicate. Some of the elements of these programmes would be worth further investigation.
- Adopting a community-based approach generates a huge range of possible activities only some of which are of proven effectiveness.
- The Government is gradually coming to accept the importance of a community-based approach to CHD prevention as evidenced by the *Health of the Nation Programme*.
- Primary health care personnel have an important role in community-based CHD prevention in supporting the activities of other agencies and as advocates for effective methods of intervention.

REFERENCES

1. Tones K. Mobilising communities: coalitions and the prevention of heart disease. Health Education J 1994; **53**: 462–73.
2. Rose G. Strategy of prevention: lessons from cardiovascular disease. BMJ 1981; **282**: 1847–51.
3. Puska P (ed). Comprehensive cardiovascular community control programmes in Europe. EURO Reports and Studies 106. Copenhagen: World Health Organization Regional Office for Europe, 1988.
4. World Health Organization. Ottawa charter for health promotion, An international conference on health promotion, November 17–21. Copenhagen: WHO Regional Office for Europe, 1988.
5. Puska P, Salonen T, Nissinen A, Tuomemilhehto J, Vartiainen E *et al*. Change in risk factors for coronary heart disease during 10 years of a community intervention programme (North Karelia Project) BMJ 1983; **287**: 1840–4.
6. Farquar J W, Fortmann S P, Flora J A, Macoby N. Methods of communication to influence behaviour. In Oxford Textbook of Public Health (ed. W Holland, R Detels, G Knox) Oxford: Oxford University Press, 1990; **2**: 331–44.
7. Gutzwiller F, Nater B, Martin J. Community-based primary prevention of cardiovascular disease in Switzerland: methods and results of the National Research Program (NAP 1A). Prev Med 1985; **14**: 482–91.
8. Abramson I H, Gofin R, Hopp C, Gofin J, Donchin M, Habib J. Evaluation of a community program for the control of cardiovascular risk factors: the CHAD program in Jerusalem. Israeli J Med Sci 1981; **17**: 201–12.
9. Heinemann L, Heine H, Eckstein M, Hellmund W. Project Schleiz-Nationales Demonstrationsproject befolkerungsweiter Prevention bei Herz-Kresilauf-und anderen nichtubertragbaren Krankheiten. Zeitschrift fur Klinische Medizin 1986; **41**: 536–59.

10. Nussel E, Scheidt R, Morgenstern W, Scheuermann W, Bergdolt H. Risikofaktoren der koronaren Herzkankheit-Ansatze zur Korrektur. In Morl H, Deiham C, Heusel G (ed.) 45 Jahre Herzinfarkt-und Fettstoffwechsel forschung. Berlin: Springer Verlag, 1988.

11. Feruglio GA, Vanuzzo D, Di Muro G *et al.*. The Martignacco project: a community study. Outlines and preliminary results after four years. Giornale di Arteriosclerosis 1983; **2**: 207–17.

12. Vartiainen E, Heath G, Ford E. Assessing population-based programs to reduce blood cholesterol level and saturated fats. Int J Technology Assessment in Health Care 1991; **7**: 315–26.

13. Farquar J W, Fortmann S P, Flora JA, Taylor CB, Haskell W L, Williams P T, Macoby N, Wood P D. Effects of community-wide education on cardiovascular disease risk factors. The Stanford Five-City Project. JAMA 1990; 264(1): 359–65.

14. Mittelmark M B, Luepker R V, Jacobs D R, Bracht N F, Carlaw R W, Crow R S, *et al.* Community-wide prevention of cardiovascular disease: education strategies of the Minnesota Heart Health Program. Prev Med 1986; **15**: 1–17.

15. Lefebvre R C, Lasater T M, Carleton R A, Peterson G. Theory and delivery of health programming in the community: The Pawtucket Heart Health Program. Prev Med; 1987; **16**: 80–95.

16. German Cardiovascular Prevention Study Research Group.The German Cardiovascular Prevention Study (GCP): design and methods. Eur Heart J 1989; **9**: 1058–66.

17. Williams K (ed). The community prevention of coronary heart disease. London: HMSO, 1992.

18. Wheeler F G, Lackland D T, Mace M L, Reddick A, Heglin G, Remington P L. Evaluating South Carolina's Community Cardiovascular Prevention Project. Public Health Reports 1991; **106**: 536–42.

19. Shea S, Basch C E, Lantigua R, Wechsler HPH. The Washington Heights-Inwood Healthy Heart Program: a third generation community-based cardiovascular disease prevention program in a disadvantaged urban setting Preventive Medicine 1992; **21**: 203–17.

20. Beurden E V, Lefebvre R C, James R. Transferring community-based interventions to new settings: a case study in heart health cholesterol testing from urban USA to rural Australia. Health Promotion International 1991; **6**: 181–90.

21. Salonen J T, Puska P, Kottke T E, Tuomilehto J, Nissinen A. Decline in mortality from coronary heart disease in Finland 1969 to 1979. BMJ 1983; **286**: 1857–60.

22. Luepker R. Community education for cardiovascular disease prevention: risk factor changes in the Minnesota Heart Health Program. Am J Public Health 1994; **84**: 1383–93.

23. Carleton R A, Lasater T M, Assaf A R, Feldman H A, McKinlay S M. The Pawtucket Heart Health Program: cross-sectional results from a community intervention trial. Abstract, 34th Annual Conference on Cardiovascular Disease Epidemiology and Prevention,Tampa, Florida, 1994.

24. Nutbeam D, Smith C, Murphy S, Catford J. Maintaining evaluation designs in long term community based health promotion programmes: Heartbeat Wales case study. J Epidemiol Community Health 1993; **47**: 127–33.

25. Vartiainen E, Puska P, Jousilahti P, Korhonen HJ, Tuohmilehto J, Nissinen A. Twenty-year trends in coronary risk factors in North Karelia and in other areas of Finland. Int J Epidemiol 1994; **23**: 495–504.

26. British Heart Foundation. Coronary heart disease statistics. London: British Heart Foundation, 1994.

27. World Health Organization. Prevention of coronary heart disease. Technical Report Series No: 678. Geneva: WHO, 1982.

28. Department of Health and Social Security. Prevention and health: everybody's business. London: HMSO, 1976.
29. Health Education Council. Coronary heart disease prevention. Plans for action. London: Pitman Publishing Ltd, 1984.
30. Department of Health. The health of the nation. A strategy for health in England. London: HMSO, 1992.
31. Health Promotion Authority for Wales. Health for all in Wales plans for action. Cardiff: HPAW, 1992.
32. The Scottish Office. Scotland's health: a challenge to us all. Edinburgh: HMSO, 1992.
33. Department for Health and Social Services Northern Ireland. A regional strategy for the Northern Ireland health and personal social services, 1992–1997. Belfast: DHSS, 1992.
34. Royal College of Physicians. Smoking and health. London: Pitman Publishing Co, 1962.
35. Royal College of Physicians. Health and smoking. London: Pitman Publishing Co, 1983.
36. Department of Health and Social Security. Diet and coronary heart disease. Report on health and social subjects No 7.London: HMSO, 1974.
37. National Advisory Committee on Nutrition Education. Proposals for nutritional guidelines for health education in Britain. London: Health Education Council, 1983.
38. Department of Health and Social Security. Diet and cardiovascular disease. Report on health and social subjects No 28. London: HMSO, 1984
39. Department of Health. Nutritional aspects of cardiovascular disease. Report on health and social subjects No 46. London: HMSO, 1994.
40. Royal College of Physicians. Medical aspects of exercise, benefits and risks. London: Royal College of Physicians, 1990.
41. Department of Health. More people more active more often. London: DH, 1995.
42. Berry J, Cavill N and King H. Take heart. Good practices in coronary heart disease prevention. London: Health Education Authority, 1990
43. Look After Your Heart—Avon Localities Project. Report of a community heart disease prevention project on the Bournville estate, Weston-super-Mare, Avon. Bristol: Look After Your Heart-Avon, 1994.
44. Longfield J and Rayner M. Preventing cardiovascular disease in Europe. London: HMSO, 1993.

17 Individual interventions and behaviour change

Theo Schofield

INTRODUCTION

The essential final step in any programme to prevent cardiovascular disease is for people to change their behaviour. This may be by adopting healthier habits and life-styles, reducing their known risk factors or adhering to any therapy that is advised. Unless behaviour changes, nothing will change. This chapter is therefore concerned with the ways that people change their behaviour and the methods that can be used to help them to do so. The questions that it will consider are:

1. **What factors influence individuals' motivation and ability to change their health related behaviour?**
2. **How does an individual's readiness to change develop over time?**
3. **What are the characteristics of interventions that are effective in promoting behaviour change?**
4. **What is the role of primary care in promoting behaviour change?**
5. **What are the tasks to be achieved in effective consultations?**

WHAT FACTORS INFLUENCE INDIVIDUALS' MOTIVATION AND ABILITY TO CHANGE THEIR HEALTH RELATED BEHAVIOUR?

Health beliefs

The *Health Belief Model* was first described by Becker in 1974[1] as a summary of the literature on patient acceptance of recommended health behaviours (Fig. 17.1). He identified the factors that influenced the likelihood of an individual taking a recommended preventive health action. These were:

- health motivation: the degree to which people are concerned about their health
- perceived susceptibility: whether people believe the disease is likely to affect them
- perceived severity: if the disease is contracted whether it would have serious consequences or could be treated easily
- benefits and barriers: a person's estimate of the benefits weighted against the cost of taking action together with other barriers involved
- cues to action: triggers such as newspaper articles, a health check, or a symptom prompting behaviour change

- modifying factors: these include people's age, sex, personality, and social circumstances
- enabling factors: these include interaction with the doctor or the nurse and their credibility.

Ten years later Janz and Becker[2] reviewed a further 29 studies which provided substantial empirical support for the health belief model. Perceived barriers proved to be the most powerful of the dimensions that predicted preventive health or sick role behaviour, and perceived severity was the least powerful. They speculated that this may be because people had difficulty conceptualizing long term threats and suggested that an attempt to induce fear is the least effective way of promoting change.

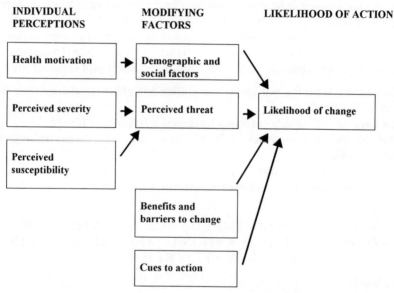

Fig. 17.1   The health belief model (After Becker M. The health belief model and personal health behaviour. Health Education Monograph 1974; **2**: 324–508.)

Self efficacy

While the health belief model concentrates on a person's beliefs about the links between behaviours and outcomes, the concept of *Self Efficacy* seeks to explore people's beliefs about their ability to change their behaviour. The concept was first described by Bandura[3] and the role of people's beliefs about their capability to achieve health related behaviour change was described by Strecher *et al.*[4] The evidence they reviewed indicated that it was their perception of the magnitude of the task and their ability to accomplish it, rather than their true abilities,that influenced behaviour. Self efficacy relates to beliefs about capabilities for performing specific behaviours in particular situations and is not a personality characteristic. It can, therefore, be influenced by training and encouragement given to people by health educators and by building on experience of success. For example, the steps required to encourage patients to take exercise after a myocardial infarction not only include explaining the procedure but also enabling patients to experience their abilities, perhaps initially in a safe environment, and then to build on their success.

Self efficacy must be distinguished from the related concepts of self esteem, locus of control and learned helplessness. *Self esteem* is a broader evaluation of self worth rather than the ability to succeed in specific situations. However self efficacy and self esteem are closely related, since success in something that a person believes to be worthwhile will enhance that person's self esteem.

People's *health locus of control* is their belief about whether their health is controlled by their own behaviour or by external forces such as chance or medical professionals. People who believe that their health is under their own control are more likely to want to adopt healthy behaviours but they still need the belief that they are capable of doing so.

Learned helplessness is a belief acquired from experience that life and health are influenced by events that one cannot control. This maybe because of a lack of personal abilities, in other words the reverse of a belief in self efficacy, but it may be because of the events themselves. It is particularly relevant in the context of health promotion when, for many people, important factors such as housing, income, employment, and educational opportunities may all appear to be beyond their control, and yet they are still expected to feel capable of adopting healthier life-styles.

Empowerment

If it is people's belief in their abilities or the control that they have over their health that determines whether they adopt healthier behaviours, then *empowerment*, the process of increasing people's sense of power and control, becomes an essential part of health promotion.

At an individual level, interventions that increase people's self efficacy will promote the choice of healthier behaviours.[4] The converse of this is the need to avoid making people unduly dependent on medical care. This is an inherent danger in a paternalistic style of communication and when the management of life-style issues, such as smoking, is medicalized.

Empowerment can also be applied to community approaches to health promotion. If environmental factors are a major determinant of people's health and they really are powerless to influence them, working with their community to increase its sense of cohesion, and its ability to take action on the environment, will not only improve the environment but also empower the individuals within it. The case for this approach is argued by Wallerstein[5], but she also goes on to discuss the great difficulties involved its evaluation.

HOW DOES AN INDIVIDUAL'S READINESS TO CHANGE DEVELOP OVER TIME?

Stages in *readiness to change* have been described by Prochaska and DiClemente.[6] They were:

- Pre-contemplation: the individual is not aware of the problem or not interested in considering change.
- Contemplation: the person becomes aware that there is a problem and is assessing its relevance and significance. It is at this stage that health beliefs affect motivation.
- Preparation: the individual is ready to change and is taking tentative steps towards doing so. At this stage belief in one's self efficacy becomes important.
- Action: changes are made and their effects are evaluated.
- Maintenance: once changes have been made they also have to be maintained and relapse avoided. At this stage recognizing the benefits and continued support become important.

This model has a number of important implications. Instruments have been developed to identify an individual's stage of change and this in turn predicts the likely eventual success. For example 21 per cent of smokers in the preparation stage were not smoking six months later, while only eight per cent of those in the pre-contemplation stage had quit.[7]

Once the stage of readiness to change has been identified, individual interventions can be tailored appropriately.

- Pre-contemplation: raise awareness of the problem
- Contemplation: explore health beliefs and enhance motivation
- Preparation: negotiate goals and specific action planning
- Action and maintenance: provide positive reinforcement and continued support.

Another implication of this model is that interventions that do not achieve immediate behaviour change may still have helped people move a stage closer to change. In evaluating a health promotion programme, its effect may be underestimated if only achievement of change is measured.

WHAT ARE THE CHARACTERISTICS OF INTERVENTIONS THAT ARE EFFECTIVE IN PROMOTING BEHAVIOUR CHANGE?

There have been many interventions which aimed to help individuals change their health related behaviours, as well as a number of reviews and meta-analyses that assess their effectiveness. Kottke *et al*[8] in their meta-analysis of 39 controlled trials of smoking cessation interventions found that the common features of successful interventions in medical practice were a team of physicians and non-physicians, using multiple interventions, to deliver individualized advice, on multiple occasions. However, the average difference in smoking cessation rates between the intervention and control groups in their trials was only 5.8 per cent. Law and Tang[9] in their analysis of the effectiveness of interventions intended to help people stop smoking found similarly low cessation rates in patients given simple advice, but argued that it remained a cost effective intervention. However, in trials involving patients at high risk of dying of ischaemic heart disease they found cessation rates between 25 per cent and 44 per cent, and a 20.5 per cent difference between intervention and control groups (95 per cent confidence interval 10.2–30.9 per cent).

Other trials of life-style advice in patients identified at increased risk of coronary heart disease have shown similar effectiveness. In the *Oslo Trial*,[10] detailed information and advice was given to middle aged men identified at screening to be at high risk. Twenty-five per cent of smokers stopped completely compared with 17 per cent in the control group, and mean serum cholesterol was 13 per cent lower in the intervention group during the trial.

Cupples and McKnight[11] however, in a randomized trial of health promotion in general practice for patients at high cardiovascular risk, found that patients who had received advice reported changes in diet and exercise, but that there were no significant differences in mean cholesterol, blood pressure, or smoking habit as a result of the intervention.

There is much less information about the effectiveness of dietary advice in primary care. The Health Education Authority Review in 1993[12] concluded that more research was required before making any recommendations. A recent study comparing the effectiveness of individual advice from a practice nurse, a dietician, or a detailed leaflet sent by post to patients with elevated cholesterol levels found no significant differences between the methods of advice in mean cholesterol, low density lipoproteins, or antioxidant levels, and the overall effectiveness was small, with a reduction of mean cholesterol of 1.9. per cent in all groups.[13]

In a controlled trial of a general practitioner intervention consisting of advice and a drinking diary given to patients with excess alcohol consumption, Wallace *et al*[14] found that in men after one year there was a drop in consumption of 18.2 units per week in the intervention group compared to 8.1 units in the controls, and a reduction in the number of excessive drinkers of 44 per cent in the treated group and 26 per cent in the controls. Similar results were found with the women in the study.

Many of these studies do not detail the educational approaches that were used to promote behaviour change. Simons-Morton *et al.*[15] in a review of 64 controlled studies of patient education and counselling for preventive health behaviours recommended adherence to certain educational principles that enhanced the likelihood of success. These principles were:

- Relevance: the content of the programme is appropriate to the patient.
- Individualization: the needs, desires, and characteristics of the patient are taken into account, and specific goals and objectives negotiated.

- Feedback: the patient is informed about goals and objectives.
- Reinforcement: the patient is given encouragement or reward for progress towards goals or objectives.
- Facilitation: materials are given to aid the patient in making behaviour changes.

Lassen[16] found the patients were more likely to report compliance with advice if the communication had been patient centred. The criteria for this were that during the consultation the doctor:

- explored the patients' expectations of the consultation
- explored the patients' ideas about their problems
- explained the nature of any advice
- explained the reasons and the relevance of the advice
- explored any obstacles to complying with the advice.

WHAT IS THE ROLE OF PRIMARY CARE IN PROMOTING BEHAVIOUR CHANGE?

It is possible to draw together our knowledge about the ways that people change their behaviour and the evidence about the attributes of successful interventions and come to some conclusions about the approaches that can be adopted in the primary care setting.

Individual life-style advice should not be seen as the sole method of attempting to achieve reductions in risk factors in the whole population. In isolation it has a very limited effect[17,18] and giving patients advice that they do not recognize that they need, and from which they are unlikely to derive much individual benefit, may not be well received.[19] In addition, the imposition on general practitioners of the responsibility to give universal life-style advice has led to understandable professional resentment[20] and had undoubted opportunity costs in diverting time and resources away from other activities in primary care. There is also risk that it can divert attention away from other issues such as advertising, employment, and social inequalities where policy changes could improve the health of the population. Focusing on the individual also runs the risk of victimizing or blaming the individual for the effects of those policies.

It is therefore important to identify the circumstances in which it is appropriate for primary care to attempt to influence people's behaviour as well as the methods that should be employed.

Empowerment in all consultations

We have shown that the ability to take control of their own health, and confidence in that ability, are very important in determining whether people make healthy choices. Therefore, every consultation should be used as an opportunity to give patients information, involve them in decisions and encourage them to take responsibility for their health.[21]

Opportunistic brief advice

Both the health belief model and the readiness to change model suggest that brief advice which prompts people to contemplate change or provides a cue to action will contribute to the likelihood of behaviour change. This is an inexpensive method and may not be much less effective than more extensive interventions. It is therefore a cost effective approach, especially for people in the earlier stages of readiness to change.

Community involvement

It is also possible for primary health care teams to work with other agencies and to contribute to the development of healthier environments and more empowered communities.[22] This may be seen as an additional burden but shifting the focus from care *in* the community to care *by* the community may relieve some of the pressures on the professionals.

Targeted care

It is then possible to focus on those patients who have been identified as having significant risk factors, and who are contemplating or planning change. Confining intervention programmes to these groups is likely to be the most cost effective approach, and they can be offered help by doctors, nurses, and others in the team and offered the time and support that they require.

WHAT ARE THE TASKS TO BE ACHIEVED IN EFFECTIVE CONSULTATIONS?

It is possible to identify a set of tasks to be achieved in individual consultations that will maximise the effectiveness of the intervention. These tasks are:

Exploration

In any consultation the first task is to establish the reasons why the patient has chosen to come, the issues that he or she wishes to discuss, and the patient's expectations of the interview. These may differ from the doctor's or nurse's understanding of the problem, but it is important to establish the patient's concerns before the agenda for the interview can be negotiated. For example, a woman visiting a nurse for a health check may regard her menopausal symptoms as her major problem and welcome the opportunity of talking to another female about them, whereas the nurse may be aiming to elicit information to complete a checklist of cardiovascular risk factors. Neither will feel satisfied unless these agendas are met and time is allocated accordingly.

The exploration must include not only the nature of the patients' problems—the symptoms, risk factors, and life-style—but also the patients' ideas, concerns, and expectations. From the models of behaviour change already described, it should be clear that this exploration should include patients' awareness and knowledge of their health problems, the factors that reward or maintain their behaviour, patients' beliefs about their susceptibility and vulnerability to ill-health, and the benefits and costs of any behaviour change.

Explanation

Having obtained this information, the explanations and information given by the health professional can build on the patients' ideas, by reinforcing positive attitudes and correct information, by supplementing incomplete information, and by countering negative ideas. Although this process may appear to be time-consuming, it has a built-in economy: it removes the need to give global explanations and allows the health professional to focus on the information that a particular patient requires. The aims of the explanations are to achieve a shared understanding about health and its problems, to allow patients to attach personal meaning to their experience, and to provide the information upon which the patient can base any decisions.

Negotiation

When a shared understanding has been achieved, it is possible to enter into a negotiation about future actions for both the health professional and the patient. This will involve exploring the options offered by both parties, and consideration of the opportunities for change, the barriers to change that may have to be overcome, and the support that is available or may be required. From these options goals can be selected and agreed by both parties. These goals must be specific and achievable. It is important that patients select their own goals and are committed to their achievement. It is easy, for example, to tell an overweight smoker to stop smoking and lose two stones in weight, or to play the classic game of 'Why don't you . . .?'—'Yes, but . . .'. The antithesis to this is: 'What would you like to do, and how can I help you achieve it?'

Support

The fourth task to be achieved is to offer appropriate support both in a single interview and over a period of time. Positive reinforcement is essential to maintain behaviour change, and the aim of health professionals must be to help people do this for themselves. This involves the patient identifying gains; for example, changes in weight from dieting, improved exercise tolerance from stopping smoking, or an increased sense of well-being from reductions in stress. The achievement of some goals depends on measurements, such as blood pressure and serum cholesterol. Consequently, feedback on progress is an essential component of follow-up.

CONCLUSIONS

- People's own beliefs both about their health and the costs and benefits of change determine their motivation to change.
- People must want to change, and believe in their own effectiveness in doing so.
- People move through stages towards making changes, and can be helped to do this.
- Interventions intended to help people change must be patient centred.
- Effective consultations will include exploration, explanation, negotiation, and support.
- Targetting interventions in primary care on those at greatest need will be more effective, give a greater yield, and be more acceptable than untargetted advice.

REFERENCES

1. Becker M. The Health Belief Model and personal health behavior. Health Education Monograph 1974; **2**: 324–508.
2. Janz NK, Becker MH. The Health Belief Model: a decade later. Health Education Quarterly 1984; **11**: 1–47.
3. Bandura A. Self-efficacy: toward a unifying theory of behavioural change. Psychological Review 1977; **84**: 191–215.
4. Strecher VJ, DeVellis BM, Becker MH, Rosenstock IM. The role of self efficacy in achieving health behavior change. Health Education Quarterly 1986; **13**: 73–91.
5. Wallerstein N. Powerlessness, empowerment, and health: implications for health promotion programs. Am J Health Promotion 1992; **6**: 197–205.
6. Prochaska JO, Di Clemente CC. Towards a comprehensive model of change. In Miller WR, Heather N (Ed.) treating addictive behaviors. Processes of change. New York: Plenum Press, 1986.
7. Di Clemente CC, Procheska JO, Fairhurst SK, Velicer WF, Velasquez MM, Rossi JS. The process of smoking cessation: an analysis of precontemplation, contemplation and preperation stages of change. Journal of Consulting and Clinical Psychology 1991; **59**: 295–304.
8. Kottke TE, Battista RN, DeFriese GH, Brekke ML. Attributes of successful smoking cessation interventions in medical practice. JAMA 1988; **259**: 2822–89.
9. Law M, Tang J. An analysis of the effectiveness of interventions intended to help people stop smoking. Archives of Internal Medicine 1995 (In Press).
10. Hjermann I, Velve Byre K, Holme I, Leren P. Effect of diet and smoking intervention on incidence of coronary heart disease: report from Oslo Study Group of a randomized trial in healthy men. Lancet 1981; **2**: 1303–10.
11. Cupples ME, McKnight A. Randomised controlled trial of health promotion in general practice for patients at high cardiovascular risk.. BMJ 1994; **309**: 993–6.
12. Nutritional Interventions in Primary Care. Health Education Authority 1993.
13. Neil HAW, Roe L, Godlee RJP, Moore JW, Clark GME, Brown J, *et al.* Randomised trial of lipid lowering dietary advice in general practice: the effects on serum lipids, lipoproteins, and antioxidants. BMJ 1995; **310**: 569–73.
14. Wallace P, Cutler S, Haines A. Randomised controlled trial of general practitioner intervention with patients with excessive alcohol consumption. BMJ 1988; **297**: 663–8.

15. Simons-Morton DG, Mullen PD, Mains DA, Tabak ER, Green LW. Characteristics of controlled studies of patient education and counseling for preventive health behaviors. Patient Education and Counselling 1992; **19**: 175–204.
16. Lassen LC. Connections between the quality of consultations and patient compliance in general practice. Family Practice 1991; **8**: 154–60.
17. Imperial Cancer Reseach Fund OXCHECK Study Group. Effectiveness of health checks conducted by nurses in primary care: results of the OXCHECK study after one year. BMJ 1994; **308**: 308–12.
18. Family Heart Study Group. Randomised controlled trial evaluating cardiovascular screening and intervention in general practice: principal results of British family heart study. BMJ 1994; **308**: 313–20.
19. Stott NCH, Pill RM. Advise yes, dictate no: patients' views of health promotion in the consultation. Family Practice 1990; **7**: 125–31.
20. Stott NCH, Kinnersley P, Rollnick S. The limits to health promotion. BMJ 1994; **309**: 971–2.
21. Pendleton D, Schofield T, Tate P, Havelock. The Consultation: an approach to learning and teaching. Oxford: Oxford University Press,1984.
22. Tones K. Mobilising communities: coalitions and the prevention of heart disease. Health Education Journal. 1994; **53**: 462–73.

18   Taking the initiative: strategies and implications

Martyn Agass and David Mant

INTRODUCTION

Medical practice has traditionally been a demand led service. Until recently, the accepted role of primary health care teams was to respond to patients' requests for help but seldom to take the initiative. This attitude is changing rapidly. The quality of clinical care is often better if health professionals are prepared to take the initiative in both the primary and secondary prevention of chronic disease. In addition, many factors which affect the health of our society, such as attitudes, unhealthy life-styles, and social inequalities, are no longer judged to be beyond the professional concern and influence of health professionals.

This chapter is about the available strategies for, and workload implications of, 'taking the initiative' in the primary and secondary prevention of cardiovascular disease. It addresses four specific issues which have proven hard to achieve in this context.

1. **How can we maximize patient involvement?**
2. **Is it possible to avoid the inverse care law?**
3. **Are there ways of avoiding an unmanageable workload?**
4. **In which ways can primary medical care teams work with others?**

It will be re-iterated throughout this and other chapters that the identification of risk is a much smaller task than its management. Although most of the strategies described were developed and assessed within the context of the British National Health Service, where everyone is registered with a general practitioner and the responsibility of each primary care team is clearly demarcated, many of the issues raised are relevant to those working within more independent systems.

HOW CAN WE MAXIMIZE PATIENT INVOLVEMENT?

Meeting patients' expectations

Most people say they would like personal advice about the avoidance of heart disease. Although men in manual occupations are least enthusiastic, the vast majority of men and women from all social classes say they would value personal life-style advice.[1] It has also been reported that, with the exception of smoking and weight reduction, patients are not receiving this advice.[2] However, the uptake of cardiovascular preventive services offered is seldom high. In primary prevention, Chazova reported that only 57 per cent of a sample of 40–59 year old males accepted an invitation to a clinic designed to provide information on risk factors for coronary heart disease, and 22 per cent of patients with coronary heart disease and 30 per cent of patients with hypertension declined to attend over an ensuing four year period.[3] Even the uptake of post-MI cardiac rehabilitation services in many parts of the UK is less than 50 per cent. Harnessing the aspirations and expectations of patients is not easy. The challenge to each practice is to provide a preventive service with much higher and sustained levels of patient involvement than has so far been achieved.

New role for receptionists

The initiation of health checks in general practice was an important move towards a structured approach to the prevention of ischaemic heart disease. The strategy capitalized on the fact that each general practitioner and primary health care team in the UK offers care to a registered population. The initial method of recruitment, developed by the Oxford Centre for Prevention in Primary Care, was that any patient attending for any appointment at the practice was also invited *by the receptionist* to make a further appointment to see the practice nurse for a health check.[4] This strategy was not only simple but revolutionary. The value of health checks may be debatable but the role of reception and other office staff is now recognized as key to almost any preventive programme. Researchers in the *MRFIT Trial* concluded that successful recruitment required identification of one or more key persons with responsibility for recruitment, repeated monitoring of recruitment rates and regular discussion of recruitment successes and problems by the whole team.[5] It is essential that office staff have a clear idea of the aims of the project and understand its organization. They must be aware of the importance of their role, and have the time and motivation to fulfil it. The success of any recruitment strategy depends on their enthusiasm and commitment.

Opportunistic approaches

Opportunistic identification means identifying patients while they are consulting for another reason. In the UK, 65 per cent of people see their general practitioner at least once a year[6] and 90 per cent every three years.[7] An opportunistic approach is particularly appropriate for dealing with smoking, blood pressure, and existing cardiovascular disease. In an American study of opportunistic screening, 97 per cent of eligible patients were invited to participate in a simple health maintenance protocol by their physicians and their acceptance varied between 77–97 per cent depending on the specific procedure (it was lowest for sigmoidoscopy!).[8] If necessary, patients found to have any significant risk factor can then be asked to return to nurse or doctor for a dedicated appointment when more time is available. Various methods can be used to cue opportunistic activity in the consultation—for example, adding a marker 'flag' or 'flow card' to the manual record. Computerized practices can use a visual or auditory prompt when the patient's record is accessed.

Systematic approaches

An opportunistic approach must be augmented by a systematic 'call-recall' system for a number of reasons:

- to identify patients who are infrequent attenders;
- to act as a 'safety-net'—opportunistic identification does not occur when health professionals are busy and behind time in their clinics;
- to identify patients with an existing condition when a new treatment or intervention becomes available;
- to identify patients discharged from hospital (e.g. post MI) who may not immediately seek primary care;
- to ensure that patients known to need surveillance or treatment are not lost to follow-up.

The key requirement for a systematic approach is a patient register. 'Call' depends on a population register and can only be implemented in countries with population registration for primary health care. 'Recall' depends on risk and morbidity registration only and is possible in all countries.

Opportunistic versus systematic approaches

These approaches must be seen as complementary. Perhaps the most important observation is that Pierce *et al*, when examining response rates to cervical screening invitations in general practice, found little difference in outcome between postal invitations and flagging records to stimulate opportunistic invitations, but both methods were significantly more effective than a control group where no action was taken in general practice.[9]

Invitation methods

The effectiveness of any specific call-recall system probably varies with the disease in question and the method of invitation. Williams and Vessey, studying attendance for mammography, found that *the inclusion of an appointment* significantly enhanced compliance compared with an open ended invitation.[10] In an American study of mammography, a *second telephone call to non-attenders* led to an improvement in attendance from 26 to 36 per cent.[11] A study of mobile breast screening in the Lothians, with a poor response of 24 per cent to opportunistic screening, reported the response to a concomitant *personal invitation from the patient's general practitioner* to women who had failed to attend an earlier screening session as 75 per cent.[12] A further study in Edinburgh showed that 33 per cent of attenders felt their decision to attend was influenced by *their doctor's interest in screening*.[13] How relevant are these studies to recruitment for cardiovascular risk factor screening? It would seem advisable always to offer patients a definite appointment with the details written on a small card. The invitation should come from the general practitioner or at least show that the general practitioner believes that the activity being advocated is very important. If the interval between recruitment and the check is unduly long a reminder, either in the form of a postcard or telephone call, is appropriate.

Family appointments

In primary care the majority of families are registered with one doctor or are in contact with a single health professional. Invitations can be extended to low and reluctant users of the service via their higher consulting relatives. Compliance may be improved by inviting patients to attend with their spouses or other family members. When conducted in this way health checks may be more effective— because the whole family can share their knowledge of risk factors, and together plan appropriate strategies (personal communication—British Family Heart Study Investigators). This may be particularly important with regard to changes in diet and exercise patterns.

Non-personal contacts

Instances of computerized multiphasic health testing have been reported where individual health risks are presented to patients via a coloured display.[14] Computer programmes are available with screen driven menus which assess patients' cardiovascular risks and provide them with a written account of this at the end of the encounter together with appropriate advice. Similarly, cholesterol testing and blood pressure measurement is available in retail outlets in a number of countries. Unfortunately, little assessment has been made of the effectiveness of such intervention, nor of the effect on patient anxiety and subsequent need and demand for personal advice and support from primary care teams. Current opinion in the UK is that until such evidence is available, anyone who is screened should have an opportunity to discuss the results with a health professional.

Patient empowerment

This issue lies beyond the scope of this chapter, but it needs to be raised at this point. The strategies discussed here are concerned with providing patients with a service they want at a convenient time and encouraging them to use it. The involvement of patients in their care is equally important. Patients have better clinical outcomes if they are encouraged to involve themselves in, and ask their doctor questions about, their clinical management. Patients are more likely to accept and act on advice if it takes account of their own situation and intentions. Other chapters in this book discuss these issues and should be read in conjunction with this chapter.

IS IT POSSIBLE TO AVOID THE INVERSE CARE LAW?

In a study in my own practice, the likelihood of an individual patient receiving preventive care was inversely related to their cardiovascular risk for all factors measured except age.[5] Attendance for preventive health care depends on the attitudes and health beliefs of individual patients and their perception of its benefit to them.[15–18] There are considerable social class differences in the priorities attached to factors affecting health[17] and these may reflect the opportunity costs involved in avoiding unhealthy habits or in making changes to life-style.[1]

How opportunism can help

Besides improving the use of time, opportunistic recruiting improves access to patients at higher risk and of lower socio-economic status. These patients tend to consult their doctors more frequently than lower risk patients—and every such visit is an opening for opportunistic health promotion.

How formal recall can help

The inverse care law operates not only for the identification of risk but for its management. Those most at risk are not only those least likely to be identified but are also among the most likely to be lost to follow-up. A formal recall system does not in itself ensure attendance for follow-up in the disadvantaged, but does make clear that appropriate follow-up and clinical care is not happening and allows a decision to be made about what should be done. This systematic decision may simply be to tag the patient record to trigger an opportunistic approach to the patient.

How a team approach can help

A well functioning, multi-disciplinary primary health care team increases the opportunities available for intervention and, by broadening the number of personalities involved, increases the chances of successful communication and the uptake of advice in areas of social deprivation. Marsh, in his practice, developed a series of interwoven strategies to document cardiovascular risk factors and increase the uptake of advice in the more deprived community within his practice.[19] Opportunistic intervention by the general practitioners and health visitors was complemented by a similar approach from the practice nurses. The reception staff too were aware of the philosophy and made quick and appropriate referrals to the nurse when indicated. Doctors and health visitors even paid joint visits to the more recalcitrant. These practical strategies were built on the foundation of meticulous management—regular progress meetings were held within the primary health care team, and both individual and collective statistics were presented in the hope of maintaining the motivation of all team members.

Liaising with other agencies

Work site health promotion programmes have become increasingly prevalent in recent years and they offer an alternative way to avoiding inverse care in the working population. In the USA, one or more programmes are to be found in two thirds of all private work sites with 50 or more employees.[20] There are several advantages in recruiting employees in their place of work. Recruits may include those people who only consult their general practitioner or other health professionals infrequently. Accessibility also enhances follow-up and further counselling about risk factors. Peer group pressure and the provision of time during working hours are incentives to compliance. Despite these advantages, there is often no commitment to obtaining comprehensive uptake (so, as usual, those at highest risk are missed) and maintaining good liaison with primary care teams can be difficult. These problems are discussed below.

ARE THERE WAYS OF AVOIDING AN UNMANAGEABLE WORKLOAD?

Preventing cardiovascular disease tests a practice's commitment, teamwork and organization to the full. Enthusiasm for identification is not enough—it is very easy to do more harm than good by identifying risk and then failing to reduce it. The rule of halves in blood pressure management is still alive and well in the UK in the 1990s.[21] The management of patients with symptomatic heart disease is less than optimal in the UK and interventions known to reduce risk of subsequent events (including life-style modification) are not being implemented. There is much to be said for setting priorities and making sure one task is achieved adequately before commencing on the next.

Potential general practice workload

A high prevalence of risk factors in the population is unsurprising, considering the high incidence of ischaemic heart disease in the United Kingdom. This has been documented in several studies but methodological problems, differing recruitment strategies and incomplete results have cast doubt on their validity for assessing the extent of cardiovascular risk in general practice.[22,23] The *OXCHECK study* was based on the entire middle-aged (35–64 years) population of five general practices, each patient being invited for a health check over a four year period. The prevalence estimates are based on the patients who were willing to attend.[24] The prevalence of risk factors in 2205 attenders in the first year (1989/90) is shown in Table 18.1. The estimates are in broad accordance with other work, although the blood pressure estimates may be low as measurements were taken on Hawksley random zero sphygmomanometers which read lower than standard clinical sphygmomanometers. It is important to notice that more than a quarter of patients aged 55–64 already had a diagnosis of ischaemic heart disease, diabetes mellitus, or hypertension and 12 per cent reported chest pain suggestive of a previous myo-cardial infarction. The implications of these prevalence data for follow-up and further care are profound. The authors of the *OXCHECK study* concluded that 73 per cent of those screened had at least one risk factor which merited some primary care intervention, more than a third of patients had two such risk factors, and a tenth of patients needed follow-up for more than two risk factors. Clearly priorities have to be set and the level of intervention tailored to resources available.

Table 18.1   Percentage prevalence of risk factors for cardiovascular disease in 2205 patients attending for health check in 1989–1990.

		Men	Women
Personal history			
Hypertension, diabetes or ischaemic heart disease		14	15
Current smoker		35	24
Chest pain		10	8
Family History			
Ischaemic heart disease in first degree relative aged < 50		6	8
Ischaemic heart disease in first degree relative aged 50–59		11	10
Dietary fat			
Low polyunsaturated fat		13	12
High total fat		31	18
Clinical measurements			
Total cholesterol (mmol/l)	⩾8.0	8	8
	6.5–7.9	30	29
Diastolic blood pressure (mmHg)	⩾100	3	2
	90–99	11	7
Body Mass Index (kg/m^2)	⩾30	10	16
	25–29.9	45	32

Staffing implications—the time involved

Tudor Hart estimated that the additional annual staff time required at Glycorrwg just to run hypertension and diabetic services for a population of 2000 was 162 hours for nurses and 12 hours for the practice manager (in addition to 72 hours of doctor time).[25] Practices do have a suitable infrastructure. By 1991, 88 per cent of practices employed one or more practice nurses, 94 per cent offered health promotion programmes, and three out of four had practice manager.[26] But have they adequate time to manage the risks identified by universal screening?

In a recent economic analysis of the OXCHECK data, it was estimated that collecting risk factor data would take about 20 minutes of nurse time for each patient and that life-style advice (including follow-up) for those 'at risk' would take approximately 100 minutes.[27] If a practice checked cardiovascular risks on 600 patients each year, and even 50 per cent needed life-style advice, this would involve a nurse in at least 700 hours work—or about 20 working weeks.

The implications of cardiovascular prevention on medical workload are difficult to assess. In the long term, there are potential gains from a decrease in morbidity. In the short term, the estimate of nine minutes/year per patient with identified hypercholesterolaemia[30] seems a gross underestimate. Merely to achieve identification will require longer routine consultations, since several studies have demonstrated a positive relationship between length of consultation and health promotion content.[28-30] Increasing the length of a routine general practice consultation by just over a minute (from seven to eight minutes) has been shown to increase the recording of blood pressure, smoking status, and alcohol consumption.[31]

But if consultation times were to be universally lengthened then, by implication, general practitioners would either have to consult for longer periods, reduce their list sizes, or (as Marsh[32] has argued) transfer some of their present clinical workload to an expanded primary health care team.

Strategy

Other chapters in this book have argued strongly that the role of primary health care teams in secondary prevention of cardio-vascular disease needs to be expanded to improve the quality of care offered to those with symptomatic disease. Improvements in available techniques for the diagnosis and management of ischaemia, heart failure, and atrial fibrillation are inevitably going to increase our existing preventive workload at a practice level. In addition, all practices need to audit and improve their management of high blood pressure so that it meets the standards we are now asking of ourselves. Both these developments are likely to become formal contractual requirements in the next few years.

The core strategy for primary prevention recommended by economic analysis is to concentrate on smoking cessation and blood pressure.[27,33] Enthusiasts may extend this strategy but should plan on the basis that the resources necessary for follow-up are approximately five times those necessary for identification of risk.

IN WHICH WAYS CAN PRIMARY MEDICAL CARE TEAMS BEST WORK WITH OTHERS?

Primary health care is only one of a number of agencies concerned with cardio-vascular disease prevention in the community, and it is important for primary care teams to be aware of their activities.

Schools

Children are a vitally important group to recruit and educate about cardiovascular risk factors. Their presence at school both makes it easier to target them and also offers the important advantage of reinforcement of knowledge by their peer group. Health education offered in an acceptable manner, and introduced at the right time for a given group of pupils, can be effective. Many such interventions have been described, which aim to prevent heart disease, strokes, cancer and drug abuse.[34–37] Aside from the immediate impact on children and their health beliefs one might hope for some influence on the family. Some programmes are run by external agencies but most rely heavily on teachers. The primary care team would do well to identify the teachers in their practice population—not only is this an effective way of disseminating health education from primary care to children outside family constraints but it may also provide a learning opportunity and point of local liaison.

Workplaces

Studies show wide variations in participation rates—reflecting differences of strategy, target population, management support, and company time available. In some of the more successful studies participation of 70–90 per cent have been achieved. At the Ford Motor Company 66–83 per cent of the workforce of four large worksites were screened for hypertension over a period of four weeks.[37] Intervention programmes for risk reduction at worksites usually have much lower participation rates, often in the range of 5–10 per cent of the at risk group over a period of one year. The degree of participation varies with the type of intervention—for instance worksite based exercise programmes have a very low recruitment rate often not exceeding 15 per cent of eligible employees. Group smoking cessation and weight management programmes fare only slightly better with rates of 20–25 per cent.[38]

The importance of effective liaison

The lack of effectiveness of liaison in the management of patients with hypertension between workplace and general practice is best demonstrated by the results of Djerassi *et al.* After identifying patients with hypertension in two factories, continuing care was arranged at the worksite in Factory A while patients from Factory B were referred back to their family physicians. After one year, the percentage of hypertensives who were controlled in Factory A had increased from 37 to 84 per cent and in Factory B from 15 to 24 per cent.[39] The results must reflect a number of issues including communication, ease of access, and quality of medical care, which need to be addressed if workplace and primary care are to be integrated effectively. They show that workplace care can reach the parts of cardiovascular prevention that general practice cannot reach and can achieve standards of care of which primary care teams would be proud.

CONCLUSIONS

- Opportunistic and systematic approaches to prevention are complementary. A formal recall system is important for follow-up of patients identified opportunistically.

- Personal invitation letters from the patient's own general practitioner, the inclusion of a suggested appointment time with an invitation, and personal telephone calls from nurses to non-attenders, all increase attendance for preventive care.
- It is important that there are adequate appointments at the right time of day and distributed appropriately throughout the week. Long intervals between the offer of an appointment and its realization will lead to defaulting.
- Patients offered a follow-up appointment should have the details written on a small card. If the interval between the invitation and the appointment is unduly long a reminder, either in the form of a postcard or telephone call, is appropriate.
- Increased attendance and compliance with advice may be improved by inviting patients to attend with their spouses or other family members.
- It is essential that the reception and office staff have a clear idea of the importance of their role, and have the time and motivation to fulfil it.
- Opportunistic recruiting improves access to patients at higher risk and of lower socio-economic status.
- A well functioning multi-disciplinary primary health care team increases the chances of successful communication and the uptake of advice in areas of social deprivation.
- The resources necessary for follow up are approximately five times those necessary for identification.
- The role of primary health care teams in the secondary prevention of cardiovascular disease will expand in the future. The basic primary care strategy for primary prevention must be to concentrate on smoking cessation and blood pressure management.
- There is much to be said for making sure one task is achieved adequately before commencing on the next.

REFERENCES

1. Coulter A. Lifestyles and social class: implications for primary care. J R Coll Gen Pract 1987; **37**: 533–536.
2. Wallace PG, Brennan PJ, Haines AP. Are general practitioners doing enough to promote healthy lifestyles? Findings of the Medical Research Council's general practice research framework study on lifestyle and health. BMJ 1987; **294**: 940–942.
3. Chazova LV, Ivanov VM, Mankian LM, Patoka NA, Sacs LM. Attitudes of district physicians and the population toward measures regarding the prevention of ischaemic heart disease. Kardiologiia 1984; **24**(11): 63–7.
4. Fullard EM, Fowler GJ, Gray JAM. Facilitating prevention in primary care. BMJ 1984; **289**: 1585–7.
5. Neaton JD, Grim RH Jr, Cutter JA. Recruitment of participants for the multiple risk factor intervention trial (MRFIT). Controlled Clinical Trials 1987; **8** (4 Suppl.): 415–535.
6. Hides D. Primary Health Care—a preview. London: HMSO, 1976, pp. 161–87.

7. Secretaries of State for Wales, Northern Ireland and Scotland. Primary health care: an agenda for discussion. London: HMSO, 1986.
8. Hahn DL, Berger MG. Implementation of a systematic health maintenance protocol in a private practice. J Fam Pract 1990; **31**(5): 492–502.
9. Pierce M, Lundy S, Palarisamy A, Winning S, Kiry J. Prospective randomized controlled trial of methods of call and re-call for cervical cytology screening. BMJ 1989; **299**: 160–2.
10. Williams EMI, Vessey MP. Randomised trial of two strategies offering women mobile screening for breast cancer. BMJ 1989; **299**: 158–9.
11. Goodspeed RB, DeLucia AG, Parravaso J, Goldfield N. Compliance with mammography recommendations at the worksite. J Occup Med 1988; **1**: 40–2.
12. Haiart DC, McKenzie L, Henderson J, Pollock W, McQueen DV, Roberts MM, Forrest AFM. Mobile Breast Screening: factors affecting uptake, efforts to increase response and acceptability. Public Health 1990; **104**: 239–47.
13. French K, Porter AMD, Robinson SE, *et al*. Attendance at a breast screening clinic: a problem of administration or attitudes? BMJ 1982; **285**: 617–20.
14. Hinohara S, Takahashi T, Vemura H, Robinson D, Steble G. The use of computerised risk assessment for personal instruction in the primary prevention of ischaemic heart disease in a Japanese automated multiphasic health testing and services centre. Med Inf London 1990; **15**(1): 1–9.
15. Pill R, Stott N. Invitation to attend a health check in a general practice setting: the views of a cohort of non-attenders. J R Coll Gen Pract 1988; **38**: 57–60.
16. Rosenstock IM. Why people use health services. Milbank Memorial Fund Quarterly 1966; **44**: 94–127.
17. Becker MJ, Maman LA. Sociobehavioural determinants of compliance with health and medical care recommendations. Medical Care 1975; **13**: 10–24.
18. Coulter A, Baldwin A. Survey of population coverage in cervical cancer screening in the Oxford Region. J R Coll Gen Pract 1987; **37**: 441–3.
19. Marsh GN, Channing DM. Narrowing the health gap between a deprived and an endowed community. BMJ 1988; **296**: 173–6
20. Fielding J. Work site practitioner and primary health care team offers care to a registered population. Health Promotion Journal 1990; **5**: 75–83.
21. Lees K, Mc Innes G, Reid J. Managing hypertension. BMJ 1992; **304**: 713–6.
22. Anggard E, Land J, Leniham C, Packard C. Prevention of cardiovascular disease in general practice. BMJ 1986; **293**: 177–80.
23. Jacobs A, Davies D, Dove J, Collinson M, Brown P. Identification and treatment of risk factors for coronary heart disease in general practice: a possible screening model. BMJ 1988; **296**: 1712–4.
24. Imperial Cancer Research Fund, Oxcheck study group. Prevalence of risk factors for heart disease in Oxcheck trial. Implications for screening in primary care. BMJ 1991; **302**: 1057–60.
25. Tudor Hart J. Rule of halves: implications for increasing diagnosis and reducing dropout for future workload and prescribing costs in primary care. Br J Gen Pract 1992; **42**: 116–19.
26. Anonymous. Medico political digest. BMJ 1991; **302**: 971.
27. Field K, Thorogood M, Silagy C, Normand C, O'Neil C, Muir J. Strategies for reducing coronary risk factors in primary care: which is most cost-effective? BMJ 1995: **310**; 1109–12.
28. Roland MO, Bartholomew J, Courtenay MJ, Morns RW, Morrell DC. The 'five minute' consultation: effect of time constraint on verbal communication. Br Med J Clin Res 1986; **292**: 874–6.

29. Morrell DC, Evans ME, Morris RW, Roland RO. The 'five minute' consultation: effect of time constraint on clinical content and patient satisfaction. Br Med J Clin Res 1986; **292**: 870–3.
30. Howie JG, Porter AM, Heaney DJ, Hopkin JL. Long to short consultation ratio: a proxy measure of quality of care for general practice. Br J Gen Pract 1991; **41**: 48–54.
31. Wilson A, McDonald P, Hayes L, Cooney J. Health promotion in the general practice consultation: a minute makes a difference. BMJ 1992; **304**: 227–30.
32. Marsh G. Caring for larger lists. BMJ 1991; **303**: 1312–6.
33. Silagy C, Mant D, Muir J, Neil A. Modelling different strategies to prevent coronary heart disease in primary care. J Clin Epidemiol 1994: 47; 993–1001.
34. Walter HJ, Wyndel EL. The development, implementation, evaluation and future direction of a chronic disease prevention program for children: the 'know your body' studies. Prev Med 1989; **18**: 59–71.
35. Wynder EL. Primary Prevention of Cancer. The case for comprehensive school health education. Cancer 1991; **67** (6 suppl.): 1820–3.
36. Perry CL. Results of prevention programs with adolescents. Drug Alcohol Depend. 1987; **20**: 13–19.
37. Foote A, Efurt JC. Hypertension control of the worksite. Comparison of screening, referral and follow-up, and on site treatment. N Engl J Med 1983; **308**: 809–13.
38. Blair SN, Piserchia PV, Wilbur CS and Cowder JH. A public health model for worksite health promotion. JAMA 1986; **255**: 921–6.
39. Djerassi L, Silverberg DS, Boldblatt H, Goldberg A, Porat V. Comparison of hypertension treatment on and off the worksite. J Hum Hypertens 1990; **4**: 322–5.

19.1 Issues in measurement: Smoking

Godfrey Fowler

There are a number of measurement issues which arise in relation to smoking and these include:

1. **Measurement of tobacco consumption—cigarettes, cigars, pipe, tobacco**
2. **Assessment of motivation to stop smoking**
3. **Assessment of nicotine dependence**
4. **Measures which predict success in smoking cessation**
5. **Biochemical validation of self-reported smoking cessation.**

MEASUREMENT OF TOBACCO CONSUMPTION

Measurement of tobacco consumption relies heavily on self-reported information. Such information includes the number and type of manufactured cigarettes or cigars smoked daily, or the amount of 'roll your own' cigarette tobacco, or of pipe tobacco used. There is no reliable way of validating this self-reported information and it is generally felt that people underestimate the amount they smoke. Blood nicotine (or cotinine) levels vary widely and are not simply related to the amount smoked but to the way smoking is carried out as well as to quantity. Various questionnaires are available to measure tobacco consumption and an example is provided in Table 19.1.

ASSESSMENT OF MOTIVATION TO STOP SMOKING

In surveys, about 70 per cent of smokers report that they want to stop smoking and make repeated attempts to do so.[1] Intention to stop smoking is the best predictor of success and assessment by the therapist of the likelihood of successful quitting is also a reliable measure.[2]

ASSESSMENT OF NICOTINE DEPENDENCE

Nicotine dependence is an important feature of smoking behaviour in many established smokers[3] and withdrawal symptoms are evident after stopping smoking. There is now much evidence of the benefits of nicotine replacement therapy in helping smokers to stop.[4,5] There is also evidence that efficacy may be related to nicotine dependence, nicotine gum being more effective in highly dependent smokers[4] and nicotine patches in those with moderate nicotine dependence.[6]

Table 19.1 Smoking questionnaire. Adapted from OXCHECK Health and Lifestyle Survey Questionnaire (ICRF Study Group. Prevalence of risk factors for heart disease in OXCHECK trial: implications for screening in primary care. BMJ 1991; **302**: 1057-60)

1 Are you now or have you ever been a smoker?	Yes .... No ....
2 At what age did you first smoke regularly (at least once a day)?	☐ yrs of age
3 For how many years altogether have you smoked/did you smoke regularly?	☐ yrs smoked regularly
4 Do you CURRENTLY smoke at least once a day?	Yes .... No ....
5 On average, how many CIGARETTES do you smoke a day?	☐ cigarettes per day
6 On average, how many CIGARS do you smoke a day?	☐ cigars per day
7 On average, how much tobacco (PIPE or ROLL-UPS) do you smoke a **week**?	☐ oz tobacco per week
8 In the last 12 months have you SERIOUSLY tried to give up smoking?	Yes .... No ....
9 In the last 12 months has a doctor or nurse advised you to give up smoking?	Yes .... No ....
10 Do you think the amount you smoke is harmful to YOUR health?	Yes .... No .... Don't know ....
11 Would you like to give up smoking?	Yes .... No .... Don't need to ....

Instruments have been developed to assess such dependence and the most commonly used one is the *Fagerström Tolerance Questionnaire*.[7] This scoring system was first published in 1978 but a revised and modified version[8] omits questions of less discriminatory value, giving greater weight to more discriminatory questions (Table 19.2).

Table 19.2   Modified Fagerström tolerance questionnaire

Questions	Answers	Points
1 How soon after you wake up do smoke your first cigarette?	Within 5 minutes 6–30 minutes 31–60 minutes After 60 minutes	3 2 1 0
2 Do you find it difficult to refrain from smoking in places where it is forbidden (eg in church, in the cinema, at the library etc)?	Yes No	1 0
3 Which cigarette would you hate most to give up?	The first one in morning Any other	1 0
4 How many cigarettes a day do you smoke?	31 or more 21–30 11–20 10 or less	3 2 1 0
5 Do you smoke more frequently during the first hours after waking than during the rest of the day?	Yes No	1 0
6 Do you smoke if you are so ill that you are in bed most of the day?	Yes No	1 0

High dependence ≥8 points
Moderate dependence 4–7 points
Low dependence < 4 points

An alternative measure of nicotine dependence is the *Modified Horn-Russell Score* (Table 19.3).[9]

Table 19.3   Modified Horn-Russell score

1 I get a definite craving to smoke when I have to stop for a while.
2 I light up a cigarette without realising I still have one burning in the ash tray.
3 I smoke automatically without even being aware of it.
4 When I have run out of cigarettes I find it almost unbearable until I can get them.
5 I find it difficult to go as long as an hour without smoking.
6 I find myself smoking without remembering lighting up.
7 I get a real hunger to smoke when I haven't smoked for a while.
8 I am very aware of the fact when I'm not smoking.
9 I would find it difficult to go without smoking for as long as a week.

Each question score a scale of 0 (not at all) to 3.
Maximum score 27.
Dependency: low ≤11; moderate 12–18; high ≥19.

PREDICTORS OF SUCCESSFUL SMOKING CESSATION

Follow-up of subjects in smoking cessation trials provides some indicators of success.[5] These include:

- lighter smoking and shorter smoking history
- older, rather than younger, smokers
- being married, rather than single
- being male, rather than female
- social factors, for example non-smoking partner or friends
- number of previous attempts
- low nicotine dependence
- smoking related health problems
- strong motivation to stop
- confidence in ability to stop.

BIOCHEMICAL VALIDATION OF SELF-REPORTED SMOKING CESSATION

Self-reported smoking cessation is generally subject to unreliability because of deception. Average deception rates of about 25 per cent are usual, but they may be higher.[10] There are a number of methods of biochemically validating smoking cessation but the two commonest and most convenient are measurement of carbon monoxide (CO) in expired air and measurement of cotinine (a nicotine metabolite with a 24 hour half-life) which can be measured in body fluids.

Carbon monoxide is an invisible, odourless, toxic gas. Each cigarette yields about 15 mg of CO and this constitutes about 5 per cent of the total gases in cigarette smoke. When tobacco smoke is inhaled, CO is absorbed and combines with haemoglobin with great affinity (200 times that of oxygen) to form carboxyhaemoglobin (COHb). The amount of CO absorbed by the smoker depends on a number of factors, including the CO yield of cigarettes and the extent of inhalation. Day time levels in regular smokers are usually at least 5 per cent COHb and sometimes reach as high as 15 per cent falling somewhat overnight. The concentration of CO in a sample of expired air correlates closely with blood COHb levels since CO in alveolar air is in equilibrium with COHb in the blood. Therefore, measurement of expired air CO level offers a non-invasive alternative to measurements of CO in a blood sample.[11] Endogenous CO production by the body and background, environmental CO levels (except in heavy traffic, for example), generally lead to expired CO levels of not more than 5 ppm and the level of 10 ppm can be safely taken as a reliable cut off point between a smoker and a non-smoker. Regular smokers may have expired CO levels of 50 ppm or more and elevation persists for some hours after stopping smoking because the half-life of COHb is about four hours. A simple, cheap CO monitor (Smokerlyzer, see

Fig. 19.1) can be used to measure exhaled CO. When using the instrument, the subject should be instructed to exhale completely, then take a deep breath, hold it for 20 seconds, and then breath out steadily into the mouth piece. The sampling system traps an end-tidal sample which diffuses into the sensor and produces an electrical signal directly proportional to CO concentration. There is some evidence[10] that demonstration of exhaled CO to a smoker may assist smoking cessation. It can certainly provide tangible proof of an immediately noxious effect of cigarette smoking.

Cotinine measurement is a less simple but more reliable validation measurement because of its longer half life and its 'invisibility' to the smoker. Measurement in saliva is now relatively simple procedure and a level less than 20 nanograms (ng/ml) is consistent with non-smoking.[12]

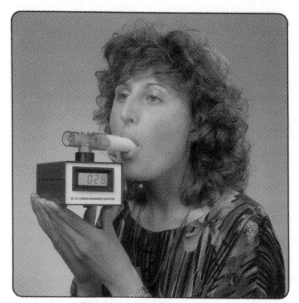

Fig. 19.1 The Smokerlyser

REFERENCES

1. Marsh A, Matheson J. Smoking attitudes and behaviour. London: HMSO, 1983.
2. Sanders D, Peveler R, Mant D, Fowler G. Predictors of successful smoking cessation following advice from nurses in general practice. Addiction 1993; **88**: 1699–705.
3. Benowitz NL. Pharmacological aspects of cigarette smoking and nicotine addiction. N Eng J Med 1988; **318**: 1318–30.
4. Tang JL, Law M, Wald N. How effective is nicotine replacement therapy in helping people stop smoking? BMJ 1994; **308**: 21–6.
5. Silagy C, Mant D, Fowler G, Lodge M. Meta-analysis on the efficacy of nicotine replacement therapies in smoking cessation. Lancet 1994; **343**: 139–42.

6. Yudkin PL, Jones L, Lancaster T, Fowler GH. Which smokers are helped to give up smoking using nicotine patches? Br J General Practice 1996 (in press).
7. Fagerström KO. Measuring degree of physical dependency to tobacco smoking with reference to individualisation of treatment. Addictive Behaviours 1978; **3**: 235–41.
8. Heatherton TF, Kozlowski LT, Frecker RC, Fagerström KO. The Fagerström test for nicotine dependence: a revision of the Fagerström Tolerance Questionnaire. British J Addiction 1991; **86**: 1119–27.
9. Russell MAH, Peto J, Patel UA. The classification of smoking by factorial structure of motives. J R Statistical Soc 1974; **137**: 313–33.
10. Jamrozik K, Vessey M, Fowler G, *et al.* Randomised trial of three different smoking cessation interventions in general practice. BMJ 1984; **288**: 1499–502.
11. Jarvis M, Belcher M, Verey C, Hutchinson DCS. Low cost carbon monoxide monitors in smoking assessment. Thorax 1986; **41**: 886–7.
12. Jarvis M. Comparison of tests used to distinguish smokers from non-smokers. Am J Public Health 1987; **77**: 1435.

19.2 Issues in measurement: blood pressure

Martin Dawes

Stephen Hals, an English clergyman, was the first to record measurement of blood pressure. This was performed in the early 1700s by connecting a main artery from a horse to a vertically held glass tube using a goose trachea. Mercury was first used by Pouseille (a French medical student) but this still required the opening of an artery. It was not until 1896, when Riva Rocci used the arm cuff for constricting the blood flow to measure systolic blood pressure, that interest in measuring blood pressure developed. In 1905 Karotkoff described the auscultatory sounds heard when releasing the arm cuff.

In measuring blood pressure there are three main issues that must be addressed:

1. **How can we avoid measurement errors due to inadequate equipment?**
2. **What procedures must be followed in taking measurements in order to achieve valid results?**
3. **Are there alternative methods of measuring blood pressure which should be considered?**

AVOIDING ERRORS DUE TO INADEQUATE EQUIPMENT

The usual screening and diagnostic tool for detecting abnormal blood pressure is now the standard mercury column manometer. It is important to take accurate measurements with good quality equipment since one must ensure that patients are really at risk from hypertension before subjecting them to pharmacological therapy for many years. There are many factors that can lead to false readings, including the following:

blocked air vent	cuff in wrong position
dirty glass	inflation valve faulty
scale not legible	patient not relaxed
badly fitting connection	poor positioning of arm
tubing perished	restrictive clothing
inappropriate bladder size	reading taken too quickly
cuff too short	parallax
velcro worn	poor stethoscope
	digit preference

The sphygmomanometer consists of a manometer (mercury or aneroid spring loaded), an inflatable cuff, and a manual inflation–deflation device. These are connected with rubber tubing which should be checked at regular intervals for leaks or obstruction. Both forms of manometer should be zeroed accurately and the aneroid should be checked more frequently as it loses accuracy over time leading to falsely low readings. The commonest fault in the inflation–deflation device is the control valve which often becomes stiff leading to sudden falls in pressure of more than 10 mm Hg. This part is cheap and easily replaceable.

The cuff bladder length should be at least 80 per cent of the circumference of the arm. If the bladder is too short then the pressure will not be evenly applied to the artery. Should this happen an artificially high reading will be obtained. If the width of the bladder is too small a similar problem will occur. The width should be 40 per cent of the circumference. In adults the range of width is usually from 12 to 15 cm. Bladder lengths advised by the British Hypertension Society are listed in Table 19.4.

Table 19.4   BHS guidelines for length of bladder in sphygmomanometer cuffs

	Bladder length (cm)
Children > 5 years	12
Usually supplied by manufacturer	23
Normal and lean arms (recommended by BHS)	35
Muscular and obese arms	42

CORRECT PROCEDURES FOR MEASUREMENT IN ORDER TO ACHIEVE VALID RESULTS

The patient should be advised about the possible discomfort of the cuff so as to reduce the possibility of raised blood pressure through anxiety. The patient should be resting—it is usually suggested that a patient should have been sitting for three minutes although there is little data that this is the optimum time. Tight or restrictive clothing should be removed from the arm and the cuff should then be applied to the arm with the tubing at the top of the cuff ensuring easy access to the area over the brachial artery. The cuff should be at the level of the heart in order to reduce baseline error. The centre of the bladder should cover the brachial artery. While palpating the artery the cuff should be blown up until the arterial pulse can no longer be felt. This both prevents the cuff being blown up too high (hurting the patient) and also avoids the examiner missing the auscultatory gap that occurs in some patients. The mercury column should be lowered at a rate of 2–3 mm/s. The options for determining the diastolic blood pressure are to use phase IV, the change from loud to muffled sound or to use phase V, the disappearance of the sound (Table 19.5). It is recommended that the fifth sound is used for assessment of blood pressure in normal clinical practice.

Table 19.5 Karotkoff Sounds

Phase	Sound
I	Consecutive beats produce sound whilst the cuff is being deflated. These sounds are of short duration.
II	Sounds or murmurs of longer duration.
III	Augmentation of sound volume due to an increased volume of blood passing through the artery as the cuff is deflated.
IV	The pressure at which the sounds become softer
V	The total disappearance of sound.

Digit preference, that is using numbers ending in 0 or 5, often leads to errors and one should try to record to the nearest 2 mm Hg. The column of mercury should be viewed horizontally to avoid any error caused by parallax. Blood pressure should be measured twice, more than one minute apart, at each visit.

Blood pressure should be measured in both arms in all patients found to have elevated blood pressure when they are first examined. If there is a difference of 20 mm Hg systolic and 10 mm Hg diastolic between the arms then blood pressure measurement should be repeated simultaneously to determine any vascular structural abnormality.

Four or more visits are needed to determine blood pressure thresholds and in mild hypertensive patients with isolated systolic hypertension, but no target organ damage, blood pressure measurements should be taken over three to six months.[1] Standing blood pressure measurements are important for elderly and diabetic hypertensive patients in whom orthostatic hypotension is common.

ALTERNATIVE METHODS OF MEASURING BLOOD PRESSURE

The Hawksley random zero sphygmomanometer has been used in most trials studying blood pressure. It was designed to reduce observer bias in blood pressure measurement. It adds a random amount of mercury to the manometer as the reading is being taken. When the mercury column has stopped falling the amount extra added can be read off and subtracted from the reading.[2] Unfortunately, it has been recognized that it reads on average 3.5 mm Hg lower than a standard mercury column when measuring diastolic blood pressure and 7.5 mm Hg lower when measuring systolic.[3] As this machine was used for most of the major hypertension morbidity and mortality studies this finding raises important issues about thresholds for treatment when using normal mercury column measurements.

It is extremely important to identify patients who have clinically significantly raised blood pressure. For 20 years, we have had evidence showing that there is a population who have raised levels of blood pressure as measured using standard sphygmomanometers but who have a normal ambulatory blood pressure (ABP) when monitoring is performed using intra-arterial catheters. The proportion of 'hypertensive' patients with so called 'white coat' hypertension maybe as much as 20 per cent.

Computerized ambulatory blood pressure monitoring machines have been produced, with a small recording unit attached to a belt fastened around the waist, using a standard cuff which is automatically inflated and then deflated to determine blood pressure. These machines have raised the issue of ambulatory monitoring in primary care. Some 1000 machines are now in use throughout the UK. As yet there have not been any long-term prospective studies into the predictive value of blood pressure measurements made using these monitors in terms of long-term mortality or morbidity. The mean diastolic blood pressure and systolic blood pressure using the ambulatory monitor is 5 and 14 mm Hg lower than using surgery readings. Equally worrying is the finding that 12 per cent of patients who have a normal blood pressure in surgery have a raised ambulatory reading. Some data suggests that a mean ABP reading of greater than 135/85 may indicate hypertensive risk.[4] However, whilst there is no consensus on the use of ambulatory monitoring, if it is used in practice a low reading should not be considered as a reliable predictor of low risk in the presence of raised surgery readings.

REFERENCES

1. Subcommittee of WHO/ISH Mild Hypertension Liaison Committee. Summary of 1993 World Health Organization-International Society of Hypertension guidelines for the management of mild hypertension. BMJ 1993; **307**: 1541–6.
2. Wright BM, Dore CF. A random zero sphygmomanometer. Lancet 1970; **i**: 337–8.
3. Conroy RM, O'Brien E, O'Malley K, Atkins N. Measurement error in the Hawksley random zero sphygmomanometer: what damage has been done and what can we learn? BMJ 1993; **306**: 1319–22.
4. Scientific Committee. Consensus document on non-invasive ambulatory blood pressure monitoring. Journal of Hypertension 1990; **8**: 135–40.

19.3   Issues in measurement: cholesterol

Andrew Neil

This section briefly reviews the most important factors that can complicate the interpretation of measurements of total cholesterol concentration. These are:

1. **Bias (inaccuracy)**
2. **Lack of standardization**
3. **Imprecision (poor repeatability)**
4. **Regression to the mean.**

BIAS (INACCURACY)

Hospital clinical biochemistry departments use conventional 'wet' chemistry enzymatic methods to measure cholesterol. In the UK they routinely participate in external quality assessment schemes which assess the accuracy of participating laboratories in relation to a consensus mean of the method group using animal-based reference materials. Good performance depends on how well a laboratory agrees with the other participants and not on how close the result is to the true value. Most laboratories track close to the consensus mean for the various schemes and probably achieve an accuracy within the recommended three per cent for the method[1] but none of the schemes in the UK are standardized to an internationally accepted accuracy base.[2]

LACK OF STANDARDIZATION

The Center for Disease Control (CDC, Atlanta, Georgia, USA) co-ordinates a laboratory reference network that enables cholesterol values to be traceable back to the definitive primary method for measurement of cholesterol—the Abell-Kendall method. Using this procedure it is possible to assess how closely laboratories agree with the 'true' value of the primary reference method. Until a national standardization scheme involving human serum or plasma based on CDC criteria is introduced in the UK, care is needed in interpreting results of specimens from the same patient measured by different laboratories. A pilot standardization scheme has been established in Scotland and Northern Ireland[2] which has reported a positive bias in cholesterol measurements of four per cent that translates into an increment of 0.3 mmol/l at 7.8 mmol/l. Until this scheme is extended to the UK as a whole, results may continue to diverge from the CDC primary reference method, and the bias will differ depending on the analyzer and kit used. This may lead to misclassification of coronary heart disease risk, although clinically the effect of a four per cent positive bias may be relatively unimportant because management of hypercholesterolaemia depends on the assessment of overall cardiovascular risk and not simply on the cholesterol concentration.

IMPRECISION (POOR REPEATABILITY)

Imprecision in measurement of cholesterol has important clinical implications for the investigation and management of patients. A single measurement of cholesterol is an imprecise estimate of the individual's true value. The degree of imprecision reflects mainly within-individual biological variation and to a lesser extent analytical imprecision—often termed laboratory measurement error. Repeat measurements on serial specimens from an individual are normally distributed around a true (mean) value, and the extent of dispersion is expressed as the coefficient of variation (which is defined as the standard deviation of repeated measurements divided by their mean).

The contribution of the biological and analytical components of variation to the total within-individual variation can be readily calculated usng the following formula:

$$cv_{tot} = \sqrt{cv^2_{biol} + cv^2_{analyt}}$$

Provided that the analytical coefficient of variation (cv) is less than the recommended limit of imprecision of 3 per cent[1], further improvement in test precision will not result in a clinically useful reduction in the total cv. The average within-individual biological variation is about 6 per cent and, if analytical variation is 3 per cent, then the total cv can be calculated to be 6.7 per cent— confirming that the analytical component contributes only a small amount to the total variation.[3,4] The precision of conventional laboratory measurement of cholesterol is therefore adequate for clinical purposes. By contrast, although desk top 'dry chemistry' analysers are accurate, with little or no bias when compared to the primary reference method, their precision (repeatability) is poorer than conventional laboratory methods. One study in general practice[5] reported an analytical cv of 5.5 per cent which would result in some clinically misleading measurements. Operator training, routine use of internal quality control, and participation in an external quality assurance scheme (often run by hospital departments of clinical chemistry) are essential if these instruments are to be used reliably in primary care.

The effect of an average within-individual biological cv of 6 per cent on repeat measurements is illustrated in Fig. 19.2. For a total cholesterol concentration of 6.5 mmol/l, 95 per cent of repeat measurements will fall within the range 5.7–7.3 mmol/l and 68 per cent of observations will fall within the narrower range of 6.3–6.7 mmol/l. The extent of biological variation means that multiple speci-mens are needed before hypercholesterolaemia can be diagnosed, and repeated measurements will be required to assess the relatively small effect expected for a therapy such as diet. To reduce test variability, account must be taken of the factors that may affect biological variation.

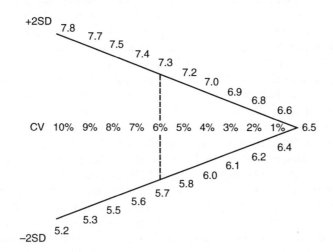

Fig. 19.2 The effect on repeat measurements of an average within-individual biological coefficient of variation of six per cent.

Factors affecting an individual's cholesterol concentration

A large number of factors can affect within-individual biological variability ;these have been reviewed elsewhere in detail and can be summarized as follows:[6]

collection	posture	diurnal variation
	exercise	seasonal variation
	venous occlusion	
others	dietary changes	acute major illness
	weight change	acute viral illness
	drugs	some chronic illnesses
	pregnancy/lactation	malignancy
	surgery	

Conditions of collection and storage make little practical difference but it is important to appreciate that serum levels are about 3 per cent higher than plasma levels. Fasting samples are only required for measurement of triglycerides, or if low density lipoprotein (LDL) cholesterol concentration is to be calculated from the total cholesterol, high density lipoprotein (HDL) cholesterol, and triglyceride concentrations using the Friedewald equation[7]:

$$\text{LDL cholesterol} = \text{total cholesterol} - \text{HDL cholesterol} - \frac{\text{triglyceride}}{2.2} \text{ mmol/l}$$

Among other factors determining cholesterol concentration diet has an appreciable effect; in general saturated fats raise serum cholesterol and polyunsaturated fats reduce it. In hypercholesterolaemic patients strict compliance with a diet containing less than 30 per cent calories as fat can reduce cholesterol levels by 10–15 per cent.[8] Intercurrent disease also affects cholesterol concentrations, and severe metabolic trauma such as surgery, acute major illnesses, or acute viral illnesses, substantially reduce cholesterol concentrations. For example, cholesterol levels are variably reduced, depending on the original level, by at least 15 per cent 48 hours or more after a myocardial infarction. However, the concentration in the first 24 hours reflects the pre-infarction level, and the changes resolve in 6–12 weeks.[9,10] Some chronic diseases appear to be associated with a fall in cholesterol; in malignancy the fractional catabolic rate of LDL cholesterol is enhanced and an unexpectedly low cholesterol level may be the first sign of an occult neoplasm. During pregnancy there is a progressive rise in cholesterol of about 1 mmol/l in the second and third trimester mainly due to an increase in oestrogens. In post-menopausal women exogenous oestrogens lower total and LDL cholesterol, but have the opposite effect in pre-menopausal women. Modern low-dose oestrogen oral contraceptives have little adverse effect on the lipid profile when combined with desogestrel or low-dose norethindrome as a progestin.[11] Other drugs can induce or aggravate hypercholesterolaemia, and the thiazide diuretics are some of the most commonly prescribed drugs to do so.

REGRESSION TO THE MEAN

One of the effects of test variability is the phenomenon of regression to the mean. If cholesterol is measured on two occasions, individuals with unusually high or low concentrations on the first occasion will, as a group, have a result nearer the average cholesterol on the second occasion. Since the underlying distribution must remain the same, there must be an opposing tendency for people with initial values close to the mean to have higher or lower repeat readings. An important effect of regression to the mean is to misclassify some individuals found to have high intial values. When recalled for futher measurements these individuals will, on average, have lower values. At least three measurements are therefore required before a firm diagnosis of hypercholesterolaemia can be made.

SUMMARY

- Repeated measurements of cholesterol are required to diagnose hypercholesterolaemia and monitor treatment.

- Allowance must be made for biological variability and analytical imprecision when interpreting results.
- Cholesterol concentrations may be substantially reduced by surgery, acute major illness, and viral illnesses.
- Care is needed in interpreting results of specimens from the same patient measured by different laboratories.
- Dry chemistry analysers should only be used in general practice with appropriate training, quality control, and participation in a quality assurance scheme.

REFERENCES

1. National Cholesterol Education Program Laboratory Standardization Panel. Current status of blood cholesterol measurement in clinical laboratories in the United States. Clin Chem 1988; **34**: 193–201.
2. Packard CJ, Bell MA, Eaton RH, Dagen MM, Cassidy M, Shepherd J. A pilot scheme for improving the accuracy of serum cholesterol measurement in Scotland and Northern Ireland. Ann Clin Biochem 1993; **30**: 387–93.
3. Mann JI, Crooke M, Hay DR, Jackson RT, Neutze JM, White HD. Guidelines for detection and management of dyslipidaemia. NZ Med J 1993; **106**: 133–41.
4. Schectman G, Sasse E. Variability of lipid measurements: relevance for the clinician. Clin Chem 1993: **39**: 1495–503.
5. Broughton PMG, Bullock DG, Cramb R. Quality of plasma measurements in primary care. BMJ 1989; **298**: 297–8.
6. Cooper GR, Myers GL, Smith J, Schlant RC. Blood lipid measurements. Variations and practical utility. JAMA 1992; **267**: 1562–660.
7. Friedewald WT, Levi RI, Fredrickson DS. Estimation of the concentration of low density lipoprotein cholesterol concentration in plasma without use of preparative ultracentrifuge. Clin Chem 1972; **18**: 499–502.
8. Ramsay LE, Yeo WW, Jackson PR. Dietary reduction of serum cholesterol concentration: time to think again. BMJ 1991; **303**: 953–7.
9. Fyfe T, Baxter RH, Cochran KM, Booth EM. Plasma-lipid changes after myocardial infarction. Lancet 1971; **i**: 997–1001.
10. Jackson R, Scragg R, Marshall R, White H, O'Brien K, Small C. Changes in serum lipid concentrations during the first 24 hours after myocardial infarction. BMJ 1987: 1588–9.
11. Godsland IF, Crook D, Simpson R, Proudler T, Felton C, Lees B, Anyaoku V, Vevenport M, Wynn V. The effect of different formulations of oral contraceptive agents on lipid and carbohydrate metabolism. NEJM 1990; **323**: 1375–81.

19.4 Issues in measurement: diet

Margaret Thorogood

Measuring a person's usual dietary intake is a challenging task. Nutritionists and epidemiologists have been working on and discussing the problems for many years, but there is still no method of collecting dietary information which is generally agreed to be accurate. There are two main difficulties in collecting such data.

1. **Is it possible to decide what dietary intake is 'usual' for any individual?**
2. **What methods are available for measuring actual intake?**

DECIDING WHAT DIETARY INTAKE SHOULD BE CONSIDERED AS USUAL FOR ANY INDIVIDUAL

Almost everybody has quite marked day to day variations, and seasonal variations, in both the type and quantity of the food they eat. Moreover, an individual's diet changes over time due to changes in personal circumstances, changes in the availability of foods, and even changes in fads and fancies. It is very difficult for subjects to remember with any accuracy what they usually ate a number of years ago, and collecting information about past dietary consumption is not really possible. Even obtaining accurate information on usual intake within the last year is difficult because of the day to day variations in a person's diet. For example, daily intake of energy varies only a little, and it has been calculated that five days of observation will be enough to obtain a fairly good estimate of energy intake whereas it will take ten days of observation to obtain the same accuracy of estimation of total fat intake, and 36 days of observation for vitamin C.[1]

WHAT METHODS ARE AVAILABLE FOR MEASURING ACTUAL INTAKE?

Eating is so much part of the every day fabric of life that it is hard for people to remember everything they ate in the last twelve hours, and virtually impossible for them to remember everything they ate two days ago. Moreover, a subject's report of what has been eaten is strongly influenced by the wider social meanings of food and eating. Food has an important social significance. It is used to reward children and to demonstrate affection and is the focal point of much social interaction. There are such strong social pressures to eat a 'good' diet that a person may often feel embarrassed or ashamed to report dietary habits they regard as 'bad' or 'unhealthy'.

Methods of collecting dietary information

While techniques of measuring dietary intake have undoubtably improved over the years, there is still no single reliable method. At one time, the 'gold standard' was considered to be a record kept by the subject over seven days, in which everything the subject ate was recorded after being weighed on a standard set of scales. Waste left over at the end of the meal was also weighed and recorded. This method, usually known as the *'seven day weighed record'* has lost its pre-eminence as a gold standard as nutritionists have come to understand more about the problems of under-reporting and non-compliance. Not surprisingly, subjects find it extremely onerous to weigh everything they eat.

Many other methods of collecting information about dietary intake have been developed. An adaptation of the seven day weighed record is an *estimated portion record* where subjects are asked to estimate the quantity of everything they eat, using either household measures or a set of photographs of portion sizes. However, this method still suffers from the disadvantage that subjects find it onerous to have to keep a record of everything eaten. Indeed, keeping a dietary record is sometimes an effective way of losing weight—it is easier to go without than to go to the trouble of recording an extra snack.

A popular method to record intake is to use a *food frequency questionnaire*, where respondents are asked how often they eat certain foods. The usefulness of such a method depends crucially on the foods included in the list. To devise a good food frequency questionnaire it is important first to decide what nutrients are of interest and then to determine which foods provide the majority of such nutrients. This is much easier for some nutrients than for others. Some nutrients are present in large quantities in a small number of foods, and hardly at all in other foods. For example, 75 per cent of the carotene in the British diet comes from carrots, butter, margarine, tomatoes, and leafy vegetables, that is, just about ten food items in all. Conversely, sodium is present in small quantities in practically all foods, and it would therefore be difficult to devise a food frequency questionnaire which adequately measured sodium intake. Diets vary a great deal between countries, and even within a country, and it is important when using a food frequency questionnaire to ensure that it has been designed for the population that it is being used with. It is no good, say, determining the fat intake of adolescents in Scotland using a questionnaire devised for elderly men in France.

In clinical practice, a dietitian will spend up to an hour carefully determining a patient's intake. This is normally achieved by asking a combination of what the patient ate in the last 24 hours (a *24 hour recall*), what the patient normally eats, and for any particular likes and dislikes. This *clinical diet history* taken by a skilled dietitian will provide both a good idea about the patients usual diet and also a basis for making any necessary changes.

A recent careful comparison of the reliability of different methods of assessing food intake has shown that a food frequency questionnaire performs poorly both in comparison with a seven day dietary record using estimated portion sizes[2] and, even more decisively, in comparison with biological markers of dietary intake, such as 24 h urinary nitrogen.[3] Results from a 24 h recall method were even more disappointing.

Apart from the doubtful reliability, most methods of collecting dietary information are far too complex and time consuming to be of value within primary care.

Dietary information in general practice

The first thing that must be understood is that it is not possible for a general practitioner, or indeed a practice nurse, to collect complete and accurate information on the food intake of a patient within the time limits of a consultation. If a good description of a patient's diet is required it is essential to refer the patient to a dietitian. What is important, therefore, for the doctor or nurse working in primary care is to decide on a very limited list of factors that are most relevant to the situation and to concentrate effort on getting the best possible information about these. In the context of reducing the risk of coronary heart disease four diet-related issues are potentially relevant. These are the intake of:

- total energy
- salt
- fat
- antioxidants

Total energy intake is only of importance if a patient is overweight or obese. If this is not the case, then no further enquiry need be made about energy intake. If weight loss is important, then, since it is not at all easy to determine a subject's total calorie intake, it would be wisest to ask a more limited range of questions targeted at consumption of high calorie foods (confectionary, cakes and biscuits, fried food, and alcohol). This information will help the nurse or doctor to give some appropriate advice.

Salt intake is also difficult to measure, because salt is present in so many foods. It is not really feasible to do more than ask about salt added to cooking and salt added at the table, which will account for only about 15 per cent of salt intake.

Saturated fat intake cannot be measured quickly with any exactitude, but it is possible to get a rough idea of whether somebody is eating a large or small amount of saturated fat. Twenty five per cent of the saturated fat in the diet comes from meat and meat products, and a similar amount from dairy produce, so questions about these foods will be particularly relevant. A food frequency questionnaire (the DINE questionnaire) designed explicitly to enable practice nurses to elicit this information from middle aged patients in England has been developed and validated by the ICRF General Practice Research Group (Table 19.6).[4] DINE will enable primary care workers to classify patients into low, medium, and high consumers of fat with reasonable accuracy.

The most important antioxidant with regard to risk of coronary heart disease is Vitamin E. The main source of vitamin E is vegetable oils and margarines, particularly sunflower oil products. Assessing intake of this vitamin would not be easy, nor would it be helpful since there is, as yet, no agreement about the desirable levels of intake.

It cannot be emphasised too much that measuring dietary intake is difficult and requires knowledge, skills, and time not readily available in general practice. When skilled dietary assessment and advice are needed referral to a dietitian would be the best solution.

Table 19.6   The Dine questionnaire

D I N E

Dietary Instrument for Nutrition Education

designed by Liane Roe, ICRF General Practice Research Group   (0865) 319121

Date of counselling session

Name of patient

Address of patient

Patient's phone number

Date of birth

Record of cholesterol measurements

Screening

Fasting

HDL   LDL   Triglycerides

Follow-up

Weight in Kg

Height in cm

Body Mass Index

| <20 under-weight | 20-25 OK | 25-30 Over-weight | 30-40 Obese | > 40 Very obese |

How do you feel about the way you are eating now? Do you follow a special diet of any kind? (slimming, vegetarian etc.)

Those intending to use the Dine questionnaire are welcome to contact Liane Roe, ICRF General Practice Research Group, (01865) 319121, for advice and assistance on its use and analysis.

Bread	less than 1 a day	1 - 2 a day	3 - 4 a day	5 or more a day
About how many pieces of bread or rolls (or chapatis) do you eat on a usual day? Are they usually white, brown, or wholemeal? (choose 1 only, if possible)				
White bread	1	4	9	13
Brown or granary bread; Mighty White, soft grain, white	2	7	15	22
Wholemeal bread or 2 slices crispbread	3	8	18	26

FIBRE SCORE

Bread score

About how many times a week do you have a bowl of breakfast cereal or porridge? What kind do you have most often? (choose 1 only, if possible)

Breakfast cereal	less than 1 a week	1 - 2 a week	3 - 5 a week	6 or more a week
Sugar type: Frosties, Coco Pops, Ricicles, Sugar Puffs Rice/Corn type: Corn Flakes, Rice Krispies, Special K	0	0	1	2
Porridge or Ready Brek *This is a source of soluble fibre* Wheat type: Shredded Wheat, Weetabix, Puffed Wheat, Fruit 'n Fibre, Nutri-Grain, Oat Krunchies, Start Muesli type: Alpen, Jordan's	1	2	5	7
Bran type: All-Bran, Bran Flakes, Sultana Bran, Team *High in sugar and calories!*	2	5	12	18

Cereal score

About how many times a week do you eat a serving of the following foods? (choose one on each line)

Vegetables etc.	less than 1 a week	1 - 2 a week	3 - 5 a week	6 or more a week
Pasta or rice	0	1	3	4
Potatoes	0	1	3	5
Peas	1	3	8	12
Beans (baked, tinned, dried) or lentils *These are a source of soluble fibre*	1	4	10	15
Other vegetables (any type)	0	1	2	3
Fruit (fresh, frozen or canned) *These are a source of soluble fibre*	0	1	3	5

Vegetables score

FIBRE RATING
Less than 30   = Low fibre intake
30 to 40   = Medium fibre intake
More than 40   = High fibre intake

TOTAL SCORE

About how many times a week do you eat a serving of the following foods?	less than 1 a week	1 - 2 a week	3 - 5 a week	6 or more a week
Cheese (any except cottage)	1	2	6	9
Beefburgers or sausages	1	2	4	6
Beef, pork or lamb (if vegetarian: nuts)	1	2	6	9
Bacon, meat pies, processed meat	1	2	5	8

FAT SCORE

Score ☐

About how many times a week do you eat a serving of the following foods?	less than 1 a week	1 - 2 a week	3 - 5 a week	6 or more a week
Chicken or turkey	0	1	3	5
Fish (**NOT** fried)	0	0	1	2
ANY fried food; fried fish, chips, cooked breakfast, samosas	1	2	6	9
Cakes, pies, puddings, pastries	1	2	5	8
Biscuits, chocolate, or crisps	1	2	4	6

Score ☐

About how much milk do you yourself use in a day, for example in cereal, tea, or coffee? What kind of milk do you usually use? (choose only 1 if possible) **Milk**	less than a quarter pint	about a quarter pint	about a half pint	1 pint or more
Full cream (silver top) or Channel Islands (gold top)	1	3	6	12
Semi-skimmed (red striped top)	0	1	3	6
Skimmed (blue checked top)	0	0	0	0

Milk score ☐

About how many pats or rounded teaspoons of margarine, butter or other spread do you usually use in a day, for example on bread, sandwiches, toast, potatoes, or vegetables? (Ask brand name)

Butter or margarine: Flora, Vitalite/Light, sunflower types, Blue Band, Golden Crown, Olivio, Krona, Stork/Light, Summer County ☐ *pats times 4 =* ☐ total

Low fat spread: Gold/Lowest, Outline, Shape, Flora Extra Light, Clover Extra Lite, Delight, Half Fat Butter, County Light ☐ *pats times 2 =* ☐ total

Spreading Fat score ☐

FAT RATING
Less than 30 = Low fat intake
30 to 40 = Medium fat intake
More than 40 = High fat intake

TOTAL SCORE ☐

UNSATURATED FAT SCORE

What sort of fat do you use: (choose one on each line)	Butter, dripping, lard, solid cooking fat (White Cap, Cookeen)	Hard or soft margarine, White Flora, Dairy Blends (Clover, Willow, Golden Crown), Half Fat Butter	Polyunsaturated/ sunflower/olive margarine or low fat spread (Gold, Outline, Shape, Flora Extra Light, Delight)	Vegetable Oil (eg sunflower, soya, corn, peanut, rapeseed, olive)	No Fat Used
on bread and vegetables?	1	2	3	4	3
for frying?	1	2	3	4	3
for baking or cooking?	1	2	3	4	3

UNSATURATED FAT RATING	5 or less	=	Low unsaturated fat
	6 to 9	=	Medium unsaturated fat
	10 or more	=	High unsaturated fat

TOTAL SCORE [ ]

SUMMARY OF DIET CHANGES AGREED

Is weight loss desired? **If no,** keep calories up with more bread, potatoes, vegetables
If yes, reduce fat, also ask about sugar, drinks, alcohol

☐ Use less spread
OR change to low fat spread
OR change to polyunsaturated spread
OR _____

Brand recommended: _____

☐ Change type of frying/cooking fat to _____

☐ Eat less fried food   Substitute _____

☐ Change to semi-skimmed/skimmed milk

☐ Eat less cheese   Substitute
OR use lower fat cheeses   _____

☐ Eat less meat   Substitute fish/pulses/poultry
OR eat leaner/trimmed meat

☐ Eat less processed meat (bacon, meat pies)
Substitute _____

☐ Eat less cakes, pies, puddings, pastries
Substitute _____

☐ Eat less biscuits, chocolate, crisps
Substitute _____

☐ Eat more bread
Or change type of bread to
_____

☐ Eat more breakfast cereal
OR change type to
_____

☐ Eat more vegetables/ pulses/ fruit/ grains

☐ Other changes
_____

Any follow-up arranged

REFERENCES

1. Bingham S. The dietary assessment of individuals; Methods, accuracy, new techniques and recommendations. Nutrition Abstracts and Reviews 1987; **57**: 705–42
2. Bingham S, Gill C, Welch A, Day K, Cassidy A, Khaw KT, Sneyd MJ, Key TJA, Roe L, Day NE. Comparison of dietary assessment methods in nutritional epidemiology. Br J Nutr 1994; **72**: 619–43.
3. Bingham SA, Cassidy A, Cole T, Welch A, Runswick S, Black AE, Thurnham D, Bates CE, Cassidy A, Key TJA, Khaw KT, Day NE. Validation of weighed records and other methods of dietary assessment using the 24h urine technique and other biological markers. Br J Nutr (in press).
4. Roe L, Strong C, Whiteside C, Neil A, Mant D. Dietary intervention in Primary Care: validity of the DINE Method for diet assessment. Family Practice 1994; **11**: 375–81.

19.5 Issues in measurement: fitness

David Mant and Paul Little

Measurement of exercise or cardio-respiratory fitness is likely to be carried out in general practice for two reasons: firstly, to assess baseline exercise levels or fitness in order to recommend an appropriate exercise programme to improve fitness; secondly, to monitor change in exercise or fitness in response to an exercise programme.

Precision in measurement is not necessary in recommending an appropriate exercise programme but it is necessary for assessing change over time. As measuring change in exercise levels or fitness is an important part of any exercise programme, poorly validated measures should be avoided. The main difficulties with fitness testing in general practice are the wide range of fitness which is likely to be encountered and the necessity for safety. The range of fitness was shown in the Allied Dunbar national fitness survey: about 30 per cent of men and over 50 per cent of women aged 55–64 years were unable to sustain walking at three miles per hour on level ground without exceeding 70 per cent of their maximum heart rate.[1] Safety implies that testing should be 'sub-maximal' and should probably not involve exercise which is likely to lead to a rate much greater than 70 per cent of estimated maximal heart rate (that is approximately 140 at age 20, 120 at age 50 and 100 at age 70)—although the Canadian home step test has been used safely in a community setting despite subjects at times exceeding this 70 per cent level.

No formal trials of the measurement of exercise or the feasibility of fitness testing in general practice have been published, but there are three options which should be considered. Item one measures activity, items two and three measure fitness.

1. **Informal questions and exercise questionnaires.**
2. **The step test.**
3. **The six or 12 minute walk.**

Both the step test and 12 minute walk have been used and validated in a community setting, and are currently being re-assessed and modified for use in general practice.

INFORMAL QUESTIONS

The informal questions recommended in the government publication 'Better living, better life' may well be adequate for recommending a safe graduated exercise programme. For example, targets suggested by the *Allied Dunbar National Fitness Survey* (ADNFS) are:

16–34 years: three or more occasions of vigorous activity lasting at least 20 minutes each week;

35–54 years: three or more occasions of a mix of moderate and vigorous activity lasting at least 20 minutes each week;

55–74 years: three or more occasions of moderate activity lasting at least 20 minutes each week.

Attainment of these targets can be assessed using the following questions:

- How many times during the past weeks have you taken any sort of physical activity at all, including walking, that lasted 20 minutes or more? (moderate)
- Which of these involved continuous movement involving the whole body, like walking, swimming, dancing? (moderate/vigorous)
- Which of these activities were vigorous enough to make you breathe hard or sweat? (vigorous)

SIMPLE EXERCISE QUESTIONNAIRES

Jacobs and colleagues evaluated 10 commonly used physical activity questionnaires in 1992.[2] The two which may be most useful in general practice are the *Lipid Research Clinic Physical Activity Questionnaire*[3] and the *Godin Leisure Time Exercise Questionnaire*.[4] The latter has achieved a commendable correlation against measured maximum oxygen intake ($r = 0.56$). They are reproduced in Table 19.7 and 19.8. No overall score is calculated for the Lipids Clinic Questionnaire, but individuals are compared both over time and against the general population on each dimension. The Godin questionnaire is slightly more complex but provides an aggregate score based on weighting episodes of activity according to intensity.

THE STEP TEST

Measuring exercise taken is an indirect method of measuring fitness, and there are advantages in direct measurement. The step test is probably the most feasible method of fitness testing for patients *without* existing cardio-respiratory disease, although formal confirmation of its successful use in general practice is awaited. It has the advantages of needing minimal equipment and of having been validated in a community population as the Canadian Home Fitness Test.[5] The Canadian test is based on the step height of a normal staircase and needs a pre-recorded cassette tape or metronome to set the stepping rate. Post-exercise pulse can be measured electronically or manually, using a watch or the cassette tape to set the time period. The test shows close correlation ($r = 0.88$) with directly measured maximum oxygen intake, which is widely used as the gold standard measure of cardio-respiratory fitness. Fig. 19.3 and the following instructions summarise the practical procedure for undertaking the test.

Table 19.7   Lipid research clinic physical activity questionnaire. From Siscovick D, Ekelund J, Hyde J, *et al.* Physical activity and CHD among asymptomatic hypercholesterolaemic men. Am J Pub Health 1988; **78**: 1428–31.)

1. Thinking about the things you do *at work*, how would you rate yourself as to the *amount of physical activity* you get compared with others of your age and sex?

    1 ☐ Much more active
    2 ☐ Somewhat more active
    3 ☐ About the same
    4 ☐ Somewhat less active
    5 ☐ Much less active
    6 ☐ Not applicable

2. Now, thinking about the things you do *outside of work*, how would you rate yourself as to the *amount of physical activity* you get compared with others of your age and sex? Would you say you are:

    1 ☐ Much more active
    2 ☐ Somewhat more active
    3 ☐ About the same
    4 ☐ Somewhat less active
    5 ☐ Much less active

3. Do you regularly engage in strenuous exercise or hard physical labour?

    1 ☐ Yes → | 4 Do you exercise or labour at least three time a week?
    2 ☐ No | „ 1 ☐ Yes   2 ☐ No

Some guidance on interpreting the results is given in Table 19.9. Obviously the test cannot be interpreted in patients taking drugs which affect heart rate (such as betablockers).

THE SIX OR 12 MINUTE WALK

This is an alternative to the step test for measuring fitness directly, and may be specifically helpful for people with ischaemic heart disease and those taking drugs such as betablockers. The test was initially described by Cooper who correlated the maximum distance covered in 12 minutes 'running preferably but walking whenever necessary to prevent excessive exhaustion' by 115 male US Air Force Officers.[6] The correlation with laboratory determined maximum oxygen consumption was 0.90. McGavin and colleagues[7] modified Cooper's test for use in older patients with chronic lung disease—again patients were asked to travel as far as possible in 12 minutes. In 1982, Butland *et al.* assessed 2, 6, and 12 minute walks, again involving patients with respiratory disease, and suggested that a 6 minute test

Table 19.8 Godin leisure time exercise questionnaire (From Godin G, Shepherd R. A simple method to assess exercise behaviour in the community. Can J Appl Sports Science 1985; **10**: 141–6.)

---

1. Considering a 7-day period (a week), how many times on the average do you do the follwoing kinds of exercise for more than 15 minutes during your free time (write in each circle the appropriate number of times per week).

TIMES PER WEEK

a. STRENUOUS EXERCISE
(HEART BEATS RAPIDLY)
(i.e. running, jogging, hockey, football, soccer, squash   ☐ ☐
basketball, cross country skiing, judo, roller skating,   30
vigorous swimming, vigorous long distance bicycling)

b. MODERATE EXERCISE
(NOT EXHAUSTING)
(i.e. fast walking, baseball, tennis, easy bicycling,   ☐ ☐
volleyball, badminton, easy swimming, alpine   32
skiing, popular and folk dancing)

c. MILD EXERCISE
(MINIMAL EFFORT)
(i.e. yoga, archery, fishing from river bank, bowling,   ☐ ☐
horseshoes, golf, snowmobiling, easy walking)   34

Considering a 7-day period (a week), during your leisure-time, how often do you engage in any regular activity long enough to work up a sweat (heart beats rapidly)? Please indicate your choice by an 'X'.

1 ☐ Often
2 ☐ Sometimes
3 ☐ Never/Rarely

Score: expressed as times/week weighted according to intensity ($3 \times$ mild $+ 5 \times$ moderate $+ 9 \times$ strenuous)

was almost as good as a 12 minute test and had the advantage of being less stressful and corresponding more closely to the usual day to day activity of moderately disabled patients.[8] Both Bittner *et al.* and Guyatt *et al.* have shown that the 6 minute walk performs adequately in patients with chronic heart failure.[9,10]

The 6 minute and 12 minute tests are little different in their ability to assess baseline fitness. However, it has been argued recently that the 12 minute test has a substantial advantage in measuring change. Correlation with baseline and change in maximum oxygen consumption for 2, 4, 6, and 12 minute walks in patients with chronic obstructive airways disease were recently reported as 0.45, 0.49, 0.48, and 0.49 and 0.53, 0.59, 0.64, and 0.77 respectively.[11] Where it is important to detect small changes in fitness the 12 minute test is better.

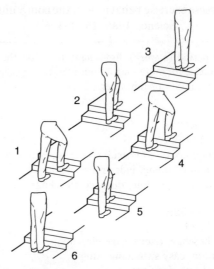

Fig. 19.3 Canadian step test protocol: stepping technique for stepping up and down two standard 10 cm steps.

The stepping tempo is should be set by a pre-recorded tape, giving 1 beat per step, which increases speed progressively; the final stepping rate (steps/minute) for each age group must be set as follows:

age	males	females
15–19	156	120
20–29	144	114
30–39	132	114
40–49	114	102
50–59	96	84
60–69	78	66

The tape can give time signals for counting an initial pulse rate after 3 minutes stepping; the test is terminated if the 10 second pulse rate exceeds the following levels:

age	pulse rate	age	pulse rate
15–19	> 29	40–49	> 25
20–29	> 28	50–59	> 24
30–39	> 27	60–69	> 23

If the pulse does not exceed these set thresholds, the individual continues for a further 3 minutes and the pulse rate is again measured.

(Adapted from Jette E M, Campbell J, Mongeon J, Routhier R. The Canadian home fitness test as a predictor of aerobic capacity CMAJ 1976: 114, 680–1 and Shepherd RJ, Bailey DA, Mirwald R. Development of the Canadian home fitness test CMAJ 1976. **114**, 675–9.)

Table 19.9 Categorization of level of fitness based on 10 second pulse rate taken 10–15 seconds after termination of exercise in Canadian step test. (Adapted from Shepherd RJ, Bailey DA, Mirwald R Development of the Canadian home fitness test CMAJ 1976; **114**: 675–9)

Age	10 second pulse rate		
	After 3 min unfit	After 6 min minimum fitness	After 6 min adequate fitness
15–19	> 29	> 26	26 or less
20–29	> 28	> 25	25 or less
30–39	> 27	> 24	24 or less
40–49	> 25	> 23	23 or less
50–59	> 24	> 22	22 or less
60–69	> 23	> 22	22 or less

Encouragement has a substantial effect on the performance of both the 6 and 12 minute tests so their conduct in this respect must be standardized. The distance covered must also be carefully measured. Most studies have utilized appropriately marked hospital corridors, but in general practice it may be difficult to find a long level area. Although the measurement of distance can be done by asking the patient to push a measurement wheel along the pavement (such instruments are sometimes seen being pushed by surveyors at the roadside), even this may not help in hilly areas. These practical issues may be resolved in current feasibility trials in general practice.

REFERENCES

1. Allied Dunbar National Fitness Survey (summary—publication SC/82/100M/6/92) London: Sports Council / Health Education Council, 1992.
2. Jacobs D, Ainsworth B, Hartman T, Leon A. A simultaneous evaluation of 10 commonly used physical activity questionnaires. Medicine and Science in Sports and Exercise 1993; **25**: 81–91.
3. Siscovick DS, Ekelund J, Hyde J, Johnson JL, Gordon DJ, LaRosa JC. Physical activity and CHD among asymptomatic hypercholesterolaemic men. Am J Public Health 1988; **78**: 1428–31.
4. Godin G, Shepherd R. A simple method to assess exercise behaviour in the community. Can J Appl Sports Science. 1985; **10**: 141–6.
5. Shepherd RJ, Bailey DA, Mirwald R. Development of the Canadian Home Fitness Test Can Med Assn J 1976; **114**: 675–9.
6. Cooper KH. A means of assessing maximal oxygen intake JAMA 1968; **203**: 201–4.
7. McGavin CR, Gupta SP, McHardy GJR. Twelve minute walking test for assessing disability in chronic bronchitis. BMJ 1976; **1**: 822–3.
8. Butland RJ, Pang J, Gross E, Woodcock A, Geddes D. Two, six and twelve minute walk tests in respiratory disease. BMJ 1982; **284**: 1607–8.

9. Guyatt GH, Sullivan MJ, Thompson PJ, *et al*. The 6 minute walk: a new measure of exercise capacity in patients with chronic heart failure Can Med Assn J 1985; **132**: 919–23.
10. Bittner V, Weiner DH, Yusuf S, Rogers WJ, MacIntyre KN, Bangdiwale SI, *et al*. Prediction of mortality and morbidity with a 6 minute walk test in patients with left ventricular dysfunction JAMA 1993; **270**: 1702–7.
11. Bernstein ML, Despars JA, Singh NP, Avalos K, Stansbury DW, Light RW Reanalysis of the 12 minute walk in patients with chronic obstructive pumonary disease Chest 1994; **105**: 163–7.

19.6   Issues in measurement: alcohol

Peter Anderson

There are three major issues that need to be considered in relation to assessing our patients' alcohol consumption:

1. **How can we best estimate the quantity of alcohol consumed by an individual?**
2. **How can we recognize when alcohol consumption is harming the individual?**
3. **Should we screen for alcohol intake and, if so, when?**

ESTIMATING ALCOHOL CONSUMPTION

Different methods have been used to measure alcohol consumption, including *quantity frequency measurement* and *description of occasions*.[1] In the *quantity frequency index*, respondents are asked about their drinking of each of three types of alcoholic beverages, namely beers, wines, and spirits (Table 19.10). For each beverage type, the usual frequency of drinking over a one month, three month, or longer period is recorded. The usual quantity of each beverage type drunk on each occasion is also elicited. Although the method is widely used,[2-4] there are some difficulties with its interpretation in terms of rate of consumption. First, it is not clear how respondents interpret the questions, which seem to require the reporting of modal rather than average frequencies and quantities. Averages will often be greater than the modes. A second difficulty concerns the effect of putting people into response categories. Under-reporting in this instance is best allowed for by providing very high response categories.

Quantity frequency questionnaires have high test re-test reliability and substantial validity.[1] As a screening instrument for hazardous alcohol consumption in general practice settings quantity frequency questionnaires have a sensitivity of 70 per cent, a specificity of 76 per cent ,and a positive predictive value of 78 per cent.[5] It is important to offer options of high alcohol intake.

A second approach, the *description of occasions* method, is based on consumption by the respondent on a number of days of the week prior to interview.[6-9] The main difficulty of this approach relates to variability of individual consumption. If week to week variation in the amount of alcohol consumed is relatively large, then the ordering of individuals by reported consumption using this method will not reflect their ordering over a longer time period.

Under reporting on questionnaire completions of alcohol consumption has been studied. Respondents tend to under-estimate frequency of drinking and to over-estimate the quantity consumed on a typical drinking occasion. Deliberate under-reporting of alcohol consumption may occur because of the stigma associated with

Table 19.10 Quantity frequency questionnaire

In the last month: have you had an alcoholic drink at all?   YES   NO

If **YES**: Please answer A and B

A. About how often have you had any of the following types of drink over the last month

Beer, lager, cider, etc.:	not at all	less than once a week	1–2 times a week	3–4 times a week	5–6 times a week	Every day
wine, sherry, vermouth etc:	not at all	less than once a week	1–2 times a week	3–4 times a week	4–5 times a week	Every day
gin, vodka, rum, brandy, whisky, etc.:	not at all	less than once a week	1–2 times a week	3–4 times a week	5–6 times a week	Every day

B. When you've had a drink over the last month how much of the following types of drink have you usually had a day (i.e. 24 hour period)

Pints of beer, lager, cider etc.:	none	½–1	1–2	3	4–5	6–7	8 or more
Glasses of wine, sherry, vermouth etc.:	none	1–2	3–4	5–6	7–9	11–14	15 or more
Measures of spirits (gin, vodka, rum, brandy, whisky etc):	none	1–2	3–4	5–6	7–9	11–14	15 or more

excessive alcohol use and its behavioural effects. There is some evidence that increased levels of reporting may be found when interviewer contact is reduced or eliminated. Computerized interviewing techniques have been shown to result in increased self-reported consumption levels when compared to personal interviews.[1]

RECOGNIZING HARMFUL ALCOHOL CONSUMPTION

Alcohol use disorders identification test

The *World Health Organization* (WHO) has developed a simple instrument, the *AUDIT questionnaire*, to screen for persons with early signs of alcohol related problems (Table 19.11).[10] The WHO core screening instrument consists of ten simple questions. Seven have been chosen as representative of the following areas:

- Alcohol dependence and black-outs (four questions)
- Negative alcohol reactions (one question)
- Alcohol problems (two questions).

Three additional questions on alcohol consumption have also been included. Each question is scored by checking the response category that comes closest to the patient's answer. A score of eight or more produces the highest sensitivity and is used as the cut off point. In general, high scores on the first three questions in the absence of elevated scores on the remaining questions suggests hazardous alcohol use. Elevated scores on questions four through six imply the presence or emergence of alcohol dependence. High scores on the remaining questions suggest harmful alcohol use.

The validity of the instrument has been calculated using hazardous alcohol consumption as the criterion for a positive case. This was defined as a mean daily alcohol intake of 40 g or more for men or 20 g or more for women. The sensitivity is 80 per cent and is higher in men than in women. The specificity is 89 per cent and is higher in women than men. The positive predictive value is 60 per cent and the predictive value of a negative result 95 per cent.

Other measures of psychosocial consequences of drinking

These include the 25 item *Michigan Alcoholism Screening Test* (MAST),[11] its shortened ten item version,[12] and the four item *CAGE questionnaire* (Table 19.12).[13] The CAGE is a more sensitive instrument than the *MAST questionnaires* for identifying the individual with drinking problems in general hospital and general practice populations. Two or more positive replies to the *CAGE questionnaire* are said to identify the problem drinker. Although it is reported in general hospital settings to have a high sensitivity (85 per cent) and specificity (89 per cent),[13] the *CAGE instrument* provides less information for intervention than the longer *AUDIT instrument*.

Table 19.11 The audit questionnaire

Circle the number that comes closest to the patient's answer.

1. How often do you have a drink containing alcohol?
   (0) Never   (1) Monthly or less   (2) Two to four times a month   (3) Two to three times a week   (4) Four or more times a week

2. * How many drinks containing alcohol do you have on a typical day when you are drinking
   (0) 1 or 2   (1) 3 or 4   (2) 5 or 6   (3) 7 or 8   (4) 10 or more

3. How often do you have six or more drinks on one occasion?
   (0) Never   (1) Less than monthly   (2) Monthly   (3) Weekly   (4) Daily or almost daily

4. How often during the last year have you found that you were not able to stop drinking once you had started?
   (0) Never   (1) Less than monthly   (2) Monthly   (3) Weekly   (4) Daily or almost daily

5. How often during the last year have you failed to do what was normally expected from you because of drinking?
   (0) Never   (1) Less than monthly   (2) Monthly   (3) Weekly   (4) Daily or almost daily

6. How often during the last year have you needed a first drink in the morning to get yourself going after a heavy drinking session?
   (0) Never   (1) Less than monthly   (2) Monthly   (3) Weekly   (4) Daily or almost daily

7. How often during the last year have you had a feeling of guilt or remorse after drinking?
   (0) Never   (1) Less than monthly   (2) Monthly   (3) Weekly   (4) Daily or almost daily

8. How often during the last year have you been unable to remember what happened the night before because you had been drinking?
   (0) Never   (1) Less than monthly   (2) Monthly   (3) Weekly   (4) Daily or almost daily

9. Have you or someone else been injured as a result of your drinking?
   (0) No   (1) Yes, but not in the last year   (4) Yes, during the last year

10. Has a relative or a friend or a doctor or other health worker, been concerned about your drinking or suggested you cut down?
   (0) No   (1) Yes, but not in the last year   (4) Yes, during the last year

* In determining the response categories it has been assumed that one drink or one unit contains 10 g alcohol. In countries where the alcohol content of a standard drink differs by more than 25 per cent from 10 g, the response category should be modified accordingly.

Table 19.12 The CAGE questionnaire

☐ Have you ever felt you should **C**ut down on your drinking?
☐ Have people **A**nnoyed you by criticizing your drinking?
☐ Have you ever felt bad or **G**uilty about your drinking?
☐ Have you ever had a drink first thing in the morning to steady your nerves or to get rid of a hang-over (**E**ye-opener)?
Any single positive answer is probably significant and two positive answers almost certainly indicate alcohol dependence

---

Biological markers

The most commonly used biological markers of excessive alcohol consumption are mean cell volume (MCV) and gamma glutamyl transferase (gamma-GT).[14] Of these, gamma-GT is a better predictor than MCV. Although the MCV is related to alcohol consumption, a raised MCV is very unreliable as a screening instrument. The proportion of heavy drinkers who have an MCV over 98 ranges somewhere between 20 per cent and 30 per cent and the false-positive rate is between 4 per cent and 6 per cent.

There is a positive relationship between alcohol consumption and gamma-GT levels. Increased gamma-GT activity in the serum can be observed after a few weeks of alcohol intake. Following reduction in drinking, serum gamma-GT levels rapidly fall, returning to normal levels within two to four weeks. The rise of the enzyme in the serum is primarily due to hepatic enzyme induction. Nevertheless, gamma-GT is not very good as a screening instrument. The proportion of heavy drinkers with a raised level, more than 50 iu/l, is about 50 per cent. The false-positive rate is 10–20 per cent. Other causes of a raised gamma-GT include other diseases of the liver, biliary, tract and pancreas. The most important use of gamma-GT is for monitoring changes in alcohol consumption.

WHY AND WHEN SHOULD WE SCREEN IN CLINICAL SITUATIONS?

The benefits of routine screening include:

1. Educating drinkers about the hazards of heavy drinking;
2. Identifying problems before serious dependence has developed;
3. Motivating patients to change their drinking behaviour; and
4. Exposing persons at risk to brief but effective interventions.

Patients tend to answer most accurately when:

1. The interviewer is friendly and non-threatening;
2. The purpose of the questions is clearly related to a diagnosis of their health status;

3. The patient is alcohol and drug free at the time of screening;
4. The information is considered confidential; and
5. The questions are easy to understand.

REFERENCES

1. Anderson P. Self-administered questionnaires for diagnosis of alcohol abuse. In (ed. RR Watson) Diagnosis of alcohol abuse. Boca Raton, Florida: CRC Press, 1989.
2. Barrison IG, Viola L, Mumford J. Detecting excessive drinkers among admissions to a general hospital. Health Trends 1982; **14**: 80–2.
3. Steissguth AP, Martin DC, Buffington VE. Test-retest reliability assessment of three scales derived from a quantity frequency variability assessment of self-reported alcohol consumption. Ann NY Acad Sci 1978; **273**: 458–62.
4. Wallace PG, Brennan PJ, Haines AP. Drinking patterns in general practice patients. J R Coll Gen Pract 1987; **37**: 354–7.
5. Anderson P. Screening for at risk drinkers in general practice. Paper submitted for publication, 1996.
6. Poikolainen K, Korkkainen P. Nature of questionnaire options affects estimates of alcohol intake. J Stud Alcohol 1985; **46**: 219–22.
7. Uchalik DC. A comparison of questionnaire and self-monitored report of alcohol intake in a non-alcoholic population. Addict. Behaviours 1979; **4**: 409–13.
8. Williams GD, Aitken SS, Malin H. Reliability of self-reported alcohol consumption in a general population survey. J Stud Alcohol 1985; **46**: 223–7.
9. Poikolainen K, Karkkainen P. Diary gives more accurate information about alcohol consumption than questionnaire. Drug Alcohol Dependence 1983; **11**: 209–16.
10. Saunders JB, and Aasland OG. WHO collaborative project on identification and treatment of persons with harmful alcohol consumption. Report on phase 1. Development of a screening instrument. Geneva: World Health Organisation, 1987.
11. Selzer ML. The Michigan alcoholism screening test. The quest for a new diagnostic instrument. Am J Psychiatry 1971; **127**: 1653–8.
12. Pokorny AD, Miller BA, Kaplan HB. The brief MAST: a shortened version of the Michigan Alcoholism Screening Test. Am J Psychiatry 1972; **129**: 342–5.
13. Mayfield D, McLeod G, Hall P. The CAGE questionnaire: validation of a new alcoholism screening instrument. Am J Psychiatry 1974; 131; 1121–5.
14. Chick J, Kreigman N, Plant M. Mean cell volume and gamma-glutamyl transpeptidase as markers of drinking in working men. Lancet 1981; **1**: 1249–51.

19.7 Issues in measurement: Diabetes

Rury Holman

This section reviews briefly:

1. **The association of diabetes and cardiovascular disease**
2. **The diagnostic criteria for diabetes**
3. **Methods of assessing hyperglycaemia**
4. **Screening for hyperglycaemia**

THE ASSOCIATION OF DIABETES AND CARDIOVASCULAR DISEASE

Diabetes mellitus is characterized by hyperglycaemia secondary to absolute or relative insulin deficiency. Around two per cent of UK subjects are diabetic with a prevalence of eight per cent in those above 60 years of age. The majority (70–80 per cent) of patients have non-insulin dependent diabetes mellitus (NIDDM) which often has an insidious onset with undiagnosed hyperglycaemia present for several years. Mortality is two to three times the normal population with a five to ten years reduction in life expectancy. Although NIDDM patients have a similar increased risk of microvascular complications (retinopathy, nephropathy, and neuropathy) as insulin dependent diabetics (IDDM) they have a strikingly increased propensity to develop macrovascular problems (see Chapter 8). Associated cardiovascular risk factors are common (high triglyceride, low HDL cholesterol, hypertension, and obesity) but explain only a small proportion of the increased risk. Diabetes related tissue damage was already evident in half of the 5102 newly diagnosed diabetic subjects recruited into the *UK Prospective Diabetes Study*.[1] As macrovascular disease and risk factors are present at the prediabetic stage of impaired glucose tolerance,[2] early identification of those at risk of diabetes is advisable so that preventative measures can be taken.

DIAGNOSTIC CRITERIA FOR DIABETES

A 1985 WHO Expert Committee agreed diagnostic criteria[3] (Table 19.3) based on epidemiological data which showed that the increased risk of retinopathy related to a fasting plasma glucose level of 7.8 mmol/l, or a level of 11.1 mmol/l two hours after a 75 g oral glucose load. In day to day clinical practice whole blood glucose levels rather than plasma levels are almost invariably used.

Table 19.13   WHO criteria for diabetes: 2 hour 75 g oral glucose tolerance test

Sample	Glucose concentration (mmol/l)	
	Fasting	2 hour
Venous whole blood	⩾6.7	⩾10.0
Venous plasma	⩾7.8	⩾11.1

If classical symptoms are present then only one diagnostic blood glucose level is needed to confirm the diagnosis whereas in the absence of symptoms two separate diagnostic blood glucose levels are required. Concurrent illness or drug therapy (for example steroids, beta blockers, thiazides that promote hyperglycaemia) may make interpretation of test results difficult. Guidelines for the diagnosis and management of NIDDM have been published by a joint working party of the British Diabetic Association, the Royal College of Physicians and the Royal College of General Practitioners,[4] and by an International Diabetes Federation working party.[5]

METHODS OF ASSESSING HYPERGLYCAEMIA

Fasting blood glucose

Day to day fasting blood glucose values are remarkably constant in non-diabetic and most NIDDM subjects.[6] Whole blood glucose values < 5.0 mmol/l should be regarded as a negative screening test, with values > 6.6 mmol/l indicative of diabetes. Subjects with blood glucose values in the intermediate range 5.0–6.6 mmol/l should be re-screened in six to twelve months time. Glucose levels should be assayed wherever possible in a laboratory with appropriate quality control procedures and which participates in a quality assurance scheme. Specimen collection should conform to the requirements of the laboratory with respect to sample size, preservatives, storage, and transport.

Oral glucose tolerance test

The oral glucose tolerance test (OGTT) is the 'gold standard' for the diagnosis of diabetes although it is poorly reproducible with a coefficient of variation of 25–30 per cent. In routine clinical practice the OGTT is only required where the diagnosis is uncertain with intermediate fasting blood glucose values *i.e.* 5.0–6.6 mmol/l. It should be performed in the morning following an overnight fast and after two to three days on a high (300 g) carbohydrate diet. Venous blood for laboratory glucose assay should be taken at baseline and two hours after a 75 g oral anhydrous glucose load. Additional interim half hourly samples may also be taken.

Random blood glucose

Random blood glucose measurements, which are subject to the vagaries of meal timing, size, and content, have proved to be a poor screening tool with a low specificity.

Glycated proteins

Glycated haemoglobin, and glycated albumin as measured by the fructosamine assay, provide an attractive approach for screening for diabetes. No specific sample time is required nor is there a need to use a glucose load. Studies on glycated haemoglobin show good sensitivity of the order of 90 per cent but somewhat lower specificity. The substantial differences in assay techniques used and the consequent differences in threshold for a positive test mean that simple ranges for screening cannot be published. Values that lie above the normal range for the laboratory concerned should be regarded as positive screening tests.

Capillary glucose

Capillary glucose assay using commercially available reagent strips, with or without a reflectance meter, is less accurate than formal laboratory assay and not acceptable for screening unless the appropriate guidelines are strictly adhered to.[7]

Glycosuria

Urine specimens should be collected into clean containers to avoid possible contamination that may interfere with the assay. Urinalysis with a glucose oxidase dip stick to detect glycosuria in an overnight fasting urine sample is fairly specific for diabetes (> 95 per cent) but has poor sensitivity (< 20 per cent) and may miss lesser degrees of carbohydrate intolerance. Sensitivity is increased following ingestion of a glucose load rising to 70 per cent at two hours after a large meal. This technique is limited by variations in the renal threshold for glycosuria (circa 10 mmol/l), as may occur during pregnancy, a tendency for the threshold to rise with age and the accuracy of the dip stick used.

SCREENING FOR HYPERGLYCAEMIA

The role of screening for unrecognized diabetes remains to be established. A recent British Diabetic Association report[8] suggests screening be restricted to adults aged 40 to 75 years particularly if there are additional risk factors such as obesity, a family history of diabetes, or an Asian/African racial origin. Subjects should be rescreened only every five years or three years if they have an equivocal test result or an additional risk factor.

SUMMARY

- Diabetes is a major risk factor for cardiovascular disease.
- Many asymptomatic cases go unrecognized for several years.
- An OGTT is not usually required since the diagnosis can be confirmed if two fasting blood glucose values are > 6.7 mmol/l.
- Random blood glucose and urine glucose measurements are of little value.
- Glycated haemoglobin is a useful screening tool.

REFERENCES

1. United Kingdom Prospective Diabetes Study (1991) VIII: Study design, progress and performance. Diabetologia 1991; **34**: 877–90.
2. Haffner SM, Stern MP, Hazuda HP, Mitchell BD, Patterson JK. Cardiovascular risk factors in confirmed prediabetic individuals. JAMA 1990; **263**: 2893–8.
3. WHO Expert Committee on Diabetes Mellitus. WHO Technical Report Series 727. Geneva: WHO, 1985.
4. Watkins PJ. Guidelines for good practice in the diagnosis and treatment of non-insulin dependent diabetes mellitus. Journal of the Royal College of Physicians of London 1993; **27**: 259–66.
5. Alberti KGMM, Gries FA, Jervell J, Krans HMJ. A desktop guide for the management of non-insulin-dependent diabetes mellitus (NIDDM): An update. Diabetic Medicine 1994; **11**: 899–909.
6. Holman RR, Turner RC. Maintenance of basal plasma glucose and insulin concentrations in maturity onset diabetes. Diabetes 1979; **28**: 227–30.
7. Price CP, Burrin JM, Natrass M. Extra laboratory blood glucose measurement: a policy statement. diabetic medicine 1988; **5**: 705.
8. Paterson KR. Population screening for diabetes mellitus. Diabetic Medicine1993; **10**: 777–81.

20 Screening policy

David Mant

Screening can never play a major role in the prevention of heart disease in the UK. By definition, screening is selective and is therefore an inappropriate general strategy to deal with a problem which afflicts the majority of the population. If it reassures people who are identified as at average relative risk, it may even prejudice a strategy to reduce the high overall risk of the entire UK population. In these circumstances, it is very important that the scientific case for screening is well founded. It is very easy for screening to do more harm than good.

The purpose of this chapter is to review the scientific evidence for including screening as an important strategic element in a general practice programme to prevent coronary heart disease (CHD) and stroke, and it will seek to answer the following questions:

1. **What are the limitations of a screening strategy?**
2. **What are the minimum criteria for screening?**
3. **For which risk factors, if any, should we screen?**
4. **For which indicators of established disease, if any, should we screen?**
5. **How does screening relate to 'multiple risk' assessment?**

In addition, where it is appropriate, for each specific indicator of cardiovascular risk or established disease, the evidence for effective intervention, the best method of identification, and the issue of who should be screened (and at what interval) will be reviewed.

WHAT ARE THE LIMITATIONS OF A SCREENING STRATEGY?

The limitations of any screening strategy in reducing the overall burden of cardiovascular disease were summarised by Rose in 1993:[1]

- treating only those at highest risk makes little impact on overall morbidity or mortality;
- the total number of people at high risk is determined by the overall distribution of risk in the population;
- achieving change in those at highest risk is largely dependent on changing attitudes in the whole population.

The first assertion—that treating only those at highest risk makes little impact on overall morbidity or mortality—is illustrated by Fig. 20.1. This shows the proportion of total deaths in the UK attributable to an individual's total blood cholesterol level. Although the absolute risk of coronary death increases with blood cholesterol (the dotted line), the distribution of cholesterol levels in the population (columns) mean that few of the deaths attributable to cholesterol (percentages above each column) occur in those at highest risk. Most deaths attributable to raised cholesterol occur in people with only moderately raised levels, simply because so many people fall into this category. A screening strategy to identify high cholesterol levels cannot make a major impact on the overall heart disease problem in the population.

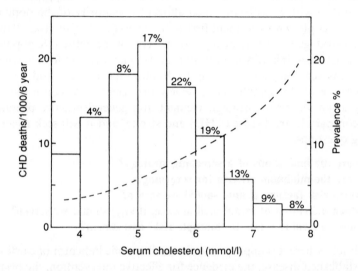

Fig. 20.1   Percentage of total CHD deaths attributable to the effect of total serum cholesterol at different levels. Data from the MRFIT study, men aged 40–59 years. Columns and right hand axis show prevalence distribution of serum total cholesterol at different levels. Broken curve and left hand axis show age adjusted CHD mortality. Percentages show proportion of deaths attributable to each level of serum total cholesterol. (Adapted from Rose G. The strategy of preventive medicine. Oxford: Oxford University Press, 1992, p. 23.)

The other two assertions are illustrated by Fig. 20.2, which shows the population distribution of the body mass index (BMI) of five groups of men and women aged 20–59 years. These groups were formed by ranking 52 population samples (from 32 different countries) and then aggregating them into five equal sized clusters. The striking feature is that the size of the 'high risk' tail of each population reflects the population mean. The coefficients of variation (the ratios of standard deviation to mean) are more or less constant. As Rose aptly observed, 'the tail of troublemakers belongs to its parent distribution'.[1] A similar effect is seen for blood pressure, for which there is a high correlation (0.85) between the proportion of the population with high blood pressure (defined as systolic blood pressure 140) and the population mean pressure.

The implication of these data is that reducing the average population risk is likely to be a very effective way of reducing the number of people at high risk—in terms of blood pressure, a fall of 4 mm Hg in mean pressure is associated with a fall of about 25 per cent in the number of people with high blood pressure (as defined above). On the other hand, an intervention targeted only at those at high risk will be constrained by cultural norms. An individual's food choice reflects popular culture, commercial advertising, retail supply, agriculture subsidy, and governmental policy on taxation. The tail and mean of the population distribution move as a whole because they are both part of a single social entity. The issue of the individual and population approaches is further considered in Chapter 21.

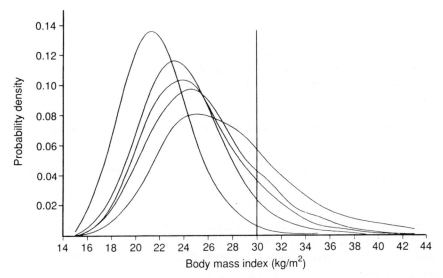

Fig. 20.2 Distribution of body mass index (BMI) in five population groups of men and women aged 20–59 years derived from 52 surveys in 32 countries. Data from INTERSALT study. The 52 population samples were ranked according to median values and then aggregated into five equal size clusters. (Modified from Rose G. The strategy of preventive medicine. Oxford: Oxford University Press, 1992, p. 59.)

WHAT ARE THE MINIMUM CRITERIA FOR SCREENING?

The residual question is whether screening has any role in reducing morbidity and mortality from cardiovascular disease in the UK at the present time. Can a population and screening strategy ever be complementary? The fact that we routinely screen for hypertension as well as trying to reduce dietary sodium intake on a population basis suggests that they can. The conditions under which screening is likely to do more good than harm are set out in Wilson's criteria, drawn up by a Civil Servant 30 years ago and reproduced below.

Wilson's criteria for screening

The disease
  should be an important problem
  there must be a recognized latent or early symptomatic stage
  the natural history must be understood (including development from latent to
    symptomatic stage)

The screen
  a suitable test or examination must be available (of reasonable sensitivity and
    specificity)
  the test must be acceptable to the population being screened
  screening must be a continuous process

Follow-up
  facilities must exist for assessment and treatment
  there must be an accepted form of effective treatment
  there should be an agreed policy on whom to treat

Economy
  the cost must be economically balanced in relation to possible expenditure on
    medical care as a whole

(From Wilson JMG. Screening criteria. In Teeling-Smith G (ed.) Surevillance and early diagnosis in general practice. 1965. OHE, London)

It is possible to reformulate the 10 criteria in a number of ways, but for our purposes it is sufficient to ask four questions. These questions focus on the intervention to be offered to patients identified as 'at risk' rather than on the screening test itself:

- Has the proposed intervention been shown to be effective?
- Is there a satisfactory way of identifying patients who should be offered intervention?
- Can we sustain effective intervention and follow-up with available resources?
- Will screening prejudice a population approach?

There is consensus in general practice that screening for hypertension meets these four criteria. Chapter 2 provides evidence that treating hypertension reduces mortality from both strokes and heart disease, that we can sustain treatment in general practice and that we can identify people at risk easily (if rather imprecisely) by routine sphygmomanometry. It also seems unlikely that screening for high blood pressure prejudices attempts to reduce population mean blood pressure by dietary intervention. We discuss below whether these criteria are equally well met for other indicators of cardiovascular risk. Unless all the criteria can be met, the best screening strategy to adopt is not to screen at all.

FOR WHICH RISK FACTORS SHOULD WE SCREEN?

Smoking

The evidence presented in Chapter 1 shows that smoking cessation advice given in primary care is effective. According to Kottke's overview, the success rate (proportion of patients who have stopped smoking for at least six months) following brief advice is unlikely to exceed five per cent—about three per cent more than would be expected without intervention.[2] General practice trials in the UK indicate that this degree of success can be achieved by brief opportunistic advice by GPs (but probably not by brief advice by practice nurses[3]) and can even be increased by targeting motivated patients, using other strategies such as nicotine replacement, and the involvement of nurses in follow-up support.

Although cessation rates are highest in motivated patients, there is little evidence about how to identify this motivated group. The best predictors of cessation are health professional assessment of likely success and number of cigarettes smoked in the period after initial cessation. Assessments of nicotine dependency do not appear to be very useful in prediction. The use of episodes of illness to define patients motivated to quit (that is targeting patients when they develop an acute respiratory illness) makes clinical sense but has been formally assessed only in relation to myocardial infarction. The recent *UK nicotine patch trial* in general practice achieved a six per cent sustained cessation rate even in the control group, although all subjects in the trial were long term heavy smokers (median consumption 25 cigarettes / day for 25 years). The recruitment of motivated subjects was achieved by writing to all patients in the participating practices offering help to those who wanted to quit.[4] This strategy could augment an opportunistic approach in routine practice, and could be offered on an intermittent basis.

There is a similar lack of evidence to help us set other screening parameters for identifying smokers and offering advice—including the target age range, screening interval, and optimal follow-up regime. Mortality risk is related both to years of smoking and number of cigarettes smoked, and absolute risk increases with age. Advice is more effective in males and in older age groups. Relapse rates are highest immediately after cessation, and continued support reduces relapse, but the optimal follow-up pattern and the trade-off between time spent giving initial advice and follow-up support have not been clearly defined.

Conclusion

Opportunistic identification of smokers by GPs and provision of brief cessation advice to those who express motivation to stop remains the first line strategy. Augmentation of this opportunistic strategy by a systematic strategy, based on contacting smokers in the practice population and offering help with cessation to those who request it, can achieve higher success rates, but the optimal interval and target age group is ill defined.

Blood pressure

Chapter 2 provides convincing evidence that both pharmacological and non-pharmacological treatment of high blood pressure effectively reduces risk of stroke and heart disease in both men and women at all ages.

Identification of hypertension is based on estimation of the patient's mean diastolic and systolic blood pressure using a sphygmomanometer. Blood pressure shows considerable variation, both between readings taken on one visit and, to an even greater extent, between visits. It is therefore good clinical practice to base this 'average' on the mean of a number of readings (see Chapter 19.2). As a measure of risk, even such an average is very imprecise and the number of treatment years necessary to prevent one event is therefore substantial (for example over 400 treatment-years were necessary to prevent one stroke in the trials of mild and moderate hypertension included in a recent meta-analysis[5]). The proponents of ambulatory measurement of blood pressure believe it will allow a more precise definition of risk to be made. It is likely to provide a better estimate of average blood pressure by taking multiple measurements over a prolonged period, but the extent to which it improves precision over surgery measurement on three occasions is not well documented. The potential improvement in predictive value from the additional information which ambulatory monitoring can provide on variability of blood pressure and on night time pressures, as well as mean daytime pressure, is also promising but remains a research issue.

The current practice of not screening (except in pregnancy) before middle age is based on the observed incidence of stroke in the UK population—annual mortality from cerebro-vascular disease is less than 10/million below age 45 years.[6] The choice of a five yearly interval reflects the rate of change in blood pressure with age documented in both cross sectional and longitudinal data.[7] Again, it would be more precise to define the appropriate screening interval for an individual on the basis of current blood pressure level and personal history, but as we have yet to move beyond the 'rule of halves' in blood pressure management in UK primary care, the simplicity of the present approach has much to recommend it. The main problem with present screening arrangements is the loss to follow-up at virtually every stage from remeasurement to treatment. A strong case can be made for a national call—recall system for hypertension screening in the UK, with the same strict quality control that is exercised for cancer screening.

Conclusion

Screening by routine sphygmomanometry at five year intervals, with no upper age limit, is still the optimal general practice strategy. Quality control criteria for screening and follow-up need to be applied much more rigorously.

Cholesterol

Chapter 3 reports evidence from clinical trials that lowering total and LDL cholesterol is effective in the prevention of CHD. Dietary advice given by trained nurses in general practice is effective in helping people to achieve a small reduction in their total blood cholesterol—in the *Oxcheck trial* a difference of about 2 per cent (3.5 per cent in women and 1.5 per cent in men) was achieved between mean levels of total cholesterol in the intervention and control groups, sustained over three years.[8] Drug treatment with statins is also an effective and feasible general practice intervention for the secondary prevention of heart disease, but high costs, limited knowledge of long term risks, and ethical considerations make the use of statins in primary prevention extremely contentious (Chapter 3, pages 42 and 46).

There is insufficient evidence to decide whether measurement of cholesterol is necessary to motivate patients to comply with dietary advice given in general practice. A strong case can be made for giving advice to reduce dietary fat without prior screening for three reasons:

(1) dietary advice is the same irrespective of individual cholesterol level;

(2) patients often request remeasurement of cholesterol after they have tried to modify their diet, and the routine measurement error for total cholesterol is greater than the mean change achieved;

(3) the opportunity cost of population screening in general practice is high.

The pressure to screen the total population for hypercholesterolaemia arises in part from the wish to identify patients at very high risk of premature coronary death from inherited metabolic defects of lipid metabolism. However, Chapter 3 concludes that levels of cholesterol that characterise polygenic hypercholesterolaemia (up to 8 mmol/l) are relatively poor predictors of individual risk. One proposed solution is to restrict screening to those with existing disease (angina, diabetes, hypertension, or previous MI). The problem with this approach is that it will not identify patients with specific metabolic defects of lipid metabolism, who have a very high absolute risk of mortality, much of which is expressed at an early age. It is important to identify and initiate treatment of these patients before irreversible arterial damage is done. It has been shown that asking all patients whether they have a family history of early CHD is a poor method of screening to detect hyperlipidaemia.[9] Therefore there are two alternatives—to screen the entire population for familial hyperlipidaemia by measuring blood cholesterol in early adult life, or to concentrate on screening the relatives of patients with hyperlipidaemia or early onset heart disease. The latter approach would require an educational programme for both doctors and patients.

Familial hyperlipidaemia is characterised by physical stigmata (such as tendon xanthoma) which in theory could be used as screening criteria. However, the ability of primary care staff to recognise these lesions has not been assessed and it is unclear how well such selective screening would operate in practice. At present, identification of stigmata of abnormal lipid metabolism should be considered a method of case finding rather than screening.

The most important factor in resolving the cholesterol screening debate is to be clear about the objective—motivation of dietary change, identification of inherited metabolic defects, or assessment of the need for drug treatment. Each objective can be legitimately defended, but the screening strategy necessary to achieve each objective is different and needs to be made explicit.

Conclusion

The first priority in general practice is to screen, and if appropriate treat, two groups of patients:
   (1) patients with recognised CHD (angina or previous myocardial infarct);
   (2) relatives of index cases of familial hyperlipidaemia or early onset CHD.

Other risk factors

A number of other primary cardio-vascular risk factors have been measured in general practice 'health checks' including body mass index, dietary intake, and physical activity. The evidence for effective intervention in general practice to reduce body mass index is extremely limited,[8,10] although there is some evidence for the effectiveness of more intensive interventions (including surgery, drugs and support groups) in obese patients. There is evidence that dietary intake can be modified to a small (but perhaps important) extent by appropriate verbal and written advice in general practice[8], but there is debate about whether this necessitates 'screening' in order to personalise the advice given. The relative effectiveness of an advice leaflet in comparison to personalized advice suggests that the marginal benefit of taking a dietary history may be small.[10] Chapter 5 provides reasonable evidence that cardio-respiratory fitness protects against cardiac death, particularly in those with existing coronary heart disease, but it provides no evidence that intervention in general practice to improve fitness is effective.

   None of these indicators of risk are used routinely for multiple risk assessment (see Chapter 15) because they are not useful independent predictors of cardio-vascular risk. Obesity is an important risk factor for NIDDM and may be important if screening for diabetes is initiated (see next section). As with cholesterol, measurement of physical fitness may be an important motivational factor to exercise, but there is no formal evidence to confirm this.

Conclusion

Evidence for the effectiveness of general practice intervention is insufficient to justify screening for body mass index or physical fitness. Formal dietary assessment in all patients is unnecessary.

FOR WHICH INDICATORS OF ESTABLISHED DISEASE SHOULD WE SCREEN?

Diabetes mellitus

The issue of screening for diabetes is raised in Chapter 19.7. There are two feasible ways of screening for NIDDM in general practice—measurement of blood glucose or glycosylated haemoglobin,[11] or urine testing 2 hours after a meal[12]—and each has its proponents. Test characteristics are probably acceptable for screening, but both blood and urine testing will identify a substantial number of patients with impaired glucose tolerance and there is considerable debate about how such patients should be managed. Screening yield can be increased by targeting older patients and by selective screening of patients with obesity and a family history of NIDDM, but data is not yet available to allow an informed choice about the most appropriate screening interval. The full results of the *UK Prospective Diabetes Study* should make clear whether early treatment influences cardiovascular outcome, and general practitioners can postpone the decision to screen until these are available.

Conclusion

The issue of screening for asymptomatic diabetes (perhaps in conjunction with screening for hypertension in patients age 70 +) should be considered when the full results of the *UK Prospective Diabetes Study* are known.

Myocardial infarction

Chapter 14 provides convincing evidence that rehabilitation programmes following myocardial infarction are effective in reducing subsequent mortality. It is difficult to isolate the effectiveness of individual components of these programmes; lipid lowering, betablockade, aspirin, anti-coagulants, smoking cessation, and exercise advice all appear to be individually effective but the synergistic effect which can be achieved is unclear. It must be stressed that success has not yet been shown in the context of UK primary care, where trained staff and resources to provide the necessary intervention are limited, although hospital rehabilitation programmes already operate in many UK centres.

Although the existence of silent myocardial infarction is well documented, the primary task for general practice is identifying patients with confirmed symptomatic infarct and auditing the quality of their follow-up care. Incident cases can be identified at hospital discharge; patients with previous infarcts can be identified from morbidity registers, repeat prescribing registers, and from hospital discharge records. This is case-finding rather than screening in its strictest sense, but it is certainly good clinical management.

Conclusion

The medical records of all patients with myocardial infarction should be identified and the quality of follow-up care audited on a regular basis.

Myocardial ischaemia

Some of the trials reported in Chapter 14 recruited patients not with established infarcts but with other evidence of arterial disease—symptomatic angina or asymptomatic arterial narrowing. If effective intervention is available, the question arises as to whether we should be screening to identify patients who would benefit. At the present time there is no logistically feasible way of mass screening for arterial narrowing, but patient-completed questionnaires to identify patients with undiagnosed angina and myocardial ischaemia have been developed. In the second *Whitehall study* the test characteristics of a patient-completed questionnaire were assessed for prediction of CHD death; the sensitivity, specificity and likelihood ratio of a questionnaire diagnosis of angina were 9.8 per cent, 96.5 per cent and 2.8 respectively.[13] The low sensitivity reflects the limitations of any risk marker for predicting mortality, and the likelihood ratio is probably too low to make screening for undiagnosed angina by questionnaire an attractive option in a community setting.

Conclusion

Screening for asymptomatic ischaemia is not recommended; as with myocardial infarction, identification of the medical records of all patients with diagnosed angina and audit of the quality of their follow-up care are recommended.

Cardiac failure

Chapter 14 again reports evidence that treatment with ACE inhibitors reduces mortality in patients with established heart failure, including impaired ventricular function after myocardial infarction. Careful symptomatic and clinical examination of patients following myocardial infarction, with a view to treatment if appropriate, is therefore good clinical practice. However, the accuracy of clinical diagnosis of heart failure in the community has been questioned[14] and screening of the elderly population by echocardiography has been suggested.[15] In addition, the *SOLVD study* suggests that echocardiographic identification and early treatment of asymptomatic left ventricular dysfunction with ACE inhibitors in elderly patients reduces both subsequent morbidity and mortality from heart failure.[16]

Although at least two practices in the UK have equipped themselves with colour Doppler echocardiographs to undertake such screening, and open access echocardiography is becoming more common, the characteristics of echocardiography as a screening instrument in relation to the clinical or biochemical (C-ANP) diagnosis of left ventricular dysfunction have not been adequately assessed.[17] In addition, the logistic feasibility of screening remains uncertain and the most appropriate target group and screening interval have not been defined. Four community based research studies are underway in the UK at present and the situation should be re-assessed when these report.

Conclusion

Screening the elderly for left ventricular dysfunction by echocardiography may be appropriate in the near future, but there is insufficient evidence to justify its use now outside a research context. Clinical assessment of post-infarct patients for evidence of cardiac failure remains important to identify those who may benefit from an ACE inhibitor.

Atrial fibrillation (see Chapter 13)

In the UK, it is estimated that about one in six strokes occur in people with atrial fibrillation.[18] The risk from atrial fibrillation appears to depend on age and on the co-existence of underlying heart disease, including heart failure. Uncomplicated atrial fibrillation in those aged under 60 years does not appear significantly to increase the risk of stroke or heart disease.[19] However, in the *Framingham study*, heart failure and valvular disease were strong predictors of atrial fibrillation, which was associated with a more than fourfold increased risk of stroke and two-fold increased risk of cardiovascular death.[20]

A formal meta-analysis of trials has now established beyond reasonable doubt that both aspirin and warfarin can reduce the risk of stroke in patients with atrial fibrillation, and that warfarin treatment reduces total mortality.[21] The number of patient-years of treatment with warfarin needed to prevent one stroke in patients aged over 65 years is 29–43—which compares very favourably with 400 plus patient-years of treatment for mild or moderate hypertension. Aspirin is not as effective as warfarin, but may be more acceptable to some patients and GPs. The safety of warfarin treatment in general practice depends on whether existing logistic problems with monitoring warfarin levels can be overcome and the quality control achieved in the clinical trials can be maintained.

Identification of atrial fibrillation in the elderly could feasibly be done in two situations in general practice: during five yearly blood pressure checks or in association with echocardiographic screening for heart failure. Echocardiography would readily identify atrial fibrillation and valvular disease as well as ventricular dysfunction. At present these remain research issues. The clinical priority in general practice is high quality clinical follow-up of patients with known atrial fibrillation to initiate appropriate investigation (including measurement of thyroxin) and treatment.

Conclusion

There is good evidence that treatment of atrial fibrillation prevents stroke. Research is currently in progress to assess the feasibility and effectiveness of a general practice screening programme.

HOW DOES SCREENING RELATE TO MULTIPLE RISK ASSESSMENT?

The relative merits of different multiple risk assessment systems, and the way in which they operate, are described in Chapter 15. In 1992, the *Coronary Prevention Group* and the *British Heart Foundation* drew up strategic guidelines for multiple risk screening, using the *Dundee Risk Disk*.[22] These guidelines are summarized in Fig. 20.3. They involve the measurement of blood pressure and the recording of smoking habit, personal history (of CHD, diabetes, hypertension, and hyperlipidaemia) and close family history (of premature heart disease before the age of

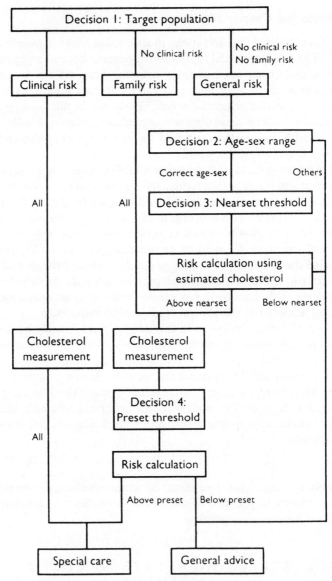

Fig. 20.3 Coronary Prevention Group—British Heart Foundation guidelines: decision flow chart. (From Randall A, Muir J, Mant D. Choosing the preventive workload in general practice: practical application of the CPG guidelines and the Dundee risk-disk. BMJ 1992; **305**: 227–31.)

50 years or familial hyperlipidaemias) in all patients aged 18–74 years. This process divides the population into three groups: those with established disease (clinical risk group), those with a family history but no established disease (family risk group), and the remainder (general risk group). All those with clinical risk are

allocated to 'special care'; allocation of other patients to 'special care' depends on whether their estimated cardiovascular risk is above a specified threshold. This threshold is set by the practice according to the amount of 'special care' it can undertake. According to the threshold set (decisions three and four in the figure), the proportion of patients needing cholesterol measurement varies from 21–80 per cent and the proportion allocated to 'special care' from 15–44 per cent.[23]

Apart from their complexity, the guidelines have also been criticized for their feasibility. Clinical audit suggests that existing clinical care of patients in the clinical risk group (that is patients already identified as suffering from hypertension, hypercholesterolaemia, diabetes, or CHD) is less than optimal. The utility of a screening strategy to identify additional patients for 'special care' is limited until practices can provide high quality care for patients already identified and can cope with their current workload. It is certain that few practices could cope effectively with the workload generated by setting a cholesterol screening threshold below a Dundee score of eight or a 'special care' threshold below a Dundee score of 12. Unfortunately, at these thresholds, 34 per cent of those with systolic blood pressure 180mm of mercury and 41 per cent of heavy smokers (> 20 cigarettes per day) will not be selected for 'special care'.[23] As the benefits of blood pressure control and smoking cessation are not restricted to cardiovascular disease, it is probably necessary to add all heavy smokers and hypertensives to the mandatory special care group. This will reduce still further the practical utility of the guidelines and their is little evidence of their application in practice.

In practice, the starting point for risk assessment in general practice is our existing commitment to screen for hypertension, to identify and advise smokers, and to manage clinically patients with symptomatic diabetes and CHD. As Chapter 15 indicates, this strategy alone will identify the vast majority of patients at high relative risk, without need for complicated multiple risk screening strategies. The first priority in offering screening or any other preventive programme is to ensure that you do not identify risk without the ability to intervene effectively and follow up assiduously. A common feature of cardiovascular disease preventive programmes in general practice has been their tendency to overreach themselves.

Conclusion

Dealing with the multiple risks that smokers and patients with CHD present to us provides a substantial clinical challenge which we have yet to meet in general practice. A multiple risk screening strategy is an unnecessary diversion.

SUMMARY

- It is essential that screening does not prejudice a population strategy to reduce overall population risk.
- Whatever screening strategy is adopted, it should be modest in its ambition. If ambition is not modest, then sustained and effective intervention will not be achieved and risk will be identified at no advantage to the individual.

- A quality controlled call-recall and follow-up procedure, similar that adopted for cancer screening, should be adopted for blood pressure screening and management.
- Smoking habit should be recorded at least once on all patients. Both opportunistic and systematic approaches to smoking cessation should be considered.
- All patients with angina, past myocardial infarct, and diabetes should be identified from medical records (including morbidity registers, repeat prescribing registers, or hospital discharge records) and the quality of their follow-up care reviewed.
- All first degree relatives of patients with familial hypercholesterolaemia or early onset CHD should be screened for hyperlipidaemia as soon as the index case is detected.
- Treatment of atrial fibrillation and asymptomatic left ventricular dysfunction has been shown to reduce morbidity and mortality from stroke and CHD respectively. The feasibility of screening for these conditions in the elderly is currently being assessed. At present, general practitioners should ensure that their management of symptomatic patients with these conditions is optimal.
- Additional screening to assess multiple risk is not necessary.

REFERENCES

1. Rose G. The strategy of preventive medicine.Oxford: Oxford Medical Publications, 1992.
2. Lottke T. Smoking cessation: attributes of successful interventions. JAMA 1988; **259**: 2883–9.
3. Sanders D, Fowler G, Mant D, Fuller A, Jones L, Marzillier J. Randomized controlled trial of anti-smoking advice by nurses in general practice. J R Coll Gen Pract 1989; **39**: 273–6.
4. ICRF Study group. Effectiveness of a nicotine patch in helping people to stop smoking in general practice. BMJ 1993; **306**: 1304–8.
5. Collins R, Peto S, MacMahon S, Herbert P, Fiebach NH, Eberlein KA, *et al*. Blood pressure, stroke and coronary heart disease. Part **2**: short-term reductions in blood pressure: overview of randomized drug trials in their epidemiological context.Lancet 1990; **335**: 827–38.
6. OPCS Mortality statistics 1992 (cause). London: HMSO, 1994.
7. Rose G. Screening for hypertension. Health Trends 1971; **3**: 2–4.
8. ICRF Oxcheck Study Group. Effectiveness of health checks conducted by nurses in primary care: final results of the OXCHECK study. BMJ 1995; **310**: 1099–104.
9. ICRF Oxcheck Study Group. Prevalence of risk factors for heart disease in OXCHECK trial: implications for screening in primary care. BMJ 1991; **302**: 1057–60.
10. Neil HAW, Roe L, Godlee RJP, *et al*. Randomised trial of lipid lowering advice in general practice: the effects on serum lipids, lipoproteins and anti-oxidants. BMJ 1995; **310**: 569–73.
11. Forrest R, Jackson C, Yudkin J. The glycohaemoglobin assay as a screening test for diabetes mellitus. Diabetic Medicine 1987; **4**: 254–9.
12. Davies M, Alban-Davies H, Cook C, Day J. Self testing for diabetes mellitus. BMJ 1991; **303**: 696–8.

13. Bulpitt C, Shipley M, Demirovic J, Ebi-Kryston KL, Markowe HL, Rose G. Predicting death from CHD using a questionnaire. Int J Epidemiol 1990; **19**: 899–903
14. Clarke K, Gray D, Hampton J. Evidence of inadequate investigation and treatment of patients with heart failure. Br Heart J 1994; **71**: 584–7.
15. Wheeldon N, MacDonald T, Flucker C, McKendrick A, McDevitt D, Struthers A. Echocardiography in the community. QJMed 1993: 86; 17–23.
16. SOLVD invesigators. Effect of enalapril on mortality and the development of heart failure in patients with reduced left ventricular ejection fractions N Engl J Med 1992; **327**: 685–91.
17. Barnett DB. Heart failure: diagnosis of symptomless left ventricular dysfunction. Lancet 1993; **341**: 1124–5.
18. Sandercock P, Bamford J, Dennis M, Burn J, Slattery J, Jones L, *et al.* Atrial fibrillation and stroke: prevalence in different types of stroke and influence on prognosis. BMJ 1992; **305**: 1460–5.
19. Kopecky S, Gersh B, McGoon M, Whisnant J, Holmes DR, Ilstrup D, *et al.* The natural history of lone atrial fibrillation; a population based study over 3 decades N Engl J Med 1987; **317**: 669–74.
20. Kannel W, Abbott R, Savage D, McNamara P. Epidemiological features of atrial fibrillation: the Framingham study. N Engl J Med 1982; **306**: 1018–92.
21. Atrial Fibrillation Investigators. Risk factors for stroke and efficacy of anti-thrombotic therapy in atrial fibrillation. Arch Int Med 1994; **154**: 1449–57.
22. Working group of the Coronary Prevention Group and British Heart Foundation. An action plan for preventing CHD in primary care. BMJ 1991; **302**: 1057–60.
23. Randall A, Muir J, Mant D. Choosing the preventive workload in general practice: practical application of the Coronary Prevention Group guidelines and Dundee coronary risk-disk. BMJ 1992; 305 : 227–31.

Part 3
Implementation

21 The population and individual strategies

Godfrey Fowler

INTRODUCTION

Health care is not the sole, nor indeed the main, determinant of a nation's health. A variety of factors—political, social, economic, legislative, and many others—contribute substantially; health measures are only supplementary and those directed at individuals are generally of relatively marginal importance.

Historically in developed countries, and currently in developing ones, improvements in economic and social circumstances which influence conditions of life have a major influence on health. They include nutrition, clean water supplies, safe sewage disposal, and living conditions generally. During the present century, an important adverse effect on health world-wide has been tobacco smoking; although this is subject to some control in developed countries and its prevalence is declining, world-wide the epidemic continues to escalate.

The objective of prevention is reduction of disability and premature death. Cardiovascular disease, and in particular coronary heart disease, is the commonest cause of death in the UK and developed countries and is becoming common in developing countries. The development of this situation during the current century and the varying and changing incidence of the disease imply preventability. The first two sections of this book concern the evidence for causation and preventability. A major challenge remains the application of the research evidence and the implementation of measures of known efficacy. It has been estimated that this could halve premature mortality from the disease.

TWO PREVENTION STRATEGIES

There are, essentially, two strategies for prevention. These are:

- a mass, population approach, aimed at reduction of risk in the whole population
- a high risk approach, involving indentifying individuals at especially high risk, with interventions targeted specifically at them.

It is now widely recognized that these strategies must be complementary. Primary care has a role in relation to both strategies; it has a public health role, reinforcing mass education and other measures; it also has a more familiar role—intervention with individuals at special risk.[1]

The introduction of the 1990 Contract in NHS general practice in the UK meant that GPs and primary care teams were required, in addition to treating sick people, to assume some responsibilty for maintaining and promoting the health of their practice populations. Public health and preventive roles were thus added to their clinical roles.

THE POPULATION STRATEGY

As eloquently expressed by Professor Geoffrey Rose[2] 'Mass diseases require population approaches for their control'. This involves shifting the population distribution of the determinants of disease in a favourable direction. An historical example of population control of common disease was the provision of clean water which contributed to the reduction in water-born diseases and the eradication of cholera in Britain in the nineteenth century. A modern example of a population measure is legislation requiring the wearing of seat belts in motor cars, which has been associated with a reduction of about a third in deaths from road traffic accidents. In relation to cardiovascular disease prevention, the population measures required are societal changes in the norms of behaviour, especially regarding smoking, eating, and physical activity.

The population strategy offers large potential for prevention in the population as a whole. This is because a large number of people, each at relatively small risk, account for a larger number of cases of disease than a small number of people at relatively high risk. This is most clearly shown by Rose's graph of cholesterol level against mortality from heart disease (see Figure 20.1, Chapter 20). The death rate from coronary heart disease rises steadily with cholesterol level; but relatively few people have high risk levels of cholesterol. So, of the coronary deaths attributed to cholesterol, less than 20 per cent occur in patients whose cholesterol level would have been likely to warrant drug treatment. It can be shown that a far greater effect on overall death rates would occur by lowering the blood cholesterol of each person a little than by attempting to achieve a larger reduction in those whose blood levels are at the upper end of the range. The same effect was shown in Chapter 2 (page 22) in relation to blood pressure lowering.

Moreover, a shift in the whole distribution of population risk in a favourable direction results in a surprisingly large reduction in the prevalence of those at the top end of the distribution curve.[2] In other words reducing the mean level of risk factor within a population also has the effect of reducing the number of individuals at high risk from that particular risk factor (Fig. 21.1).[3] This was shown very clearly in the *INTERSALT study* for this and other risk factors (Fig. 21.2). The prevalence of a condition in a community—that is the number of people at high risk—rises linearly with the mean within that community. The strength of the population approach is illustrated by the calculation, for example from Framingham and other data, that a 10 per cent lowering of cholesterol distribution as a whole would correspond to a 20–30 per cent reduction in coronary heart disease mortality.

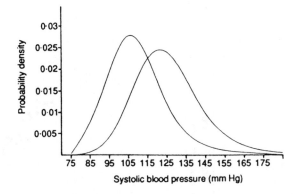

Fig. 21.1 Distribution of systolic blood pressures for averages of the five populations with the lowest mean values and the five with the highest. (From Rose G, Day S. The population mean predicts the number of deviant individuals. BMJ 1990; **301**:1031–4.)

One of the frustrations of preventive medicine is that action by many is required to achieve benefits for a few. This is particularly true when one applies a population strategy. There will be only a small benefit for the great majority of individuals, especially short-term, and only a small minority achieve significant gain. This has been described as the Prevention Paradox: a preventive measure which brings much benefit to the population offers little to each participating individual. An example is provided by seat belt legislation: about 400 drivers must wear seat belts on every journey throughout their adult lives to avoid the death of one of them.[3]

Because of these considerations, the population strategy suffers from the disadvantage that:

• It is hard to develop motivation of individuals when benefits are small and long-term
• It is hard to motivate health professionals, when the improvement for individuals is marginal.

The 'high risk' strategy

Because doctors, other health professionals, and also those outside the health care professions tend more easily to focus on individual people rather than populations, it is usually also easier for them to associate prevention with individuals. It is certainly more consistent with normal medical practice. The high risk strategy for prevention seeks to achieve a truncation of risk distribution in the population by identifying and 'treating' those in the upper tail of the distribution curve of disease determinants (Fig. 21.3). This is intuitively attractive because identification of those who 'have a problem' appears to make sense and intervention with them seems clearly justifiable both to the individuals and their doctors. Moreover, as

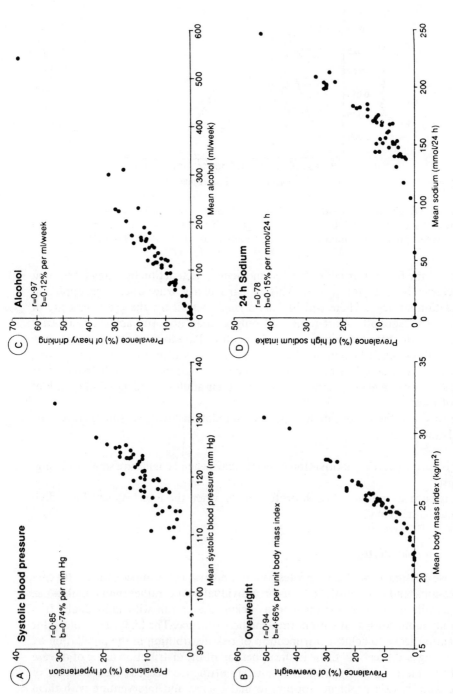

Fig. 21.2 Relationship between population mean and the prevalence of deviant (high) values across 52 population samples from 32 countries, men and women aged 20–59. Systolic blood pressure (A); body mass index (B); alcohol intake (C); urinary 24 h sodium excretion (D). (From Rose G, Day S. The population mean predicts the number of deviant individuals. BMJ 1990; **301**:1031–4.)

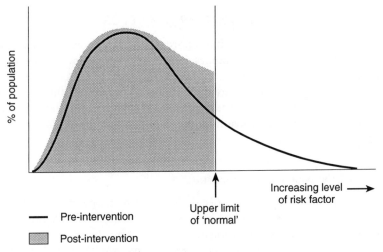

Pre-intervention

Post-intervention

Upper limit
of 'normal'

Increasing level ⟶
of risk factor

Fig. 21.3 The high risk strategy.

demonstrated in Part 1 of this book, there is often research based evidence that, if individuals are identified as being at increased risk, they benefit from having that risk reduced. For example, identification and treatment of those who have an elevated blood pressure level has been clearly demonstrated to reduce the likelihood of them suffering heart disease or stroke. So, in contrast with the population strategy, the high risk approach is likely to:

- encourage motivation in individuals;
- encourage motivation of health professionals.

But, as already pointed out, such indivduals are likely to be relatively few in number, and represent only the top end of the risk distribution curve. If intervention is confined to these 'high risk' patients, then the potential for a major effect on the health of the population is limited.

There are also a number of other problems which can limit the scope for benefit from a high risk approach. These include:

- poor discrimination between those at high risk and others;
- problems of 'labelling';
- unwarranted reassurance of those not identified as at high risk;
- side effects of intervention since, although benefits of intervention are greater in this group than in the general population, more patients are subjected to pharmaceutical interventions than gain benefit.

High risk screening is seductive to patients because most people look to it for reassurance, rather than 'trouble finding'. Screening is also more 'comfortable' for health professionals because it is more closely allied to traditional medical care than population educational initiatives. This is especially so if high risk identification implies the need for medication or some other medical intervention, rather than just life-style advice. High risk strategies are therefore associated with 'medicalization'.

SETTING PRIORITIES

Clearly the population and individual approaches must be complementary—the population approach because changes in the mean risk levels for the whole population have the greatest potential for saving most lives, as well as reducing risk for those at high risk: the individual approach because of the clear evidence that identifying and managing certain patients at high risk significantly increases their chances of a longer and healthier life. But practices have limited resources, and so must set priorities.

Priorities and the population approach

Primary care teams firstly have to decide how much energy they can spend on a population approach. Since policy here largely relates to the exemplar role, to supporting other groups, and to using influence to lobby, the effort does not have to be excessively time consuming or to compete for time with the practices' initiatives using the high risk strategy. Many ideas are set out in Chapter 23.

Priorities and the individual approach

The prevalence of risk factors in the UK middle age population is well illustrated by data from two large general practice-based cardiovascular intervention trials, the *OXCHECK*[4] (Table 21.1) and *Family Heart*[5] studies. Over three quarters of men and two thirds of women have at least one cardiovascular risk factor at a level justifying advice and follow-up and over a third have a combination of risk factors. The workload implications of offering individual interventions to such a large proportion of the population are huge (Chapter 15).

Table 21.1   Prevalence of risk factors for cardiovascular disease in patients aged 35–64 yrs. (From ICRF OXCHECK Study Group, 1991)

Risk factor	Male (%)	Female (%)
Current smoking	35	24
DBP		
$\geqslant 100$	3	2
90–99	11	7
Total cholesterol		
$\geqslant 8.0$	8	8
6.5–7.9	30	29
Body mass index		
$\geqslant 30$	10	16
25–29.9	45	32

Using mortality statistics, hospital admission rates, and health and life-style survey data, it has been shown that a hypothetical practice of 10 000 patients in the North of England could expect approximately the following numbers within the practice population:[6]

> myocardial infarctions, 23/year
> myocardial infarction survivors, 350 at any one time
> patients with angina, 175 at any one time
> patients with diabetes, 165 at any one time
> coronary artery bypass operations, 3/year
> strokes, 20/year
> TIAs, 4/year
> patients with hypertension, 1150 at any one time
> smokers, 2700 at any one time
> obese patients (BMI > 30), 2785 at any time
> patients taking very little exercise, 6900 at any time.

Figure 21.4 illustrates these data as an iceberg, with those having overt disease 'above the water line' and the many more people with raised risks 'below the surface'. The figure demonstrates the need for establishing priorities, working first with those having overt disease, who are relatively few in number and for whom

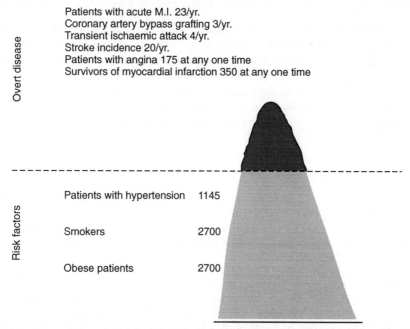

Fig. 21.4 The coronary heart disease and stroke iceberg. Expected numbers in a hypothetical population of 10 000 patients are given. (Modified from Charlton BD *et al.* Health promotion priorities for general practice: constructing and using 'indicative prevalences'. BMJ 1994; **308**:1019–22.)

there is good evidence of benefit for intervention; then with those having risks (such as hypertension or smoking) where the numbers are still manageable and for which there is proven benefit from interventions; both these groups having priority over the large number with raised risk factors for which there is poor evidence of the effect of intervention in practice.

The evidence set out in the first part of this book has made it clear that preventive intervention for certain groups of patients with established disease produces clear benefit. Such patients include:

- patients with established heart disease (angina, myocardial infarction, coronary artery bypass graft, or angioplasty)   Chapter 14
- patients following stroke or transient ischaemic attack   Chapter 13
- patients with diabetes   Chapter 8
- patients with atrial fibrillation   Chapter 13

It has also been shown that intervention can benefit certain patients either at high risk or where there is a clear beneficial intervention for those with a specific risk. Such patients include:

- hypertensive patients   Chapter 2
- smokers   Chapter 1
- those with familial hyperlipidaemia or very high cholesterol   Chapter 3
- post-menopausal women who have had a hysterectomy   Chapter 10

For such patients the evidence suggests that practices should be considering systems to provide individual care. Such systems are outlined in Chapter 23.

It has also been considered whether patients should have special care on the basis of a high multiple risk score. It has been shown that there are few such patients who are not already managed on the basis of one of the criteria listed above; and that the effectiveness of intervening with such patients is unproven (Chapters 15 and 20). Implementation of such a programme will not be considered further.

REFERENCES

1. Fowler G, Gray M, Anderson P. Prevention in general practice. Oxford: Oxford University Press, 1993.
2. Rose G. The strategy for preventive medicine. Oxford: Oxford University Press, 1992.
3. Rose G, Day S. The population mean predicts the number of deviant individuals. BMJ 1990; **301**: 1031–4.
4. ICRF OXCHECK Study Group. Prevalence of risk factors for heart disease in OXCHECK trial: implications for screening in primary care. BMJ 1991; **302**: 1057–60.
5. Family Heart Study Group. British Family Heart study: its design and method, and prevalence of cardiovascular risk factors. Br J Gen Pract 1994; **44**: 62–7.
6. Charlton BD, Calvert N, White M, Rye GP, Wlasislaw C, van Zwanenberg T. Health promotion priorities for general practice: constructing and using 'indicative prevalences'. BMJ 1994; **308**: 1019–22.

22 Preparing the practice

Martin Lawrence

THE QUALITY PRACTICE

Prevention of cardiovascular disease (CVD) is a major task for any general practice. Many of the practice staff are involved—whether receptionists making appointments and giving results, nurses doing health check clinics, or doctors making management decisions. Unless the practice is well prepared and organized, the whole exercise is likely to fail. It is much better to take a little longer to plan well and to prepare everyone involved before embarking on a programme of CVD prevention than for a start to be made piecemeal, or by individuals without adequate consultation.

The theory of improving practice quality and preparing practices to introduce change is largely borrowed from industry. Several American quality experts, notably Edward Deming, developed theories which played a large part in turning Japanese industry from shoddy to high quality output over twenty years.[1] These theories have been adapted for medical care, especially by Donald Berwick, of the Institute for Health Care Improvement in Boston, and are now being adapted and incorporated into Primary Health Care planning.

Development of any organization involves working on two areas—the culture of the organisation and the techniques and skills needed for running the required programme. By the culture is meant the leadership, teamwork, interaction, openness, and morale. If the culture of a practice is not well developed then it will not be possible to use the techniques and the delivery of high quality care is unlikely to occur.

THE QUALITY PRACTICE

CULTURE
Leadership
Team working
Training
Reward

TECHNIQUES
Organisation
Implementing guidelines
Record keeping
Audit

THE CULTURE

Leadership

A healthy practice needs to know its objectives, and have a commitment to attaining them.[2] It is important that everyone in the practice wants to achieve high quality care, but it is the leaders who must take the decisions on priorities, convince other members of the team, and set in place the necessary organization. If the leaders are committed to improving quality then the morale and determination of the whole team will be raised; and if the leaders are accessible and open their decisions and vision become clearer to the rest of the practice. They need to be committed to change and to improvement, beginning with the assumption 'health care is very good today; together we intend to make it better'.[3]

The leaders in practice may be the partners, but preferably include key people from other disciplines in the team—manager, practice nurse, health visitor, receptionist, midwife, and others if appropriate. They listen to all the members of the practice, assess the needs of the practice and its patients, and decide on direction. Above all it is important that no key member of the practice appears to disagree with the agreed direction and plan; Deming, a leading developer of quality improvement in the USA, would never even visit a company if any member of the board was absent; without that endorsement he knew that change was highly unlikely. Of course in general practice it may be that some partners are less enthusiastic than others. This can be managed, as long as they do not *oppose* change, but are willing to endorse those who are undertaking development.

Teamwork

No longer is it true that the care process just involves one doctor and one patient. CVD prevention—with appointments, call/recall, screening, recording, and management—requires 'faithful, clear, mutually respectful collaboration among workers with many different credentials'.[4] Yet hierarchy persists, team members frequently feel inhibited when doctors are in the group, and this inhibits our ability to work together effectively.

Primary health care professionals have increasingly to learn and to be willing 'to work in teams, share responsibility, and relinquish absolute professional autonomy in the interests of attaining a shared purpose'.[4] The practice needs time together to plan its objectives and to ensure that everyone knows and agrees the plan. This may require an occasional 'away day' when the whole team meets in protected time away from the pressures of the job. There needs to be open communication—by meetings or by open availability between team members—to enable team members to continue to share any concerns over planned developments. There needs to be a method of communicating success, failures, and progress—perhaps by a notice board for practice projects.

There is an extensive literature to help practices achieve this, both generic[5] and aimed at primary care.[6] In addition, local tutors and facilitators, often employed by health commissions, can advise and support practices on methods for teamwork development.

Training

Of Deming's 14 key points in quality development, two were to 'institute training and retraining' and to 'institute a vigorous programme of education and retraining'.[7] This emphasises how importantly he regarded the education and training of the whole work force. In introducing new staff members it is important that they are properly trained, and do not just pick up the job from a colleague—with all the in built errors; and once the organization begins to change and introduce new processes, then it is equally important to educate and train everyone appropriately.

The introduction of a CVD prevention programme will require training at several levels. The nurses and doctors will need education on the modern management of CVD, ranging through risk factor measurement, drug therapy, counselling methods, and implementation systems for guidelines. It will be necessary to check diagnostic technique, such as taking blood pressure or measuring blood lipids, and learn to interpret the results. Education may take place 'in-house', with the help of literature such as this book, or may require external educational facilities.

It is certainly important that such management systems are understood by others in the practice, partly so that they all feel 'ownership' and are therefore determined to succeed, but partly because even receptionists need to know what they are asking patients to sign up to. And receptionists need training on their own special skills, for instance call–recall or communication skills.

Rewards

Maslow, in his hierarchy of needs, demonstrated that once we have met basic needs—such as food and shelter—which can be bought for money, then other needs become more important than finance (Fig. 22.1).[8] So in a well motivated practice

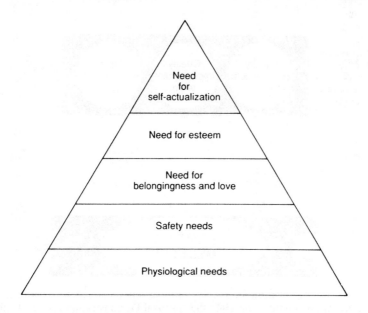

Fig. 22.1 Maslow's hierarchy of needs.

it is not only pay that is important, but good working conditions, and especially companionship, recognition, and acknowledgement. Leaders in a practice must remember that thanks, acknowledgement, and rewards such as social activities and personal recognition, can be as important as financial reward.

TECHNIQUES

Organization

A practice may be committed to working as a team but it needs an organizational structure to enable it to perform. One helpful structure is illustrated in Fig. 22.2. The practice 'quality executive' should include leaders from some or all of the key disciplines in the practice—doctor, manager, practice nurse, etc. It may contain all the partners but must at least be endorsed by all the partners; it will contain many

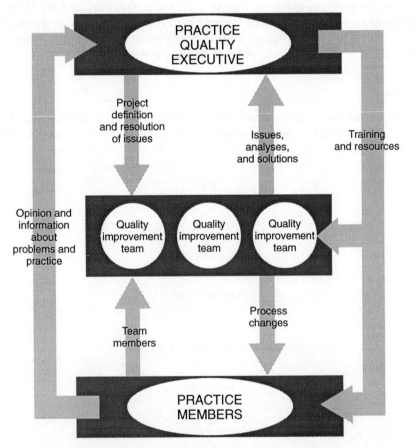

Fig. 22.2   Practice organization for quality improvement. (Adapted, with permission, from *Improving health care quality*, copyright the National Demonstration Project, Institute for Healthcare Improvement, 135, Francis St, Boston, Mass., USA.)

practice leaders. The executive hears the views of all the practice—using meetings or away days—and develops strategy. It then appoints small groups to work on projects, one of which may be CVD. Without a committed group or 'executive' to brief the teams, set the timetable, expect results, and provide support and education, the work of individual teams is likely to slip behind or lack focus.

The project team, or the team appointed to work on the CVD prevention, are the key to success. They need a clear brief (for instance should the project include care from the time the patients leave the hospital? Should it only concern the long-term management of patients with previous heart disease? Is there an age cut off point?). They should also know what resources are available, especially in terms of professionals' time; there is no point in suggesting a special nurse clinic if there is not money to pay for it.

The team need not be large, for CVD prevention it should include a doctor and practice nurse, but could include a receptionist, an audit clerk and a district nurse—depending on who is involved. There needs to be some prior agreement on empowerment: if the team draws conclusions it should be allowed to implement them unless there is an overriding objection.

Implementing guidelines

Guidelines can be considered as aids to decision taking. A widely accepted definition is 'systematically developed statements to assist practitioner and patient decisions about appropriate health care for specific clinical circumstances'.[9] Guidelines are a bridge between research evidence of good practice and day to day clinical behaviour. Not only is research evidence often difficult to find, it is not straightforward to put the findings into practice. Despite studies showing the benefits of life-style change or of drug treatments, patients and doctors are often reluctant to implement them, whether because of lack of understanding, or because of the disadvantages of the proposed changes. People are more likely to change if they are in possession of a succinct and set of guidelines indicating the steps required in a given situation. Satisfactory guidelines should be:[10]

- Valid – *following the guidelines leads to the health gain predicted.*
- Reproducible – *given the same evidence, another group would make the same recommendations.*
- Reliable – *different health professionals interpret them in the same way.*
- Representative – *key affected groups should participate in their development.*
- Clinically applicable – *the patient groups to which they apply should be clear.*
- Clinically flexible – *They should show where variation is acceptable for different circumstances and patients.*
- Clear – *they should be unambiguous, precise, and user friendly.*
- Meticulously documented – *they must document assumptions made and evidence used.*
- Scheduled for review – *A firm date for review should be stated.*

The principles for the development and implementation of clinical guidelines in general practice have been clearly summarised by the Royal College of General Practitioners.[11] This document makes clear the paradox of guideline development and implementation—that the development of rigorous guidelines, in accordance with the list of criteria above, requires time and expertise that is probably not available in practice, but needs to be done on a national scale; and yet the likelihood of a guideline producing change is much greater if it is developed locally. Indeed the likelihood of guidelines achieving change is summarized in the Table 22.1.[12]

Table 22.1 Factors influencing the likelihood of guidelines producing change

Likelihood of change	Development strategy	Dissemination strategy	Implementation strategy
High	Internal	Specific educational intervention	Patient specific reminder at consultation
Average	Local	Continuing medical education	Patient specific or general feedback
Low	National	Publication in journal	General reminder of guidelines

The paradox can be resolved by emphasizing the distinction between guideline development and guideline implementation. External guidelines are never appropriate or precise enough to be used in practice without being adapted and detailed. They need adaptation both in respect of the social and the health needs of the local practice population, although the adapting group must be reluctant to adapt items which have strong evidence to support them, as opposed to those which are based on weaker evidence or consensus. The guidelines will also need adapting to be appropriate for the characteristics and facilities of the practice, as well as having details added to enable their practical use—items such as recruitment method; who will run the clinic and when; what recording method will be used; or who is responsible for evaluation. In this way an *external guideline* can be used for a practice to develop its own policy, and implement its own *practice protocol*.[13] The advantages of external expertise in development can in this way be harnessed to the implementation of local policies and protocols.

This book is, in effect, the basis for guidelines for CVD prevention. The evidence is documented in Parts 1 and 2. The statements in Chapter 23 are supported by that evidence and form a basis on which practices can develop their own policy and implementation protocol.

Record keeping

Recording systems have two main functions: to prompt professionals into making and recording examinations, and to provide data for use in clinical care and audit.

The 'prompt' function is part of implementing guidelines, since one of the proven characteristics of an effective implementation programme is a (local) prompt.[12] For this reason practices need to develop reminder systems, either paper cards in the patients' records, or more usefully a template on an on-desk computer screen—which is used when a consultation is taking place.

Two types of prompt are required—one for general opportunistic screening, and one for the more detailed examination of a patient specifically for CVD prevention. Thus, an opportunistic screening template should include reminders regarding data which we have shown should be recorded on all patients in the target age group—blood pressure, smoking habit, and family history of CVD. For patients who are being particularly targeted for CVD prevention (see Chapter 23), special templates need to be drawn up to include the criteria listed in that chapter: thus for instance there should be a template for patients with existing CVD or for patients with diabetes.

Once recorded, such data can be used for management, especially to ensure that cardiac risks are addressed according to the agreed practice protocol. And a further advantage of keeping such structured records on computers is that they are readily available for audit.

Audit

Any systematic programme of care introduced into a practice (and CVD prevention is one such) needs to be associated with a regular evaluation programme to ensure that high standards of care are being maintained, and to provide accountability both to patients and to authorities.

Audit is usually seen as being carried out as a cycle (Fig. 22.3).[14] The key first step is to define the criteria that are expected of professionals in carrying out care—and from these criteria, target standards of care can be established (Fig. 22.4).[14] Thus, for example a criterion for opportunistic screening could be that all patients aged 30–74 should have their blood pressure measured every five years. We can then set a target that 90 per cent of the practice's patients should satisfy this criterion. Target standards for care can be derived from the criteria of care set out for each category of patient in Chapter 23.

By setting up suitable recording templates, data for audits can easily be provided on a regular and systematic basis. But the key stage in audit is to plan care or implement change if performance is not measuring up to the target set. So, if blood pressure recording is inadequate, the plan might be for partners to try harder during consultations, and if that were not successful then a recall system might be introduced for those whose blood pressure has not been measured for over five years. The less time the practice has to spend doing data analysis (much of which can be done automatically by computer), the more time is available for the stage of discussion and planning change.

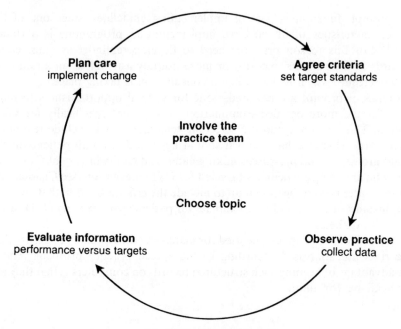

Fig. 22.3   The audit cycle.

Other aspects of audit

We should not forget that there are other important aspects of audit than analysis of computer recording:

- Critical incident analysis. This is a process by which a significant event (anything from a patient defaulting follow-up, to a patient having a stroke when the blood pressure had not been measured) is discussed by all those involved. The aim is to identify failures in the process of care, and to alter those processes to try and ensure that it doesn't happen again. Critical incident analysis is a powerful form of audit: it may highlight an area of deficiency not previously noticed; it makes practitioners concentrate on areas that they might prefer to forget; and it raises morale in the practice by showing that problems are not being forgotten.
- Qualitative audit. Descriptive audits of individual cases, perhaps coming from focus groups, can illustrate vividly areas of good or deficient care. This raises issues of patients' needs, so enabling the practice to target care appropriately. And if extended to the issue of patient satisfaction it can ensure that care remains patient focused and sensitive, and not merely doctor centred.

INFLUENCING THE PRACTICE POPULATION (CHAPTER 16)

It is harder for a practice to develop a population than an individual strategy in reducing cardiovascular disease risk, because it is quite different from the usual approach to risk reduction in general practice.

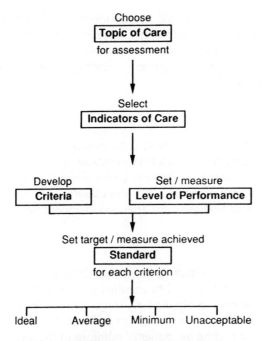

Choose
Topic of Care
for assessment

Select
Indicators of Care

Develop
Criteria

Set / measure
Level of Performance

Set target / measure achieved
Standard
for each criterion

Ideal   Average   Minimum   Unacceptable

Target standards reflect *intended* quality of care.
Achieved standards reflect *delivered* quality of care.

Fig. 22.4 The definition of a standard for an element of care. Target standards reflect intended quality of care; achieved standards reflect delivered quality of care.

There is a danger of the 'population approach' being interpreted as the offering of a 'high risk' approach to every member of the practice population. This would be costly (Chapter 18) and time consuming because many healthy individuals will be accorded a one-to-one consultation which is not justified on the basis of their low risk. 'Population approach' means applying health promoting intervention for the practice population in the hope that everyone will change a little.

There is a limit to the extent that practice teams should expect to become health promotion advocates by outreach into the community when they are frequently already severely stretched in undertaking practice based tasks and satisfying their contracts and terms of service. There are however ways in which practices can both provide health education within their own premises and co-operate with local activities.

Posters and leaflets

Wall space can be used effectively to inform patients with a variety of displays. Controversial or shocking material is not the best way to encourage a positive approach to good health in any area, including cardiovascular disease, and should usually be avoided (Chapter 17, p222). The local Health Promotion Unit can help with advice, posters, and information on the dates of national campaigns.

One person in the practice should be responsible for the appearance of display material, but it is often more interesting if the responsibility is rotated amongst the staff as each individual will bring his or her style to a display. It is important that all the staff from the practice are equipped to answer questions or comments that displays may provoke.

Audio visual aids

If the space and opportunity is available in the practice, video and audio equipment can be used to give information and advice to patients and staff. Practical issues such as security and maintenance will have to be considered. Health Promotion Units usually have a catalogue of video and audio cassettes and are a useful source of advice and help in assessing the most appropriate recordings for patients.

Patient groups

Developing a patient participation group can help to ensure that the service provision is appropriate. Care will be required to ensure that the patients form a truly representative group, and in the early stages it is helpful if at least one partner is enthusiastic and involved. The group can assist in spreading awareness of new clinics and policies; in finding out patients' opinions of the service and suggestions on how it could be improved; or in the development of a newsletter.

Practice health promoting policies

Members of the practice can influence the patients by implementing policies in keeping with a healthy life-style. For example by instituting a non-smoking policy on the premises applicable to both patients and staff; by adopting a healthy eating policy, for instance when they go out for a practice party; and by advocating and even patronising local sports facilities.

Links with community initiatives (Chapter 16)

There are usually health promoting activities taking place in the practice area which are grateful for support from the primary health care team. It is important to consider all the dimensions of health, and remember people learn best when they are enjoying themselves. The following organisations and groups are just a few of the many which may exist in your local community:

Schools	Churches
Sports clubs	Slimming clubs e.g. Weight Watchers
Leisure centres	Stop Smoking groups
Youth clubs/Scouts/Guides	Alcoholics Anonymous
Mothers' groups	Look After Your Heart (LAYH)
Older people's societies	Local work place initiatives

It is important to blend the resources of the practice and the community. Knowing what sort of activities are available within the community can often save time at a consultation. Or it may be necessary to make simple changes, such as the time of a clinic to coincide with a bus timetable, in order to help patients attend and thus become motivated.

It may well be possible to influence behaviour in the local area. The workplace is an area where health promotion can have a major impact, and general practitioners may well be able to influence local firms. There is opportunity for the introduction of non-smoking policies, healthy canteen menus, exercise facilities for use in break periods or out of work time, and to alter working practices to reduce stress. Or it may be possible to influence local restaurants; many areas have introduced healthy eating awards for local restaurants, which may also include credit for the introduction of non-smoking policies.

SUMMARY

- A practice embarking on a cardiovascular risk prevention programme (or any other systematic programme) needs to concentrate on areas of culture and technique.
- Leadership is crucial. In particular, it is important that uninvolved partners endorse the activity and do not obstruct it.
- The practice needs an organization structure to oversee progress towards an objective, while enhancing team work.
- All primary health care team members embarking on a new project require consideration of their training and educational needs.
- The practice will benefit by taking external guidelines and then implementing them as a practice protocol according to practice circumstances.
- On-desk computers can provide both reminder systems and data for audit.
- A practice can influence the community both by provision of health promotion displays, and by its exemplar role in adopting healthy life-style behaviours.
- It can be as effective for members of the practice to co-operate with local health promoting initiatives as to start their own new projects.

REFERENCES

1. Deming WE. Out of the crisis. Cambridge Mass: Massachusetts Institute of Technology, 1986.
2. Stewart R. The reality of organisations. London: MacMillan Pan, 1972.
3. Berwick DM. Continuous improvement as an ideal in health care. N Engl J Med 1989; **320**: 53–6.
4. Berwick DM, Enthoven A, Bunker JP. Quality management in the NHS: the doctors' role. BMJ 1992; **304**: 304–8.
5. Sholtes P R. The team handbook. Madison Wisconsin: Joiner Associates. 1988.
6. Pritchard P, and Pritchard J.Teamwork for primary and shared care. Oxford: Oxford University Press, 1994.

7. Walton M. The Deming management method. London: Mercury, 1989.
8. Maslow A. Motivation and personality. London: Harper, 1954.
9. Field MJ, Lohr KN (ed.) Institute of Medicine Guidelines for clinical practice: from development to use. Washington DC: National Academic Press, 1992.
10. Grimshaw J and Russell I. Achieving health gain through clinical guidelines: I. Developing scientifically valid guidelines. Quality in Health Care 1993; **2**: 243–8.
11. Royal College of General Practitioners. The development and implementation of clinical guidelines: Report from general practice 26. London: RCGP, 1995.
12. Grimshaw J, Russell I. Achieving health gains through clinical guidelines: II. Ensuring that guidelines change clinical practice. Quality in Health Care 1994; **3**: 45–52.
13. Clinical Outcomes Group. Clinical audit in primary health care. London: Department of Health, 1994.
14. Lawrence MS, Schofield TPC. Medical audit in primary health care. Oxford: Oxford University Press, 1993.

23 Principles of patient management

Martin Lawrence, Andrew Neil, David Mant, and
Godfrey Fowler

In developing guidelines for clinical management, any recommendation should be based, so far as possible, on evidence. The first two parts of this book provide the evidence for and against intervention in the prevention of cardiovascular disease. This chapter lists recommendations for activity in practice, referencing back to Parts I & II of the book where appropriate. External recommendations or guidelines are not appropriate for direct incorporation into practice (see Chapter 22, page 313–4), but need to be adapted by practices according to their particular clinical circumstances. The statements in this chapter, and the evidence in the book which supports them, are intended to help practices formulate their own policies and protocols for the prevention of cardiovascular disease.

In drawing up a practice policy for prevention and clinical management of cardiovascular disease, each activity must be important in terms of:

1. Its potential to reduce substantially the number of premature deaths from cardiovascular disease;
2. Its proven effectiveness in a general practice setting;
3. Its feasibility within the resources available to most general practices.

Where the supporting evidence suggests the recommended activity meets all three criteria it is marked with a solid bullet point, ● or ◆. Where the supporting evidence suggests the recommended activity meets one, but not necessarily all of these three criteria, it is marked with an open bullet point, ○ or ◇. In addition, the nature of the supporting evidence is indicated with a letter, A, B, or C:

A—based on well designed randomized control trials, meta-analyses, or systematic reviews;
B—based on well designed cohort or case-control studies;
C—based on other evidence or consensus.

ASSIGNING PRIORITIES

In Chapter 21, p308, it was argued that there are two categories of patients warranting intervention in order to prevent cardiovascular disease. Firstly, there are those who already have established disease, and, secondly, there are those without established disease but where intervention has been demonstrated to produce benefit.

Those with established disease should be identifiable from the practice records or disease register, they include:

- patients with angina, previous myocardial infarction, coronary artery bypass grafting (CABG), or angioplasty
- patients following stroke or transient ischaemic attack
- patients with diabetes
- patients with atrial fibrillation.

Those without established disease but in whom there is a clear benefit from intervention include:

- smokers
- patients with hypertension
- patients with familial hypercholesterolaemia (FH)
○ heavy drinkers of alcohol
○ post-menopausal women who have had a hysterectomy.

Such individuals require identification, effective intervention, follow-up arrangements, and audit of coverage and quality of care. The practice needs an agreed, written protocol for diagnosis, management, follow-up and audit. It will be noticed that the risks to be identified, the screening procedures, and the age bands recommended for screening differ from those currently required by the UK general practitioner contract, but the recommendations here are those supported by evidence.

IDENTIFYING THE PATIENTS AT HIGH RISK WITHIN THE PRACTICE POPULATION (CHAPTER 15)

The practice population should be screened for:

- smoking (Chapter 1)
  Smoking increases mortality from CHD about threefold (B), as well as causing many other diseases. Stopping smoking rapidly reduces that risk (B). Primary care teams are effective in helping smokers to stop (A).
- blood pressure (Chapter 2)
  There is a linear relationship between mortality and morbidity due to CHD and stroke (B),and this risk is reduced by treatment (A). Hypertension can be effectively managed in general practice (C).
○ alcohol consumption (Chapter 6)
  Mortality and morbidity rise in heavy drinkers of alcohol (B). Primary care teams and other agencies can be effective in helping patients to control their drinking (A).

The following should also be identified:

◇ relatives of patients with familial hypercholesterolaemia or early onset CHD (Chapter 3).
Relatives of patients with familial hypercholesterolaemia or early onset CHD may have an inherited disorder of lipoprotein metabolism, and so should be screened to exclude this (B). Asking all patients whether they have a family history of early onset CHD is a poor method of screening to detect hyperlipidaemia (B) (Chapter 20, p289).

○ obesity (Chapter 4)
Obesity is a marker of cardiovascular risk, although not an independent risk factor (B). There is little evidence that obesity can be reduced by management in primary care. It is valuable to identify patients who are obese in order to attend more carefully to other risk factors (C). There is no evidence of the benefit of recording the weight of patients who are not obese.

Age limits for screening

The ages at which screening should start and cease are not clearly established.

○ The benefits of systematic screening from adolescence are uncertain.
There is no evidence that smoking, obesity or alcohol intake can be modified by systematic screening of young adults. There is no evidence that systematic screening of young adults for family history of heart disease (as opposed to the screening of relatives of index cases) is effective in detecting FH at a young age. Morbidity due to CHD and stroke is negligible before the age of 35 (B) (Chapter 2).

● Systematic screening for smoking and blood pressure should start at age 35.
At this age morbidity/mortality rises, and there is evidence that intervention in primary care is effective (A) (Chapters 1 and 2).

● Blood pressure should be recorded at least once every five years (B) (Chapter 2).

● Screening for smoking, hypertension, atrial fibrillation, and cardiac failure should continue in the elderly indefinitely, subject to the quality of life of the individual.
Studies in the elderly show that the effects of these risk factors, and the benefits from controlling them, continue to operate at all ages studied (A) (Chapters 1, 2, 13, and 14).

MANAGEMENT OF PATIENTS WITH ESTABLISHED HEART DISEASE (CHAPTER 14)

Such patients include those with stable angina, previous myocardial infarction, or with angiographically proven CHD including those who have had CABG or angioplasty.

The practice needs (Chapter 22):

- a register of patients with established cardiovascular disease
  Screening for patients with undiagnosed disease is not recommended (Chapter 15).
- a protocol for management and follow-up.

Preventive interventions include:

- life-style counselling and advice on:
  - smoking avoidance/cessation
    Observational studies show the mortality of those who continue to smoke after myocardial infarction is more than twice that of those who quit (B) (Chapter 14). Intervention in primary care is effective in helping patients to stop smoking (A) (Chapter 1).
  - dietary behaviour
    Reducing saturated fat intake and blood cholesterol reduces mortality in patients with established CHD (A) (Chapter 3). Increasing consumption of fish oils (C) (Chapter 4) and dietary antioxidants (C) (Chapter 12) reduces mortality.
  - physical activity
    Exercise rehabilitation following MI reduces mortality and increases well-being (A) (Chapter 5).
  ◇ alcohol consumption
    An intake of one to two units of alcohol per day is associated with up to 30 per cent reduction in CHD mortality (B). Consumption of over three units per day is associated with increased total mortality compared to abstinence (B) (Chapter 6).
  ◇ coping with stress
    Certain stresses, especially lack of control, are associated with increased mortality (C) (Chapter 7).
- drug therapy
  - low dose aspirin
    Meta-analysis of clinical trials demonstrates 12 per cent reduction in mortality. 75 mgs aspirin daily should be taken unless there are contraindications (A) (Chapter 14).
  - lipid-lowering drug therapy
    The Simvastatin Survival Study shows that patients with established CHD and total cholesterol at any level greater > 5.5 mmol/l after diet benefit from statins (A) (Chapter 3).
  - beta blockers
    Meta-analysis of clinical trials shows 20 per cent reduced mortality. Beta blockers should be considered for patients in whom there are no contra-indications (B) (Chapter 14).
  - ACE inhibitors
    Clinical trials show reduced mortality and morbidity in patients using ACE

inhibitors when there is evidence of cardiac failure following myocardial infarction (A) (Chapter 14).
- ◆ blood pressure controlled at least to 160/90 mm Hg
  This is the optimum level for reduced mortality (B) (Chapter 2).
- ◇ consider anticoagulants
  If there is a risk of thromboembolism (A) (Chapter 14).
- management of other known existing diseases, especially diabetes (C) (Chapter 8)
- referral for consideration of revascularization if the cardiac condition worsens, especially if angina worsens (C) (Chapter 14).

MANAGEMENT OF PATIENTS WITH PREVIOUS STROKE OR TRANSIENT ISCHAEMIC ATTACK (CHAPTER 13)

The practice needs:

- a register of patients
- a protocol for follow-up of such patients.

Preventive interventions include:

- life-style counselling and advice on:
  - ◆ smoking
    Recurrence of stroke is more frequent in persisting smokers (B) (Chapter 13).
  - ◆ alcohol consumption
    While low consumption may be protective, high alcohol intake increases stroke (B) (Chapter 6).
  - ◇ physical activity
  - ◇ coping with stress
  - ◇ dietary advice to avoid obesity
    The above three items reduce CHD but have not been shown specifically to prevent recurrence of stroke (C).
- drug therapy
  - ◆ consideration of anticoagulation if patient is in atrial fibrillation
    Anticoagulation is more effective than aspirin unless there are contraindications (A) (Chapter 13).
  - ◆ low dose (75mgs daily) aspirin
    Aspirin reduces recurrence of stroke by 20 per cent and should be taken unless there are contraindications (A) (Chapter 13). Not to be used for haemorrhagic stroke.
  - ◆ control of blood pressure at least to 160/90 mm Hg (B) (Chapter 2)
- management of other known existing diseases, especially diabetes (B).

MANAGEMENT OF PATIENTS WITH DIABETES (CHAPTER 8)

The practice needs:

- agreed criteria for identification
  It is not recommended to screen for diabetes except in groups at high risk—such as the obese (C) (Chapters 8, 19.7 and 20).
- a register of patients with diabetes
- a protocol for management and follow-up.

Preventive interventions include:

- ◆ regular diabetes follow-up including control of blood glucose and screening to identify complications of diabetes
  Maintenance of optimal glycaemic control has been shown to reduce the development of microvascular complications (A) (Chapter 8). It has not been shown to reduce the incidence of CHD although it may do so. Because CHD is so prevalent in diabetic patients it is particularly important to control other risk factors (C).
- ◆ smoking avoidance/cessation (Chapter 1)
- ◆ control of blood pressure at least to 160/90 mm Hg (Chapter 2)
- ◆ dietary and drug therapy to correct any abnormal lipid profile (Chapter 8)
  There are no trials to establish the optimal threshold for intervention with drugs.
- ◆ physical activity (Chapter 5).
  Exercise also increases insulin sensitivity.
- ◇ alcohol consumption (Chapter 6).
  Alcohol exacerbates hypertriglyceridaemia which is the characteristic lipid abnormality in non-insulin dependent diabetes (NIDDM).

MANAGEMENT OF PATIENTS WITH ATRIAL FIBRILLATION (CHAPTER 13)

The practice needs:

- a decision to check the pulse rhythm when measuring blood pressure routinely
- a register of patients with the condition
- a protocol for management and follow-up.

Potential interventions include:

- use of anticoagulants or low-dose aspirin.
  Warfarin reduces the risk of stroke further when compared to aspirin, but it also increases the risk of haemorrhage(A)(Chapter 13).

MANAGEMENT OF PATIENTS WITH HYPERTENSION (CHAPTER 2)

The practice needs:

- an agreed method of identification (Chapters 15, p288, and 19.2)
- a register of patients with the condition
- a protocol for management and follow-up.

Preventive interventions include:

- life-style counselling/advice on:
    - smoking avoidance/cessation
      The effect of this added risk factor is more than additive (B) (Chapter 15).
    - alcohol consumption
      Low intake is protective against CHD (B), but alcohol increases blood pressure (A) and high intake increases overall mortality (B) (Chapters 2 and 6).
    - dietary behaviour to lower lipids and avoid obesity
      Obesity increases blood pressure (B) (Chapter 2). The effect of the added risk factor of raised lipids is more than additive (B) (Chapter 15). Increasing fish oils and dietary antioxidants (C) (Chapters 4 and 12) should also be considered.
    - maintaining/increasing physical activity
      Exercise reduces mortality (B) and so is particularly important in the presence of hypertension (C) (Chapter 5).
    - coping with stress
      Stress is associated with CHD, and managing stress can reduce blood pressure (C) (Chapter 7).
- drug therapy
- blood pressure control at least to 160/90 mm Hg (A)
- consideration of lipid-lowering drug therapy if appropriate.
  The risk factors of hypertension and raised cholesterol are more than additive (B) (Chapter 15). The optimal level for intervention and therapy is not established.

MANAGEMENT OF PATIENTS WITH FAMILIAL HYPERCHOLESTEROLAEMIA (CHAPTER 3)

Although there will be relatively few such patients in any one practice, those who have been identified warrant priority attention because of their high risk of premature coronary heart disease. Most will also be under specialist supervision, but the practice needs to ensure maintenance of treatment and no lapse from follow-up. The practice therefore needs:

- An agreed method of identification
  See identifying patients at high risk, p322.
- A register of patients with the condition
- A protocol for management, follow-up and screening of other family members.

Preventive interventions include:

- ◆ Lipid lowering management using diet and drug therapy
  Essential and normally requires specialist care (B) (Chapter 3).
- ◆ A policy of screening of all first degree relatives
  This is the most efficient way of detecting undiagnosed cases (B) (Chapter 20, p289).
- ◆ Review and management of associated risks such as smoking, hypertension, or diabetes
  The effect of further risks are more than additive (B) (Chapter 15).
- ◇ Advice on lifestyle such as physical activity and stress
  All measures which can reduce cardiovascular disease are of increased importance in the presence of FH (C).

MANAGEMENT OF PATIENTS WHO SMOKE
(CHAPTER 1)

Almost a third of adults smoke cigarettes and this is an important contributor to cardiovascular disease, especially in those who are, on other grounds, identifiable as being at particular risk.

The practice needs:

- an agreed method of identification (Chapter 19.1)
- a register of smokers and their smoking status
- a protocol for smoking cessation/counselling.

Briefly, the clinical tasks are to:

- ◆ assess the motivation of patients to give up (C) (Chapter 17)
- ◆ offer appropriate information and advice
  Brief advice from general practitioners produces sustained cessation in up to 5 per cent (A) (Chapter 1).
- ◆ assist those who want to stop by counselling, support, provision of self-help literature, and recommendation of nicotine replacement therapy, where appropriate
  The provision of leaflets and nicotine replacement both increase the cessation rate in smokers who are motivated to give up(A) (Chapter 1).
- ◆ assess and manage associated risks, for example blood pressure, diabetes
  The effect of further risks is more than additive (B) (Chapter 15).

◆ arrange follow-up and continued support of those trying to quit.
   More extensive counselling and follow-up, including by nurses, increases the
   cessation rate (A) (Chapter 1).

MANAGEMENT OF HEAVY DRINKERS OF ALCOHOL (CHAPTER 6)

Moderate alcohol intake protects patients against heart disease, but patients consuming over 21 units of alcohol weekly have some increase in total mortality, and those consuming over 50 units per week have a significantly increased risk of mortality and especially stroke (B).

In relation to heavy drinkers the practice needs:

● an agreed method of identification of heavy drinkers of alcohol (Chapter 19.6)
● a register of alcohol intake in all adult patients
● a protocol for management of heavy drinkers.

The clinical tasks are to:

◆ assess organ damage if appropriate (Chapter 19.6)
◆ assess the motivation of patients to change (C) (Chapter 17)
◆ offer appropriate information and advice
◆ general advice under 35 units per week
◆ more specific counselling over 35 to 50 units per week
   Counselling in primary care is effective in helping patients to control their
   drinking (A) (Chapter 19.6)
◇ assist those who want to stop by counselling, support, and liaison with other agencies.
   More intensive support, including prolonged support in a dedicated setting, is
   more effective than brief support in maintaining control of alcohol consump-
   tion (A).

MANAGEMENT OF POST-MENOPAUSAL WOMEN WHO HAVE HAD HYSTERECTOMY (CHAPTER 10)

Although women are at lower risk than men, the risk increases after the menopause, and there is now strong observational evidence that hormone replacement therapy (HRT) reduces all cause and CHD mortality in women who have had hysterectomy.

The practice needs:

● a register of women who have had hysterectomy. This register should identify those who have had bilateral oophorectomy
● a protocol for management and follow-up.

Potential interventions include (unless there is contra indication to HRT):

- Advising HRT for at least 10 years for any women below menopausal age who have had hysterectomy and oophorectomy
  Premature menopause leaves the woman liable to earlier osteoporosis and cardiovascular disease (B).
- Offering HRT for at least 10 years to women reaching menopausal age who have had hysterectomy
  There is strong observational evidence of reduction in CHD with no significant increase in breast cancer in patients taking HRT for up to 10 years (B).

Index

Action on Smoking and Health (ASH) 216
adolescents 323
Adventist Health study 58–9
Aerobics Centre Longitudinal study (Dallas study) 69, 70, 73
Afro-Caribbeans 27
AIRE study 180
alcohol consumption
  biological markers 277
  'description of occasions' 273
  estimating 273
  haemostatic factors 144–5
  hypertension 31
  intervention 87–8, 225
  quantity frequency measurement 273
  recognizing harmful 275–7
  reduced risk of CHD 81–2
    at population level 86–7
    explanation for 85–6
    individual implications 86
  screening 277–8, 322
  stroke and 82–4
  tobacco smoking 85
  total mortality 84–5
  under-reporting 273, 275
alcohol use disorders identification test 275
Allied Dunbar National Fitness survey (ADNFS) 77, 266–7
ambulatory blood pressure monitoring 252, 288
angina
  personality type 95
  screening
    hypercholesterolaemia 289, 290
    undiagnosed 291–2
  secondary prevention 177, 179, 181, 322, 325
angioplasty 181, 322
angiotensin converting enzyme (ACE) inhibitors
  in blacks 27
  in diabetes 27, 114
  secondary prevention 180, 292, 324–5
  side effects 30

antioxidants 54, 59, 112, 178, 260
antiplatelet agents, 162–3, 178–9; see also aspirin, warfarin
Antiplatelet Trialists' Collaboration 162–4, 178–9
apolipoproteins 38–9
arterial narrowing, screening 291–2
artificial heart valves 179
Asians 115
ASPECT study 179
aspirin
  mortality after MI 178–9, 324
  non-rheumatic atrial fibrillation 165, 293
  stroke prevention 162–4
  versus warfarin 165–6, 168
aspirin plus dipyridamole 163–4
aspirin plus warfarin 179
Asymptomatic Carotid Surgery trial 170
atherogenesis 18, 41, 60, 143–4
atrial fibrillation, see non-rheumatic atrial fibrillation
audit
  clerk 313
  critical incident analysis 316
  cycle 316
  qualitative 316
AUDIT (alcohol use disorders identification test) 275, 276
Australian Therapeutic Trial in Mild Hypertension 24, 28–9

Bedford study 114
Belgian Physical Fitness study 70
beta blockers
  in blacks 27
  in diabetes 114
  hypertension 26, 30
  secondary prevention after MI, 179–80, 324
  side effects 30
beta carotene 54, 59
bezafibrate 150
Black Report 127
blood glucose 280–1

blood pressure
  diabetics 108–9
  exercise and 71
  level of treated 29, 325
  measurement 311
    ambulatory monitoring 252, 288
    equipment-related errors 249–50
    frequency 28
    Hawksley random zero sphymomanometer 251
    historical review 249
    Karotkoff sounds 251
    mercury column manometer 249, 250
    procedure 250–1
    sphygmomanometer 250, 288
  population distribution 284–5
  systolic/diastolic 27–8
blood viscosity 144
body mass index
  population distribution 284–5
  screening 290
  see also obesity
breast cancer
  fat intake 61
  HRT and 138
British Doctors study 5–6, 8
British Family Heart study 195, 234
British Health Food Shop Users study 59
British Heart Foundation 293
British Hyperlipidaemia Association guidelines 49
British Hypertension Society 178, 250
British Regional Heart study
  coronary prone personality 95
  exercise 72
  HDL cholesterol and CHD 38
  multiple risk score 190
  obesity and cholesterol level 60
  smoking cessation 81
  social class 122, 123, 125

Caerphilly and Speedwell
Collaborative Heart Disease
study 39, 95, 125, 147, 149
Caerphilly and Speedwell
Prospective studies 39
CAGE questionnaire 275, 277
calcium channel blockers 30, 180
call-recall system 233–4, 235
Canadian step test 267–8, 270,
271
cardiac catheterization 181
cardiac death, sudden 5, 71, 74
cardiac failure
ACE inhibitors 180
hypertension 22, 26
screening 292, 293
cardiac rehabilitation
programmes
effectiveness 291
overall benefit 75, 78
sudden cardiac death 74
uptake 232
cardio-respiratory fitness
CHD and 73
measurement 268–71
screening 290
carotid artery stenosis 171–2
carotid endarterectomy 170–1
CASANOVA study 171
catecholamines 71, 101
Centers for Disease Control
(CDC) 253, 254
cervical screening 233
CHAD Program (Israel) 205
children
early growth and CHD 125–7
lowering cholesterol levels 46–7
tobacco smoking 4
Chinese 11, 44
cholesterol 35, 57, 59–60
in diabetics 107
genetic variation 40–1
haemostatic factors 145
Keys dietary score 57, 60
lowering
benefits 43
in children 46–7
clinical trials 41, 195
drug indications 50
in elderly 48
high risk 61–2
J-shaped curve 44
mildly elevated risk 63
pre-clinical cancer effect 44
primary prevention 41–2
risks 44–6

secondary prevention 42,
177–8
in women 47–8
management guidelines 49
measurement 311
bias 253
diet 256
Friedewald equation 256
imprecision 254–6
individual factors 255
regression to mean 256
retail outlets 234
standardization 253–4
mortality and total blood 284
screening 288–90
summary 50–1
see also lipoproteins
cigarette smoking 5–6
age of first 4
alcohol consumption 85
cessation
benefits 8–10
biochemical validation 246–7
intervention policies 11–13,
195, 224–5
motivation 243
nicotine replacement
therapy 12–13, 14
patient management
principles 328–9
predictors of successful 246
protocol 14
public policy measures 212–
13
readiness to change 224
secondary prevention of
CHD 176–7, 324
social class and 127
diabetes 108, 111
exercise and 71
government action 216
haemostatic factors 144–5, 148
lung cancer 3, 5
measurement 243
mechanisms of action 7–8
nicotine dependence 243–5
oral contraception 5
passive 10–11
prevalence 3
screening 287, 322
social class 3–4
cigar/pipe smoking 7
ciprofibrate 150
clofibrate 44, 149
clotting factors 71
Committee on Medical Aspects

of Food Policy (COMA) 216
community-based interventions
203–20
definition 203
effectiveness 204–7
and government action 209,
216–17
health education 203
healthy public policy
measures 203–4
population/high-risk strategies
203
range of possibilities 207–9,
210–15
role of primary care 217
settings 203
community initiatives 318–19
computerized health tests 234
CONSENSUS II trial 180
consultation
effective 227–8
length of 238
Copenhagen AFASAK study 165
coronary artery bypass grafts 6,
181, 322, 323
Coronary Prevention Group 293
cotinine 243, 246, 247
critical incident analysis 316
CT scan 164
cuff bladder length 250

Dallas study (Aerobics Centre
Longitudinal study) 69, 70, 73
DART trial (diet and
reinfarction trial) 62
decision latitude hypothesis 96–8
depression 95–6
description of occasions method
273
Diabetes Control and
Complications trial 110
diabetes mellitus 110–14, 279
blood pressure 27, 108–9, 251
cigarette smoking 108
diagnostic criteria 279–80
frequency of CHD 105–6
independent effect on CHD
109–10
insulin-dependent 27, 279
insulin resistance syndrome
114–16
non-insulin dependent 27,
279, 280, 290–1
obesity 109, 290
patient management
principles 326

plasma lipid and lipoproteins 107–8
screening 289, 290, 290–1
diet
  atherogenicity/thrombogenicity 60
  blood lipid levels and 59–60, 178, 256, 289
  and CHD 54–9
  diabetics 112–13
  fibrinogen 150
  government action 216
  healthy, promotion of 210–11
  intervention 60–3, 324
    high risk groups 61–2
    mildly elevated risk 63
    in primary care 225
    secondary prevention 177–8
  lipid-lowering 40, 41, 45, 48, 49
  measurement
    in general practice 260
    individual variation 258
    methods 55, 258–60
  Mediterranean 59
  screening 290
dietitian 113, 259, 260
diet records 55
diet and reinfarction trial (DART trial) 62
DINE questionnaire 260–4
dipyridamole plus aspirin 163–4
diuretics
  in diabetes 114
  hypercholesterolaemia 256
  hypertension 24–5, 30
Donolo-Tel Aviv study 38
Dundee Risk Disk 191–2, 198, 293
Dutch civil servants 28
Dutch TIA trial 164

Eberbach Weisloch Project 205
echocardiographic screening 180, 292, 293
eicosapentaenoic acid 57
elderly
  atrial fibrillation 166, 293
  blood pressure 24–5, 251
  cardiac failure 292
  cholesterol 48
  exercise 75
  screening 323
empowerment 223, 226, 234
energy intake, 260, *see also* fat
European Atherosclerosis study group 49

European Atrial Fibrillation trial (EAFT) 165
European Societies of Cardiology, Atherosclerosis, and Hypertension Task Force risk chart 188–9
European Working Party on Hypertension in the Elderly (EWPHE) 24–5
exercise 67–80, 324
  bias 70
  fitness studies 73
  haemostatic factors 144–5, 145
  measurement 69–70
  minimum level for fitness 73–4
  physiological basis for benefit 71
  promotion of 75–8, 214–15
  protective effect 68–9
  questionnaires 267
  screening 75, 290
  sudden cardiac death 74
  target pulse rate 77
  vigorous 71–3
  see also cardio–respiratory fitness

factor II–VII–X, 143, 145, 146
factor VII:C 143, 146
factor VII 109, 143, 146
Fagerstrom Tolerance Questionnaire 244, 245
Family Heart study 63
fasting blood glucose 280
fat intake 54, 56–7, 260
fibrates 149–50
fibre 57
fibrinogen 71, 109, 143, 149–50
  lowering
    in clinical practice 150
    dietary methods 150
    drugs 149–50
    effect on CHD 150
  other risk factors 7, 144, 145, 146, 148–9
fibrinolytic activity 109, 143, 144–5, 146
Finland
  diet and CHD 56
  lipid risk factors and gender 108
  North Karelia Project vi, 43, 194, 204, 205–7
  social class and CHD 126

fish oils 57
fitness, *see* cardio-respiratory fitness
food frequency questionnaires 55, 259, 260–4
food labelling 204, 207
Framingham study
  age 48
  atrial fibrillation 166, 293
  blood pressure and diabetes 108
  cholesterol 36, 38, 39, 302
  diabetes 106, 109
  epidemiology and prevention programmes 204
  exercise 67
  filter/non-filter cigarettes 8
  haemostatic factors 145, 147, 148, 149
  HRT 135, 136, 137, 139
  hypertension and morbidity 19, 20
  multiple risk effect 186
  obesity 57–8
  psychosocial stress 100
  risk score 192, 199
France 59, 109, 110
free radicals 7
Friedewald equation 256
fruit 59, 112

gamma glutamyl transferase (gamma–GT) 277
general practice
  audio visual aids 317
  community links 318–19
  dietary advice 63
  on-site healthy policies 318
  patient groups 318
  population strategy 316–17
  posters and leaflets 317
  protocol 314
  quality
    audit 315–16
    implementing guidelines 313–14
    leadership 309–10
    organization 312–13
    record keeping 314–15
    rewards 311–12
    teamwork 310
    training 310–11
  social class 127, 128
general practitioner 311, 312
  opportunistic intervention 232, 235

smoking cessation 4, 11, 12, 287
see also general practice; primary care
genetic factors 40
German blue collar worker studies 98
German Cardiovascular Prevention study 205, 206, 207
glucose tolerance, impaired 114–16
glycaemic control 110–11
Godin Leisure Time Exercise Questionnaire 267, 269
Gothenburg study 39
    haemostatic factors 145, 146, 147, 149
    multiple risk factors 194
    obesity 58
    tobacco smoking in diabetics 108
Gottingen Risk, Incidence and Prevalence study (GRIPS) 147, 148, 149

haemorrhagic stroke
    alcohol consumption 83
    antiplatelet agents 162–3, 164
    reduced cholesterol 44
    tobacco smoking 5
    warfarin and 166–7
haemostatic factors
    biological plausibility 143–4
    cardiovascular disease outcome 145–9
    and clinical practice 150
    diabetes and CHD 109–10
    and other risk factors 144–5
    reversibility 149–50
Harvard alumni study 67, 68, 69, 72
Hawksley random zero sphymomanometer 251
health beliefs 221–2
health checks
    invitation methods 233–4
    non-personal contacts 234
    occupational programmes 236, 239
    opportunistic approach 232–3
    potential practice workload 236–7
    recruitment 232
    schools 238–9
    team approach 235–6

workplace-general practice liaison 239
health locus of control 223
Health of the Nation 216, 217
Health Promotion Unit 317, 318
health-related behaviour
    effective consultation 227–8
    factors influencing 221–3
    readiness to change 224
    successful interventions 224–6
health visitors 235, 310
Heartbeat Wales 205, 206, 207, 209
high density lipoprotein (HDL) 35, 37–8
    diabetes 107
    exercise 71
    obesity 60
HMG CoA reductase inhibitors (statins) 42, 113, 177, 289, 324
hormone replacement therapy (HRT) 48, 131–42, 132
    breast cancer 138
    coronary heart disease 134–7
    combined therapy 133–4, 180
    mechanisms of cardioprotection 132–4
    osteoporosis 139
    patient management 330
    stroke 137–8
    unopposed oestrogen 180
Horn–Russell Score, modified 245
hypercholesterolaemia
    drugs and 256
    familial 40, 46–7, 50, 327–8
    monogenic disorders 40–1
    polygenic 40, 47, 50, 289
    screening 289, 323
    see also cholesterol; lipoproteins; triglycerides
hyperfibrinogenemia, 149–50; *see also* fibrinogen
hyperlipidaemia, familial 289, 290
hypertension
    continuum of risk 20–2
    definition 20
    in diabetics 27
    in elderly 2426
    ethnic groups 27
    haemostatic factors 145
    health promotion 239
    J-curve phenomenon 29

obesity 30
patient management principles 327
potassium intake 31
salt intake 31
screening 322
    hypercholesterolaemia 289
    Wilson's criteria 286
secondary prevention after MI, 178
summary 31–2
treatment
    non-pharmacological 30–1
    rule of halves 22
    side effects 30
white coat 27, 250, 252
in women 26–7
see also blood pressure
hyperglycaemia
    assessment 280–1
    screening 281
Hypertension Detection and Follow Up Programme (HDFP) 23, 178
Hypertension in the Elderly Project (HEP) 24–5
hypertriglyceridaemia 47

ICRF General Practice Research Group, DINE questionnaire 260–4
insulin resistance syndrome (syndrome X) 114–16
international normalised ratio (INR) 167
INTERSALT study 284–5, 302
in utero events 40, 125–7
inverse care law 235–6
Ireland–Boston study 56–7
ISIS-2 trial 178
ISIS-4 trial 180

Japan 10, 36, 44, 56

Karasek workplace hypothesis 96–7
Karotkoff sounds 251
Karvonen method 77
Keys dietary score 57, 60

laboratory measurement error 254
lifestyle advice
    patients' expectations 231–2
    in primary care 225, 226, 324–9

uptake of services 231–2
see also health checks; health–
related behaviour
Lifestyle Heart trial 178
Life-style study 61, 62
Lipid Clinics Prevalence study
46
lipid levels
epidemiology 59–60
fish oils 57
obesity 60
lipid-lowering agents
atherosclerotic regression 42
benefits 43
in children 47
diabetics 113–14
guidelines 49–50
risks of 44–6
trials evidence 41–2, 324
in women 47–8
Lipid Research Clinic Physical
Activity Questionnaire 267,
268
Lipid Research Clinic
Prevalence study, The
Follow-up study 38, 48, 69,
73
lipoprotein lipase 71
lipoproteins 35, 39, 108
high density 35, 37–8, 60, 71,
107
low density 35, 40, 71, 107,
255–6, 256
very low density 35, 107
London bank clerks and bus
drivers study 57, 67
Look After Your Heart
Programme 205, 216, 217
low density lipoprotein (LDL)
35, 255–6
diabetes 107
exercise 71
familial hypercholesterolaemia
40
in malignancy 256
oestrogens 256

Martignacco Project (Italy) 205
Maslow's heirarchy of needs
311–12
Mayo Clinic trial 170
Mediterranean diet 59
mercury column manometer
249, 250
Miall and Chinn hypertensive
study 28

Michigan Alcoholism Screening
Test (MAST) 275
migrant studies 55, 56
Minnesota Heart Health
Program 194, 205, 206
MRC/BHF Heart Protection
study 177
MRC European Carotid
Surgery trial (ECST) 170
MRC study on lifestyles and
health in the UK 87
MRC trial of mild hypertension
19, 24, 30
MRC trial of treatment of
hypertension in older adults
26
multiple risk
British Regional Heart study
risk score 190
comparison of methods 193
Dundee risk disk 191–2, 198
effectiveness of interventions
194–5
Framingham score 192, 199
relative or absolute 188
usefulness in clinical care 192,
195–6
visual charts 188–9
weight and cholesterol levels
188
Multiple Risk Factor
Intervention Trial (MRFIT)
24, 36–7, 44, 48, 186–7, 194,
232, 284
myocardial infarction
cholesterol levels affected by
256
and depression 95–6
familial hypercholesterolaemia
40
screening 322
angiography 181
and cardiac failure 292
hypercholesterolaemia 289
secondary prevention
ACE inhibitors 180
angioplasty 181
antiarrythmic drugs 181
antiplatelet agents 162–3,
178–9
beta blockers 179
calcium channel blockers
181
diet 62
evidence for 175–6
HRT 180

recommendations 182
surgical intervention 181
warfarin 179

National Advisory Committee
on Nutrition Education
(NACNE) 216
Netherlands
diet 56, 57
Dutch TIA trial 164
hypertension 28
stress 100
in utero deprivation 126
nicotine 243–5
mechanism of risk 7
pipe smokers 8
nicotine chewing gum 12, 243
nicotine patches 12, 243
nicotine replacement therapy
(NRT) 12–13, 14, 243
NI-HON-SAN study 36, 56
non-rheumatic atrial fibrillation
aspirin 165
patient management
principles 326
screening 293
stroke risk off treatment 166–
7
warfarin versus aspirin 165–6,
168
North American Symptomatic
Carotid Endarterectomy trial
(NASCET) 170
North Karelia Project (Finland)
43, 194, 204, 205–7
Northwick Park Heart study 58,
145, 146, 147, 149
Norwegian Cardiovascular
Disease studies 60
Nurses' Health study 137
nutrition, *see also* diet

obesity
CHD and 57–9, 178
diabetes 109
haemostatic factors 144–5,
145
lipid levels 60
screening 290, 322, 323
total energy intake 260
waist-to-hip ratio 58
occupational health promotion
programmes 236
oestrogen, *see also* hormone
replacement therapy; oral
contraceptives

olive oil 56
OPCS longitudinal study 122, 124
opportunistic health promotion 232, 233, 235, 315
oral contraceptives
    cholesterol level 256
    haemostatic factors 144–5, 146
    tobacco smoking 5
oral glucose tolerance test (OGTT) 280
oral hypoglycaemic agents 111, 114
Oslo trial 194, 225
osteoporosis 139
Ottawa Charter for Health Promotion 204
OXCHECK trial vi, 63, 192, 195, 236–8. 244, 289, 306
Oxford Centre for Prevention in Primary Care 232
Oxfordshire Community Stroke Project 145–6
Oxford study (alcohol consumption) 88
Oxford Vegetarian study 59, 60

Paris Prospective study 109, 110, 114
patient management
    atrial fibrillation 326
    diabetics 326
    established CHD 323–5
    familial hypercholesterolaemia 327–8
    heavy alcohol drinkers 329
    hypertension 327
    identifying high-risk patients 322–3
    post-menopausal women with hysterectomy 329–30
    previous stroke or TIA 325
    tobacco smokers 328–9
Pawtucket Heart Health Program 205, 206
personality
    coronary prone types
        evidence for 93–5
        modification 101–2
        type A concept 93–5
    summary of findings 102
Physicians' Health study 39
pipe smoking 8
plasma viscosity 143, 144

plasminogen 143, 145, 146
platelets 7, 71, 101, 109
Postmenopausal Estrogen-Progestin Interventions (PEPI) trial 134
potassium intake 31
practice guidelines
    development 314
    features 313–14
    implementation 314
    and protocol 314
    record keeping 315
practice manager 310, 312
practice nurse 12, 310, 311, 312, 313
practice protocol 314
pregnancy 256
Prevention and Health: Everybody's Business 209
Prevention Paradox 303
prevention strategies
    individual approach 301, 303–5
        priorities 306–8
    population approach 301
        disadvantages 303
        potential effect 302
        priorities 306
primary care
    advice on exercise 75–8
    alcohol consumption 87–8
    effective consultation 227–8
    health promotion, see health checks
    role in CHD prevention 217–18
Prospective Cardiovascular Munster study (PRO–CAM) 147, 149
prothrombin time ratio (PTR) 167
psychosocial factors
    haemostatic factors 148–9
    see also personality; stress

quantity frequency index 273, 274

Rancho Bernardo study 57, 136
receptionist 232, 235, 310, 311, 313
record keeping 314–15
regression dilution bias 19
Review Panel on Coronary-Prone Behaviour and Coronary Heart Disease 93

risk, relative or absolute 188
rule of halves 22, 288

St Thomas' Atherosclerosis Regression study (STARS trial) 62
salt intake 31, 113, 260
SAVE study 180
Scandinavian Simvastatin Survival study 42, 177, 182, 324
Schleiz Project (GDR) 205
schools 238–9
Scotland 22, 145
Scottish Heart Health study 145
screening
    body mass index 284–5, 290
    cholesterol 288–90
    exercise 75, 290
    high risk 301, 303–5
    hypertension 286, 288
    limitations 283–5
    minimum criteria 285–6
    multiple risk assessment 293–5
    opportunistic 232–3, 233, 315
    practice population
        age limits 323
        alcohol consumption 322, 323
        atrial fibrillation 323
        blood pressure 322, 323
        cardiac failure 323
        family history 323
        obesity 323
        smoking 322, 323
    smoking 287, 322, 323
    Wilson's criteria 286
self efficacy 222–3
self esteem 223
Seven Countries study 36, 56
seven day weighed record 259
Seventh Day Adventists diet 58–9, 60
simvastatin 42, 177, 182, 327
Smokerlyser 247
smoking cessation clinics 12, 13
social class 119–22
    attitude to health checks 235
    British Regional Heart study 122, 123, 125
    cigarette smoking 3–4
    definition 124
    haemostatic factors 144
    intervention strategies 127–8
    in utero/early childhood events 125–7

military records 123–4
OPCS longitudinal study 122, 124
selection effect 124
traditional risk factors 125
Whitehall study 122–3, 124, 125
SOLVD study 180, 292
sphygmomanometer 250, 288
Stanford Heart Disease Prevention Program's Five-City Project 194, 195, 205, 206
Stanford Heart Disease Prevention Program's Three Community study 194, 195, 204, 205
statins 42, 113, 177, 289, 324
step test 267–8
Stockholm Prospective study 39
stress
    at work 96–9, 102
    haemostatic factors 145
    management techniques 101–2, 103, 324
    mechanisms for inducing CHD 99–100, 102, 103
stroke
    alcohol consumption 82–3
    antiplatelet agents
        atrial fibrillation 165
        primary prevention 162–3
        secondary prevention 163–5
    atrial fibrillation 166–7, 165
    carotid endarterectomy 170–1
    fibrinogen levels 145–6
    haemostatic factors 146
    and HRT 137–8
    hypertension 18, 19, 20, 21, 23–4, 26
    patient management principles 325
    tobacco smoking 5–6
Stroke Prevention in Atrial Fibrillation study (SPAF) 165, 167, 168
suicide 44
sulphinpyrazone 163
Swedish Aspirin Low-dose trial (SALT) 164
Swedish Trial of Old Patients with Hypertension (STOP) 26
syndrome X (insulin resistance syndrome) 114–16
Systolic Hypertension in Elderly Persons (SHEP) 25

teachers 239
tendon xanthoma 289
β-thromboglobulin 109
thyroxin 293
ticlopidine 150, 163
tobacco smoking, *see* cigarette smoking
training 310–11
transient ischaemic attack (TIA) 162
    fibrinogen levels 145–6
    patient management principles 325
    secondary prevention 163–4
    see also stroke
triglycerides 35, 39–40, 60, 107, 255

UK
    alchohol consumption 87–8
    CHD mortality rate 36
    CHD prevention programmes 205–7
    cholesterol 59, 253–4
    diabetes and CHD 109
    diet 54, 57, 59, 62
    exercise 75–6, 77
    lung cancer 10
    psychosocial stress 100
    social class
        British Regional Heart study 122, 123, 125
        military records 123–4
        OPCS longitudinal study 122, 124
        Whitehall study 122–3, 124, 125
UK Civil Service study 67, 69, 71–2, 75, 76
UK nicotine patch trial 287
UK Prospective Diabetes study (UKPDS) 109, 110, 111, 114, 291
UK TIA aspirin trial 164
University Group Diabetes Program (UGDP) 110
urinary nitrogen 259
USA
    CHD prevention programmes 204, 205–7
    cholesterol 57, 253
    diet 56, 57–8
    dietary fibre 57
    exercise 69–70, 72, 74, 75
    health promotion programmes 232, 236

passive smoking 10, 11
sudden cardiac death 74, 75
tobacco smoking in diabetics 108
working environment 97
US Railroad study 69–70, 71

vegetables 58–9, 112
verapamil 181
very low density lipoprotein (VLDL) 35, 107
Veterans Administration Co-operative study group 18
Veterans Affairs Co-operative study 170, 171
visual risk charts 188–9
vitamin C 59
vitamin E 54, 59, 260

walking 76
warfarin
    atrial fibrillation 165, 293
        versus aspirin 165–6, 168
    mortality after MI 179
    risk of haemorrhage 166–7
warfarin plus aspirin 179
Warfarin Re-Infarction study 179
Western Collaborative Group study 93, 95
Western Electric study 57
West of Scotland Coronary Prevention study 42
white coat hypertension 27, 250, 252
Whitehall study 28, 122–3, 124, 125, 148, 292
WHO (World Health Organization)
    alcohol use disorders identification test 275, 276
    Cooperative Trial on Primary Prevention of Ischaemic Heart Disease 44–5
    diagnostic criteria for diabetes 279–80
    European Collaborative Group study 193
    Factories trial 194
    on health promotion 204
    Multinational study of vascular disease in diabetics 105–6, 109

Wilson's criteria for screening
    286
women
    abdominal adiposity 39
    alcohol consumption 81
    cholesterol 43, 47–8

haemostatic factors 145
hormone replacement therapy
    329–30
hypertension 26–7
lipids 38, 108
stroke and alcohol

consumption 83, 84
triglycerides 39
working environment 30, 96–9,
    236, 319

Zutphen study 57